BOOKSBOOKSBOOKSBOOKSBOOKSBOOKSBOOKS

UNIVERSITY OF OSTEOPATHIC MEDICINE
AND HEALTH SCIENCES

Presented to
UOMHS Library
by
Anonymous

BOOKSBOOKSBOOKSBOOKSBOOKSBOOKSBOOKS

Dates in Medicine

Dates in Medicine

A chronological record of medical
progress over three millennia

Edited by
Anton Sebastian

The Parthenon Publishing Group
International Publishers in Medicine, Science & Technology

NEW YORK   LONDON

Published in the USA by
The Parthenon Publishing Group Inc.
One Blue Hill Plaza
PO Box 1564, Pearl River
New York 10965, USA

Published in the UK by
The Parthenon Publishing Group Limited
Casterton Hall, Carnforth
Lancs. LA6 2LA, UK

British Library Cataloging in Publication Data

Sebastian, A.
  1.Medicine - History - Chronology
  I.Title
  610.9

  ISBN 1-85070-095-8

Library of Congress Cataloging-in-Publication Data

Sebastian, Anton.
  Dates in medicine / by A. Sebastian.
    p. ; cm.
  ISBN 1-85070-095-8 (alk. paper)
   1. Medicine--History--Chronology. I. Title
  [DNLM: 1. Medicine--Chronology. WZ 30 S443d 1999]
  R133 .S33 1999
  610'.9--dc21

                                               99-052481

Typesetting by H&H Graphics, Blackburn, UK
Printed and bound by Bookcraft (Bath) Ltd., Midsomer Norton, UK

Foreword

This volume provides a brief overview of the progress of medicine throughout the ages by noting, in chronological order, many of the important milestones in the development – since antiquity – of modern medicine.

Although medicine has been practiced from time immemorial, the Chinese were probably the first to document it around 5000 years ago. The Egyptians followed and several of their papyri contain medical information that can be dated to about 3000 BC. The Sanskrit manuscripts of the Atharaveda in India were written over 1000 years ago. Greek medicine became established by 600 BC, most particularly in the later works of Hippocrates. The Romans started treating medicine as a respectable profession 400 years later. A description of Roman surgery was provided by Celsus at the beginning of the first millennium, and the death of the Roman physician Galen in AD 200 virtually brought to an end new learning until the rise of Arab medicine in the 7th century.

The outlook for medicine was bleak at the start of the present millennium. The Arab physicians collated and expanded Egyptian and Greek medicine and made further discoveries. Some such notable physicians were Rhazes who gave the first description of smallpox and measles in AD 900; Avicenna whose *Canon of Medicine* remained a standard work for nearly 700 years; Albucasis who wrote the first illustrated work on surgery around AD 980; Avenzoar who discovered the itch mite of scabies in 1070; and Ibn al-Nafis of Cairo who wrote a commentary on the works of Avicenna around 1250. The Christian church during this time upheld the works of Galen, however erroneous, and subjected those with different ideas to the Inquisition. The dissection of human bodies was banned by Muslims and Christians and anatomy continued to be based on the dissections of pigs and apes, as performed by Galen 1000 years previously.

From the twelfth to the fifteenth centuries European scientists obtained most of their medical knowledge from translations of Arab texts into Latin, which themselves were based on earlier writings. The beginning of the Renaissance in Italy in the fourteenth century followed the founding of universities in the twelfth century and provided a new impetus to medicine. The school of Salerno in Italy, founded in the ninth century, became a source of surgical knowledge in the second half of the twelfth century. In the thirteenth century the schools at Montpellier, Padua and Bologna gained prominence. The defiant Italian anatomy professor at Bologna, Mondino de Luzzi, was the first person since the Alexandrian period to carry out human dissections in public, around 1315. Other surgeons such as Guy de Chauliac of France, Theodoric of Bologna, Roger of Palermo, Henri de Mondeville, Lanfranc, and John of Arderne in London practiced and wrote on surgery. Around this time Europe was thrown into disarray by the arrival of bubonic plague, first in Provence in France in 1347; it is estimated to have killed a third of the population of Europe by 1350. This was followed by epidemics of syphilis and influenza in the next century. These led to the establishment of hospitals, quarantine restrictions, and some improvements in public health and hygiene.

The advent of the printing press, invented by Gutenberg of Mainz in 1455, helped to disseminate medical knowledge, and a Latin translation of Avicenna's work was one of the first medical books to be printed, in 1473. The technology came to America nearly a century later and one of the first books in the New World, *Opera Medicinalis* by Francisco Bravo, was printed in Mexico in 1570. Meanwhile, in Europe Leonardo da Vinci, around 1490, started questioning the validity of Galen's teachings through observation of his own human dissections. The Flemish founder of anatomy Vesalius followed, and the Swedish physician Paracelsus went further and publicly burnt Galen and Avicenna's works. The church, meanwhile, continued its repression of new ideas. Michael Servetus, who described pulmonary circulation in his thesis of 1546, was burnt at the stake as a heretic. Girolamo Fracastoro, a physician of Verona, despite his revolutionary publication in 1546 of a possible infectious etiology for disease, escaped the wrath of the church. Around 1560 the French surgeon Ambroise Paré did away with cauterization of wounds with boiling oil and introduced dressings and sutures. This new scientific culture paved the way for the British physician William Harvey's experiments leading to his discovery of blood circulation in 1628. Marcello Malpighi of Bologna completed the discovery with his description of capillary circulation in 1661. At the same time, quinine was introduced from Peru for treatment of malaria.

The next three hundred years saw an exponential rise in discovery and invention. Sanctorio Sanctorius of Padua did the first scientific study of metabolism in humans around 1600 and invented a clinical thermometer. In 1674 the Dutch microscopist, Antoni van Leeuwenhoek used microscopes to describe protozoans. English scientist, Robert Hooke, also an early microscopist, in 1667 demonstrated artificial respiration with the use of bellows. London architect, Sir Christopher Wren, inaugurated the first intravenous administration of a drug by injecting opium and crocus into the veins of dogs using a quill in 1656. English clergyman, Stephen Hales, measured arterial blood pressure in a horse in 1733. Postmortem examination was introduced and John and William Hunter collected many autopsy specimens. Thomas Willis of London initiated neurology as a specialty in 1664. A hundred years later Benjamin Rush wrote the first American textbook on psychiatry. Richard Lower of Cornwall gave the first blood transfusion, from one animal to another, in 1665. Bernardino Ramazzini of Padua published the first systematic work on occupational diseases in 1700. A professor of anatomy at Padua, Battista Morgagni, in 1761, published a work based on over 600 postmortems and established pathological or morbid anatomy. William Withering published an account of the benefits of foxglove in dropsy in 1776. In 1774 an English farmer Benjamin Jesty inoculated his wife and two sons with the material taken from cowpox and this paved the way for Edward Jenner's successful vaccination against smallpox in 1796.

The nineteenth century brought more revolutionary thinking. In 1803 an English clergyman Thomas Robert Malthus, suggested the survival of the fittest by pointing out that the only limits to expansion of population were space and food. Charles Darwin, partly inspired by his work, pursued the theory and published his work on evolution in 1859. The spinal sensory and motor nerve roots were discovered in 1810 by the Scottish surgeon in London, Charles Bell, and their role in nervous reflex was demonstrated by a French physiologist, François Magendie in 1822. The French physician René Laennec revolutionized clinical medicine with his invention of the stethoscope in 1816. A professor of anatomy and physiology at Liège, Theodor Schwann, proposed the cells as the basic units of all living things in 1839, and Rudolph Virchow explained pathology on the basis of cells in 1858. The French chemist Louis Pasteur proved his germ theory of disease in 1842. In America Crawford Long gave a successful demonstration of surgical anesthesia with ether in 1842. James Young Simpson introduced chloroform for obstetric anesthesia in 1847 and it became widely accepted after John Snow administered it to Queen Victoria in 1853. The Augustinian monk, Gregor Mendel, commenced his epoch making work on genetics at his monastery at Brünn in 1856. His publication in a local journal in 1865 went unnoticed until the British geneticist William Bateson revived it in 1902. The German bacteriologist, Robert Koch, established the principles of bacteriology and discovered the tuberde bacillus in 1882. Asepsis was proposed in 1847 by Hungarian physician, Ignas Semmelweiss, and the idea was revived in 1865 by the English surgeon, Joseph Lister. The identification of *Anopheles* mosquito as the vector of malaria in 1897 by the British physician, Ronald Ross in India provided the final link in the struggle against the biggest killer since Roman times. Aspirin was first marketed in 1899, and Konrad Röntgen provided a fitting finale for the end of the nineteenth century with his discovery of X-rays in 1895.

More lives have been saved during the present century than ever before making it the most important era for mankind. The Austrian-born American pathologist Karl Landsteiner in 1900 discovered the A-B-O blood groups making blood transfusions safe. Marie Stopes opened the first birth-control clinic. Wilhelm Einthoven introduced the ECG. Alexis Carrel's successful experiments on cardiac and renal transplantations in animals in 1905 paved the way for transplantation medicine and culminated in the first successful renal transplant in 1954.

The battle against tuberculosis started with the introduction of BCG vaccine by Albert Calmette and Alphonse Guérin of France in 1924. Although Alexander Fleming observed the bactericidal effect of penicillin mold *in vitro* in 1928 it was left to Howard Florey and Ernst Chain to make penicillin therapy a reality and save thousands of lives during the Second World War. The German bacteriologist Paul Ehrlich founded modern chemotherapy with his side-chain theory and concept of the 'magic bullet' in 1911, and discovered the first antimicrobial, Salvarsan, used against syphilis. He also contributed to hematology through his staining methods in 1877. In 1943 Selman Waksman discovered the antibiotic, streptomycin, while sulphonamides were developed ten years earlier.

The discovery of insulin in 1922 by Frederick Banting and Charles Herbert Best brought hope to thousands with diabetes. William Kolff in The Netherlands offered new life to those in end-stage renal failure by establishing long-term survival in a patient using his kidney dialysis machine in 1938. Cardiac surgery became one of the most advanced fields of this era, starting with the development of the heart–lung bypass machine by the American surgeon, John Gibbon in 1951 and culminating in heart transplant by Christiaan Barnard of South Africa in 1967. Helen Brooke Taussig of Johns Hopkins Hospital brought hope to children with congenital heart diseases with her first operation for Fallot tetralogy in 1944. Cardiac defibrillation combined with external compression for cardiac resuscitation developed by William Kouwenhoven of Johns Hopkins in the 1950s continues to save thousands of lives. Ultrasound in clinical medicine was also developed at this time. This was followed by the development of the CAT scanner in the 1970s and MRI in the 1980s.

Immunology moved on from its application to infectious diseases and made leaping progress in relation to autoimmune disease and transplantation medicine. Jonas Salk developed a vaccine against polio in 1955 and measles vaccine was introduced in 1963. The discovery of the structure of DNA by James Watson and Francis Crick in 1953 opened the doors to genetic engineering and the immense possibilities of cloning, biotechnology, and gene therapy. However, a further threat to the well-being of mankind was discovered in 1981 with the first clinical description of AIDS.

Much of the story of medicine is marked and documented by the extensive chronological listing contained in the pages of this book. Of course, it would never be possible to list all the significant milestones in the advance of medicine, nor could there ever be general agreement about what have constituted the most important points of progress over the centuries. Nevertheless, without any claim to being completely comprehensive, this volume does record an extraordinary and impressive story about the growth of man's understanding of the human body and the mechanisms and management of human disease.

Anton Sebastian
January 2000

circa
8000BC
Trephining of the skull with the use of stone tools practised by the Neolithic man.

circa
4000BC
Sumerian records report euphoric effect of the poppy plant.

circa
2900BC
The ancient Chinese medical text, *I Ching*, was attributed to Emperor Fu Hsi. He developed a system representing all the yin–yang combinations and which is still extant.

circa
2720BC
Shen Nung born. A Chinese emperor, physician and reformer who experimented with plants and discovered their medicinal values. He originated acupuncture, and the great herbal Pen Tsoa, which describes over 365 medicinal plants is attributed to him.

circa
2698BC
Huang Ti, the Yellow Emperor, born. An ancient Chinese physician who originated the Nei Ching, the oldest treatise of internal medicine, in which he gave the first description of asthma (referred to as 'noisy breathing') and included five forms of therapeutic care; spiritual cure, pharmacology, diet, acupuncture, and treatment of respiratory diseases.

circa
2650BC
Imhotep born. An Egyptian physician, architect and astrologer during the third dynasty, who designed the first pyramid at Saqqara and was deified as the god of healing.

circa
2000BC
The Kahun Papyrus written. An Egyptian treatise which dealt with gynecological diseases, mentioned contraceptive methods, and also dealt with veterinary medicine. It was discovered by Sir William Flanders Petrie in 1919 and is dated between 2000–3000 BC.

circa
1700BC
The Code of Hammurabi was commissioned in Babylon, providing the first laws which regulated medical practitioners and dealt with physicians responsibilities and fees.

circa
1700BC
The Smith Papyrus written. An Egyptian medical treatise thought to be copied from a manuscript dating from about 3000 BC. It contains descriptions of surgical procedures, examination, diagnosis, treatment, prognosis and drugs, in addition to descriptions of the heart and large blood vessels and the first record of the nervous system. Acquired by Edwin Smith an American Egyptologist in 1862 and presented to the New York Historical Society on his death in 1906.

circa
1550BC
The Ebers Papyrus written. A collection of Egyptian medical texts containing descriptions of 'hardening of the limbs', probably

arthritis deformans, and suggesting remedies to 'make the joints limber'. It contains over 700 remedies for various ailments and shows that at least a third of the medicinal plants used in modern pharmacy were known to the ancient Egyptians; and a relatively accurate description of the circulatory system and the heart's function. Acquired in 1873 by George Maurice Ebers, a German Egyptologist and novelist.

circa
1450BC
The Berlin Papyrus written. An Egyptian text which concentrates on the treatment and protection of mothers and babies.

circa
900BC
The Hindus identified the human uterus, tubes and ovaries.

circa
800BC
Midwives in Greece began to gain high status in society. Traditional birth attendants worked in the same way for 2000 years or more.

circa
624BC
Thales born. A Greek philosopher, astronomer and geometer from Miletus in Asia Minor, who proposed that water was the essence and origin of all things.

circa
600BC
An early treatise on the pulse was written by Pien Ch'iao of China.

circa
540BC
Heraclitus of Ephesus born. A Greek philosopher who proposed that fire and water were fundamental to the balance of the world. He explained breathing as a regular alternation between the proportions of elements within an organ.

circa
520BC
Alcmaeon of Croton, a Greek philosopher and physiologist is reported to have been the first person to dissect human bodies. He recognized that the brain, not the heart, was the main organ of sensation and intellect, discovered the optic nerve, suggested the presence of the Eustachian tube and distinguished veins from arteries.

circa
490BC
Empedocles of Agrigentum born. An Italian physician who considered the heart to be the center of the system of blood vessels through which the blood (life) distributed innate heat to other parts of the body.

circa
470BC
Socrates born. An Athenian philosopher regarded as the instigator of inductive reasoning and abstract definitions who left no writings, although most of his works were made known through Plato and Xenophon.

circa
460BC
Democritus born. A Greek philosopher from Abdera who first stated that everything in nature, including the body and soul, consisted of atoms. He wrote several monographs on medicine and anatomy.

circa
460BC
Hippocrates born. A physician in ancient Greece, regarded as the father of medicine. The *Corpus Hippocraticum*, a collection of many texts on various areas of medicine including the treatment of fractures, ulcers, surgery, asthma, allergies and diseases of the skin is attributed to him.

circa
431BC
Brahmanic hospitals established in Sri Lanka.

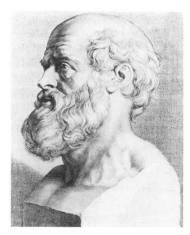

Hippocrates

circa **428**BC

Plato born. An Athenian philosopher who proposed the Doctrine of Ideas. He was a student of Socrates for 8 years, then travelled extensively before retiring near Athens where he founded the Academy for the pursuit of philosophical and scientific teaching and research.

circa **384**BC

Aristotle born. A Greek philosopher and scientist who studied under Plato and wrote three great biological dissertations, *Historia Animalorum*, *De Generatione Animalorum* and *De Partibus Animalorum*, translated into Latin in the 15th century.

circa **372**BC

Theophrastus born. A Greek physician and philosopher who wrote several treatises including *Peri phyton historia*, *Peri phyton aition* and *Charakteres*. He laid the foundations for botany through his work on plant pathology, anatomy and physiology.

circa **340**BC

Erasistratus born. One of the first anatomists at the Alexandrian school, where he dissected cadavers. He is regarded as the founder of physiology and is noted for his studies of the circulatory and nervous systems and accurate descriptions of the convolutions and ventricles of the brain.

circa **335**BC

Herophilus of Chalcedon born. A Greek physician from Asia Minor who, while working in Alexandria, pioneered the study of anatomy, wrote books on midwifery and the eyes, and described the brain, veins, arteries and pulse. He was the first to recognize the brain as the center of the nervous system and seat of intelligence.

circa **273**BC

Ashoka born. Emperor in the Mauryan dynasty of India and humanist Buddhist who built many hospitals where people were given herbal treatment as well as physical therapy. His edicts were engraved on rocks and pillars such as those at Girnar, near Juna.

circa **124**BC

Asclepiades born. A Greek physician from Bithynia who worked in Rome where he established a medical school. He advocated safe, speedy and agreeable treatment of disease and pioneered humane treatment for mental disorders.

circa **100**BC

The Romans established hospitals (valetudinaria) to treat sick and injured soldiers.

circa **14**BC

Aulus Cornelius Celsus born. A Roman physician who described the four cardinal signs of inflammation (calor, rubor, dolor and

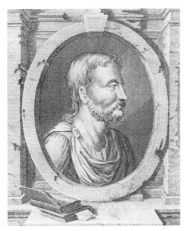

Aulus Cornelius Celsus

turgor), surgical operations, plastic surgery, skin grafting, the use of antiseptic substances, dyspnoea, asthma, the vulva, vagina and uterus. He wrote *De Medicina* around AD 30, a treatise divided into three parts, dietetic, pharmaceutical, and surgical. It contained the first accounts of heart disease, the use of ligatures to stop arterial bleeding, descriptions of hydrotherapy, lateral lithotomy, and insanity.

23 AD   *Gaius Plinius Secundus (Pliny The Elder)* born. A Roman naturalist and prolific writer who wrote *Historia Naturalis*, an encyclopedia on natural history, which provided a valuable insight into the culture, science and medical knowledge of earlier Roman and Greek times.

40   *Dioscorides* born. A Greek physician and pharmacologist who served as a surgeon in the Roman Emperor Nero's army. He studied the medicinal properties of many plants and minerals and described nearly 600 plants including cannabis, colchium and peppermint in his *De Materia Medica*. This text, written around the year AD 77 as five books, dealt with approximately 1000 simple drugs and was a leading pharmacological text for 16 centuries.

70   *Rufus of Ephesus* born. A Greek anatomist, physician and surgeon who studied in Alexandria and worked in Rome. He was author of a treatise on the nomenclature of parts of the human body, advocated a form of fever therapy, and gave a description of plague.

81   *Aretaeus of Cappadocia* born. A Greek physician who practiced in Alexandria and Rome. He distinguished between spinal and cerebral paralysis, and described pneumonia, asthma, pleurisy, diphtheria, tetanus and epilepsy in his manuscripts *On the Causes and Indications of Acute and Chronic Diseases* (4 volumes) and *On the Treatment of Acute and Chronic Diseases* (4 volumes). He also gave diabetes its name.

98   *Soranus of Ephesus* born. A Greek gynecologist, obstetrician and pediatrician who practiced in Alexandria and Rome and is considered to be the father of obstetrics. He wrote *On Midwifery and the Diseases of Women*, a text in four parts which dealt with conception and pregnancy, contraception, labor and birth, women's maladies, and complications of childbirth. His writings influenced gynecology for 1500 years. He described nervous disorders and their treatment in *On Acute and Chronic Diseases.*

115 *Hua Tu* born. A Chinese surgeon who used cannabis and other narcotics as anesthetics during his operations, which included laparotomy and excision of the spleen.

129 *Claudius Galen* born. The most famous of the Roman physicians who founded the Galenic system

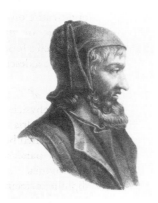

Claudius Galen

of medicine, which was followed for 1500 years until the Renaissance when it was questioned by Andreas Vesalius and Paracelsus.

354 *Augustinius Aurelius (St Augustine)* born. A North African physician who taught in Milan. His book *Confessions*, a text on introspective psychiatry, is considered to be one of the earliest contributions on psychiatric self-analysis.

370 The first Christian hospital was built at Caesarea by St Basil.

390 Fabiola, a wealthy Roman woman, founded one of the first hospitals

in Rome, following which several more were founded in Byzantium.

ca 480 *St Benedict* born. A monk who founded a monastery and infirmary at Monte Cassino, from which the medical school of Salerno, ultimately grew.

502 *Aetius of Amida* born. A Greek physician in the Court of Byzantium who advocated cutting back to healthy tissue when excising a tumor and cauterizing the wound to staunch blood flow. He wrote a compilation of the medical practice of his celebrated predecessors.

525 *Alexander of Trailles* born. A Greek philosopher and physician noted for his *Libri duodecim* (Twelve Books of Medicine) which included a description of parasitic worms. He promoted rhubarb as a laxative and also used exotic remedies such as live beetles.

560 *Isidorus, Archbishop of Seville*, born. He published *Etimologiarum libri XX*, an encyclopedia of human and divine subjects which was an important reference book on science, medicine and theology during medieval times.

625 *Paul of Aegina* born. Alexandrian physician and surgeon famed for his encyclopedia *Epitomae medicae libri septem*, which contained almost all the medical knowledge of his time; including descriptions of lithotomy, trephining, tonsillotomy, paracentesis, and mastectomy and also dealt with pediatrics and obstetrics, apoplexy and epilepsy, and pulses associated with various diseases.

643 *Chen Chuan* born. A Chinese physician who observed the symptoms of thirst and production of sweet urine (diabetes).

777 *Johannes Mesue the elder, or Johannes Damascenus*, born. A Christian and an important physician in Greek–Arabic medicine, he was director of the hospital at Baghdad. His brother, Johannes Mesue the younger, also a physician, wrote *Mesue Opera*, illustrated with pictures of medicinal herbs.

809 *Hunayn Ibn Ishaq* born. An Arab Nestorian Christian physician who studied in Baghdad and translated many Greek texts, including the works of Galen, into Arabic and Syriac. He drew the first detailed diagram of the eye in *Kitab al-'ashr maqalat fi l-'ayn* (Book of the Ten Treatises on the Eye).

850 *Rhazes* born. A Persian physician, considered the greatest physician of the Islamic world. He wrote

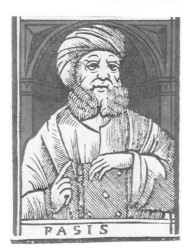

Rhazes

many medical texts, among them *Liber Continens*, an encyclopedia of medical practice and treatment, and his famous, *De variolis et morbillis* (A Treatise on the Smallpox and Measles) in which he gave the first accurate description of the two diseases and distinguished between them.

930 *Haly Abbas* born. A Persian physician whose principal work, *Kamil al-sina'a al-tibbiya* (The Complete Medical Art) was divided into two sections on theoretical and practical medicine. Each section contained 10 tracts on specialised topics.

936 *Albucasis (Abu 'l-Quasim)* born in El-Zahara near Cordoba. A physician, and reputed to be the greatest Islamic surgeon of the Middle Ages. He wrote Al-Tasrifan an illustrated encyclopedia of medicine and surgery, in which surgical procedures for bladder stones, wound cauterization, obstetrics, dentistry, fractures and dislocations, abscesses and eye surgery were described.

965 *Alhazen* born. An Arabian mathematician and physicist from Basra who made significant contributions to optical theories. His treatise *Kitab Al-Manazir* (Book of Optics) included theories on refraction, reflection and the study of lenses and gave the first accurate account of vision. His theories formed the basis for the invention of spectacles and microscopes.

980 *Avicenna* born. A famous and influential Iranian physician and philosopher-scientist who wrote a vast scientific and philosophical encyclopedia, *Kitab-ash-shifa* (The Book of Healing) and a treatise on medicine, *al-Quanum fil-Tibb* (The Canon of Medicine) in five volumes and ranked among the most famous books in the history of medicine.

997 *Abengnefil or Aben-Guefit* born. An Arabian physician who wrote a medical treatise which was translated as *De Virtuitibus Medicinarum et Ciborum* and printed in Venice, Italy in the late 16th century.

1010 The medical school of Salerno, Italy became prominent. The earliest in Europe, it attracted students from Europe, Asia and Africa and was the parent school of those founded at Montpellier, Paris, Bologna and Padua.

1074 *Ibn Jazla* born. A physician from Baghdad who wrote *Taqwim al-abdan fi tabdir al-insan* (The Proper Assessment of Bodies for the Pursuit of Man's Well-being), which was translated into Latin in the 16th century.

1091 *Avenzoar* born in Seville, Spain. A pioneering physician and clinician who was the first to describe a tracheotomy operation and who initiated direct feeding through the gullet in cases where normal feeding was not possible. His *Kitab al-Taisir fi al-Mudawat wa al-Tadbir* (Practical Manual of Treatments and Diet) contained detailed discussions of pathological conditions and their treatment. In

1150, he described the causative agent of scabies (the itch mite *Sarcoptes scabei*). Medical practice in Christian Europe was greatly influenced by his teachings.

1099 A hospital which specialized in treating eye disease was established in the Holy Land by the Knight Hospitalers of the Order of St John, an order which has survived through the centuries as the St John's Ambulance Corps.

1123 St Bartholomew's Hospital in London was founded by Rahere, a courtier of Henry I. The oldest general hospital in the UK, it was given a Royal Charter in 1546.

1132 *Hsu Shu-Wei* born. An early Chinese physician who wrote on treatment for spermatorrhea, hypogonadism and impotence.

1135 *Moses Maimonides* born. A Jewish physician who fled from Cordoba during the Muslim persecution of Jews and eventually settled in Cairo. He wrote a book on diet and personal hygiene, *Tractus de regime sanititis*, and a treatise on asthma, *Tractus contra Passionem Asmatis*.

1140 *The Antidotarium* by Nicolas of Salerno – the first formulary to be printed – appeared.

1145 The Hospital of the Holy Ghost was founded at Montpellier in France. It established a high reputation and later became one of the most important centers in Europe for training doctors.

1161 *Abdul-Latif* born. An Arab scientist and traveler in Egypt, credited with 166 treatises (some on medical topics), who studied human osteology and found that many of Galen's writings on the subject were inaccurate.

1170 Use of seaweed for treatment of goiter was advocated by Roger of Palmero.

1180 *Gilbertus Anglicus* born. An English medical writer who taught at Salerno and wrote *Rosa Anglicana*, his famous compendium of medicine, in which he suggested a 'safe' treatment for goiter and described leprosy and smallpox, recognizing the contagious nature of the latter.

1181 The medical school at Montpellier, France, founded.

1193 *Albertus Magnus* born. An early German physician who recommended hog testes for impotence, and powdered hare womb for infertile women.

1210 *William of Saliceto* born. An Italian cleric, physician and surgeon who wrote *Chyrurgia*, an extensive treatise on surgery. He was experienced in human dissection, differentiated between arterial and venous hemorrhage, described the suture of severed nerves, and gave one of the earliest accounts of dropsy resulting from kidney disorder (Bright disease).

1213 St Thomas' Hospital in London was founded, near the Roman bridge of Southwark, as the infirmary of the Augustinian Priory of St Mary.

1222 The University of Padua in Italy, which rose to prominence during the Renaissance as an important pioneering centre of anatomy, was founded.

1247 The Hospital of St Mary of Bethlehem (Bethlem Royal Hospital also known as Bedlam), the first asylum for the insane in England, was founded by Simon FitzMary, Sheriff of London. It accommodated permananent patients in 1403 and was given a Royal Charter in 1547.

1250 *Peter of Abano* born. An Italian physician and philosopher who proposed the revolutionary idea that the brain was the source of nerves, and the heart was the source of blood vessels.

1250 *Lanfranc of Milan* born. An Italian surgeon who worked in Paris and wrote *Chirurgia Magna*, which contained sections on anatomy, embryology, ulcers, fistulas, fractures, and other pathological conditions in addition to a section on herbs and pharmacy. He was the first to describe concussion of the brain, and also wrote on cancer of the breast.

1260 *Henri de Mondeville* born. A surgeon to the French royal family who advocated simple bathing of wounds and dry healing without pus formation. He was one of the first to write on abdominal injuries.

1265 The study of optics was introduced into Europe by Vitello of Silesia in Poland who wrote *Opticae Libri-decem* (Ten Books Of Optics).

1267 Immediate closure of penetrating chest wounds was advocated by Theodoric in his *Chyrurgia*.

1270 *Mondino de Luzzi* born. An Italian physician and anatomist who wrote *Anathomia Mundini*, the first anatomy textbook written since antiquity, and which was based on the dissection of human cadavers. It remained a standard text for over 200 years. He reintroduced systematic teaching of anatomy and performed dissections at public lectures.

1276 The Al-Mansur Hospital in Cairo founded, one of the earliest hospitals of the Middle Ages.

1298 *Guy de Chauliac* born. An eminent 14th century French surgeon who described surgical procedures for hernia and cataract, as well as

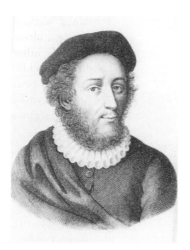

Guy de Chauliac

numerous other pathological conditions, in his *Chirurgia Magna*, which was a standard surgical text book until the 17th century. He recommended a wide excision to remove cancer where the growth seemed operable and also distinguished between bubonic and pneumonic plague.

1307 *John of Arderne* born. The first great English surgeon, noted for the revival of successful corrective surgery for ischiorectal abscess and fistula. His two main written works were *Surgery and Treatment of Anal Fistulas*.

1330 *Hu Ssu-Hui* born. A Chinese physician who wrote *Yin Shan Cheng Yao*, detailing vitamin deficiency disease, and seaweed as a cure for goiter.

1340 Bile stones, or gallstones, were first observed by Italian professor Gentile da Foligno.

1347 The Black Death broke out, killing a quarter of the European population.

1368 A master surgeon's guild was formed in London.

1386 Heidelberg University, the oldest continuously surviving university in Germany, was founded.

1443 *Antonio Benivieni* born. A Florentine surgeon and pathologist who described diseases such as fibrinous pericarditis, diseases of the hip, ruptured intestines, and cancer of the stomach in his classic work *De Aditis Causis Marborum*. He carried out 15 autopsies where his findings correlated with prior symptoms in the deceased.

1452 The first known professional association of midwifery was formed at Regensburg in Germany.

1452

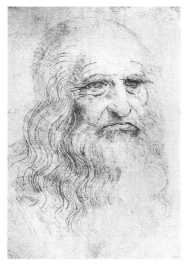

Leonardo da Vinci

Leonardo da Vinci born. A Renaissance artist, inventor, engineer and anatomist from Northern Italy who produced some 750 detailed and accurate anatomical drawings based on his own dissections. He accurately depicted the fetus in utero, the uterus with its blood supply, and produced a wax cast of the ventricles of a human brain. His work predated that of Vesalius by some 30 years, but was undiscovered until 1794, hence its medical importance only became apparent many years after his death.

1460 *Jacopo Berengario da Carpi* born. An Italian anatomist who described appendix vermiformis, the thymus, valvular heart disease and dilated heart, and was the first to perform a vaginal hysterectomy. He was noted for his use of mercurial ointment to treat syphilis. He published *De fractura calvariae sive cranii* (On fracture of the cranium) (1518), *Commentaria super anatomia Mundini* (Commentary on the anatomy of Mondino) (1521), and his noted, *Isagogue* (1522), an anatomical compendium.

1463 *Alexander Achillini* born. A celebrated Italian anatomist who described the function of the small bones in the ear and gave the names 'hammer' and 'anvil' to two of the auditory bones.

1474 The earliest printed book on ophthalmology, *De Oculis eorumeque egritudinibus et curis*, was written by Benvenuto Grassi of Salerno, Italy.

1475 *Wang Hsi* born. An early Chinese physician who wrote *I Lin Chi Yao*, describing the thyroid gland position in the body, and used animal gland as a treatment for this.

1478 *Girolamo Fracastoro (Fracastorius)* born. An Italian physician who proposed a scientific germ theory of disease more than 300 years before those proposed by Pasteur and Koch. He made an intense study of epidemic diseases and outlined his concept in *De contagione et contagiosis morbis* (On Contagion and Contagious Diseases). He introduced the term syphilis in his work *Syphilis sive morbus Gallicus.*

1489 The first European pharmacopeia, *Ricettario Florentino*, was published in Florence, Italy.

1493 *Paracelsus (Philippus Aureolus Theophrastus Bombastus von Hohenheim)* born. A German–Swiss physician, alchemist, philosopher and astrologer who publicly denounced the ideas of Galen and was the founder of chemical therapeutics. He published a clinical description of syphilis in 1530 and a surgical textbook *Dergrossen Wundartzney* (Great Surgery Book) in 1536.

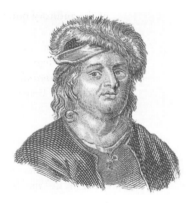

Paracelsus

1494 *François Rabelais* born. A French priest, physician and writer who published his own editions of *Hippocrates' Aphorisms* and *Galen's Ars parva* (The Art of Raising Children).

1497 *Jean François Fernel* born. An eminent French physician who invented the terms physiology and pathology and published *Universa*

Medica (a standard textbook for over a century). He observed that the spinal cord was hollow, and was one of the first to suggest syphilitic origin of aortic aneurysms and to give a clear description of appendicitis and the peristaltic action of the alimentary canal.

1498 The first Spanish treatise on syphilis was written by Francisco Lopez de Villalobos, a physician to King Charles I.

1499 Excision of a herniated gangrenous lung following a chest wound was carried out by Rolandus.

1500 *Chu Chen-Heng* born. An early Chinese endocrinologist who wrote on the use of the placenta and urine extracts in infertility and dysmenorrhea.

1500 *Guido Guidi (Vidius of Pisa)* born. A professor of medicine at the University of Pisa who first described the nerve of the pterygoid (Vidian nerve) and its artery (Vidian artery).

1500 *Thierry de Hery* born. A French physician who wrote a treatise on syphilis in which he recommended guaiacum from resin of the guaiacum tree, to be taken internally, or mercury for injection or fumigation.

1504 An iron hand prosthesis was used by German pirate, Gotz von Berlichingen.

1505 *Pierre Franco* born. A French surgeon who introduced suprapubic cystotomy for the removal of stones, and published one of the first monographs on hernia.

1510 *Ambroise Paré* born. A French surgeon, regarded by some as the father of modern surgery. who wrote *La Méthod de traicter les playes faites par les arquebuses et autres bastons a feu* (1545) in which he described an improved method for treating gunshot wounds. He reintroduced the application of a ligature for bleeding after amputation instead of searing vessels with hot irons, and described podalic version of the fetus in utero, artificial limbs and eyes, teeth implantations, and the use of the truss for hernia.

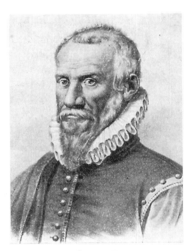

Ambroise Paré

1510 *Josephus Struthius* born. A Hungarian physician who wrote *Ars sphigmica*, an important work on the action of the heart and diseases of the blood vessels.

1510 *Giovanni Filippo Ingrassia* born. An Italian surgeon who gave the largest compilation of diseases ever chronicled, in a treatise on tumors which also included ulcers, furuncles, scabies and hernias.

1510

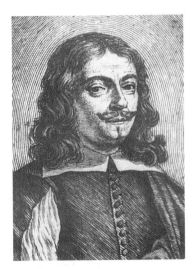

Bartolommeo Eustachio

Bartolommeo Eustachio born. A professor of anatomy in Rome who discovered the Eustachian tube, the Eustachian valve in the fetus, the thoracic duct, the suprarenal bodies and the abducent nerve. He wrote *Opuscula anatomica* published in 1564, which contained specialized studies on the kidney, the ear and the venous system.

1511 *Michael Servetus* born. A Spanish physician and theologian who described the pulmonary circulation of the blood from the right chamber of the heart to the lungs in his *Christinaismi Restituto*, published in 1553. He stated that the blood did not pass through the central septum of the heart, as had previously been believed, but did not suggest that there might be a systemic circulation. The publication of *Christinaismi Restituto*, led to him being burned at the stake for heresy.

1512 A parliamentary act was passed in England during the reign of Henry VIII which helped in the supervision of midwives.

1513

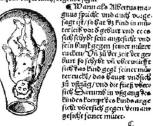

Rosengarten

Rosengarten, Der Schwangern Frauen und Hebammen roszgarten published. A classic illustrated treatise on obstetrics, written by Eucharius Rösslin, a German physician, which was translated into several languages and numerous editions until the 18th century. An English version entitled *Byrthe of Mankinde*, written by Richard Jonas, was published in 1540.

1514 *Andreas Vesalius* born. A Flemish physician who revolutionized the study of medicine with his detailed

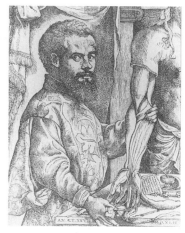

Andreas Vesalius

descriptions of the anatomy of the human body, based on his own dissections of cadavers. He is considered the 'father of anatomy' and demonstrated the first endotracheal intubation to maintain life in an animal. He wrote and illustrated the first comprehensive textbook of anatomy, whilst at the University of Padua. *De humani corporis fabrica libri septem*, commonly known as *de Fabrica*, his major work, printed in 1543.

1515 *Valerius Cordus* born. A German physician who wrote the first real pharmacopoeia, *Pharmacorum Conficiendorum Ratio*.

1516 *Matteo Realdo Colombo* born. An Italian anatomist and surgeon who outlined the pulmonary circulatory system and noted that blood emerged from the lungs a brighter red after being mixed with a 'spirit' in the air. His only formal written work, *De re anatomica*, published in 1559, included the best descriptions to that time of the mediastinum, pleura and peritoneum. He also correctly stated that blood was received into the ventricles when the heart muscle was relaxed (systole) and expelled from the heart by contraction of the heart muscle (diastole).

1518 *Li Shih-Chen* born. A Chinese physician to the Imperial Medical Academy who is considered the father of modern Chinese herbal medicine, and whose *Pen T'sao Kang Mu* (Great Pharmacopeia), completed in 1578, described more than 2000 drugs and directions for more than 8000 prescriptions.

1518 The Royal College of Physicians in London was established by an Oxford physician, Thomas Linacre, under the patronage of Henry VIII. The College was empowered to decide who should practice medicine in London, had authority to examine and licence physicians throughout the kingdom, to examine prescriptions and drugs in apothecaries' shops, and to impose fines and imprisonment on those who broke the laws. Graduates of Oxford and Cambridge Universities were exempt. Linacre was the first president of the new college.

1519 *Andreas Cesalpino* born. An Italian physician from Arezzo who affirmed that the heart was the origin of blood vessels and that blood moved from the vena cava through the heart to the aorta then through the body. His work on the anatomy and physiology of blood circulation predated that of William Harvey.

1520 *Giulio Cesare Aranzi* born. An Italian physicist and anatomist at the University of Bologna who described the choroid plexus, foramen ovale (1557), ductus arteriosus (1564), and named the hippocampus of the brain.

1521 *Christopher Langton* born. A London physician who wrote on madness and afflictions of the mind, and published *An introduction into phisyke, wyth an universal dyet* and several other works.

1521 Description of arytenoid cartilage was given by the Italian anatomist, Berengarius of Carpi .

1522 *Isagogue* (1522) by Jacopo Berengario da Carpi, an Italian anatomist, published. A medical compendium it contained illustrations of the heart.

1523 *Gabriele Falloppius* born. An Italian anatomist who described the ear and cerebral arteries, the

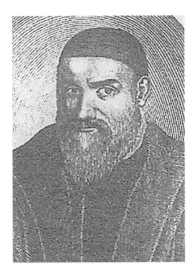

Gabriele Falloppius

Fallopian tubes, the circular folds of the small intestine, the inguinal ligament, the semicircular canals of the ear, the chorda tympani, the lacrimal duct and the trigeminal, auditory, and glossopharyngeal nerves, in his *Observationes Anatomicae*, published in 1561. His *Opera omnia* was published in 1584, twenty years after his death.

1524 The first hospital in North America was built in Mexico City in 1524 by Cortés; the structure still stands.

1525 *Banckes Herbal*, the earliest English printed herbal, was published by Rycharde Banckes. It was followed in 1526 by *The Great Herbal*, the first illustrated English herbal. These, and earlier French and German works, were important in beginning the codification of herbal medicines, the basis of therapeutics before the modern era.

1527 French physician, Jacques de Bethencourt, described the new disease syphilis as morbus venereus.

1530 *Hieronymus Mercurialis (Geronimo Mercuriale)*, born. A professor of medicine in Italy who wrote the first systematic treatise on skin diseases and the first Italian book on obstetrics (1586), in which he advocated cesarean section in cases of contracted pelvis. He also wrote texts on the ear and children's speech. (1584)

1530 Paracelsus made the first attempt at mechanical respiration. He inserted the nozzle of fireside

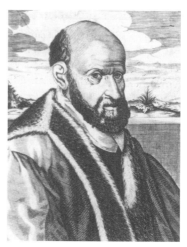

Hieronymus Mercurialis

bellows into the nostrils of the patients, but his method was not successful.

1531 The first recorded human dissection in England was performed by Davis Edwardes, who also published the first anatomy book in England.

1534 *Volcher Coiter* born. An Italian physician and endocrinologist who showed that the ovary is not a source of sperm, and described the corpus luteum.

1535 *Santo de Barletta Mariano* born. A Neapolitan surgeon who described the perineal median operation for stone in the bladder.

1535 *François Rousette* born. A French physician and contemporary of Ambroise Paré, who advocated cesarean section and published a series describing 15 successful cesarean sections.

1536 The first book devoted entirely to the anatomy of the head, *Anatomia Capitis Humani*, was written by Johannes Dryander.

1536 *George Bartisch* born. An ophthalmologist from Dresden regarded as the founder of modern ophthalmic surgery, who removed a bulbous cancer of the eye. He was author of *Ophthalmodouleia*, the first book on eye surgery.

1536 The wormian bones or ossa suturarum (Andernach ossicles) were described by Johann Winter von Andernach, professor of medicine at Louvain.

1536 *Felix Platter* born. A physician in Basel, Switzerland who was the first to distinguish between various mental disorders. He wrote extensive accounts of psychiatric disorders in his *Praxis Medica* and *Observationum* published in 1602 and 1614, respectively. He described cretinism and goiter, recognized hypertrophy of the thymus as a cause of infant death and described asthma due to obstruction of the small pulmonary arteries or nerve disturbances.

1537 *Hieronymus Fabricius ab Aquapendente (Geronimo or Girolamo Fabrizio or Fabrici)* born. A distinguished Italian anatomist and embryologist at the University of Padua, where William Harvey, the English anatomist, was one of his pupils. He described semilunar valves in veins, accommodation of the eye, the larynx, and made important contributions to comparative embryology, repro-

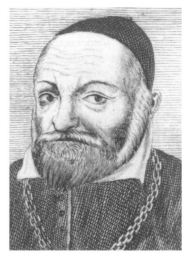

Girolamo Fabrizio

duction, childbirth and the anatomy and physiology of the fetus. His most important written works were *De Formato Foetu* (1600) and *De Venarum Ostiolis* (1603).

1538 *Guillaume de Baillou* born. A French physician and founder of modern epidemiology who wrote *Epidemiorum* and was the first to describe whooping cough (1578). He also described plague, diphtheria, and measles, and distinguished between gout and rheumatic fever, referred to as acute polyarthritis, and distinguished acute gouty arthritis and rheumatoid arthritis.

1539 An early account of neurosyphilis was given by an Italian professor from Venice, Niccolo Massa.

1540 Andreas Vesalius named the axis (second vertebra on which the atlas pivots). During a visit to the

University of Bologna, Vesalius challenged Galen's teachings and demonstrated that Galenic anatomy was based on animal dissections which had then been applied to the human form.

1540 Valerius Cordus from Simsthausen in Germany, synthesized sweet oil of vitriol from sulfuric acid and alcohol. This was renamed ether in 1730 by Frobenius. Cordus wrote *Dispensatorium*, the first European pharmacopeia which contained descriptions, recipes, strengths, standards of purity and dosage for drugs. He presented it to the city council of Nuremberg in 1542 and they published it in 1546, two years after Cordus died.

1540 Guild of Surgeons merged with the Barbers by Act of Parliament, to form the Barber–Surgeons Company. The first Master of the United Company of Barber Surgeons was Thomas Vicary, chief surgeon to the king.

1542 Leonhard Fuchs, a Bavarian physician and botanist, published *Historia Stirpium*, a botanical work in which the medicinal properties of plants were described. It contained precise and accurate descriptions and illustrations of plants, their form, habitat and what he called their temperament and powers. Among those described were *Digitalis purpurea* (common foxglove) and *Cannabis sativa*.

1543 *Constanzio Varolius* born. An Italian professor of anatomy at Bologna and Rome who described the fluid in the brain and the pons (1573) the latter being named pons varoli in his honor.

1543 *De Fabrica Humani Corporis*, Vesalius' text on anatomy, was published. It contained more accurate and extensive descriptions of the human anatomy than any previous texts.

1546 The valves at the orifices of hepatic veins were first detected by Charles Estienne of Paris, who also described the central canal of the spinal cord and published *De dissectione partium corporis humani*.

1548 Thomas Vicary, an English surgeon, wrote the first anatomy book in English, *A Treasure for Englishmen, containing the Anatomie of Man's Body*. The text was reprinted in 1571 by his colleagues at St Bartholomew's Hospital and remained a classic text until the 17th century.

1549 Vertigo was described as a symptom of brain disease by Jason Pratensis, a physician from Zealand, Denmark.

1549 *Gasparo Tagliacozzi* born. An Italian professor who specialized in plastic surgery, revived rhinoplasty (a procedure practiced by the ancient Hindus), and whose work was opposed by Falloppius and Paré on religious grounds.

1550 Andreas Vesalius differentiated the hard and soft palate between the oral and nasal passages, referred to the carotid artery as arteriae sopariae and described the carpus, the eight carpal bones of the hands.

1550 *Jacques Guillaume* born. A French obstetrician who recommended podalic version, practiced cesarean section in a dead mother to save the child, and published *L'Heureux Accouchement des Femmes*.

1550 *Andreas Baccio* born. An Italian physician from Ancona and physician to Pope Sextus V, he wrote two classic treatises *De Thermis Libre Septem* and *Tabula Simplicium Medicamentorum*.

1550 The origin of the optic nerves in the brain was described by Italian professor and anatomist, Bartolommeo Eustachio.

1550 *Peter Lowe* born. A British surgeon who wrote *A Discourse of the Whole Art of Chirurgerie* (1597) reputed to be the first textbook of surgery written in English. He founded the Faculty of Physicians and Surgeons of Glasgow, Scotland in 1599.

1552 Asthma caused by feather in pillows was discovered by French physician, Jerome Cardan.

1552 *Giulio Casserio* born. An Italian who was assistant to Fabricius and instructor of William Harvey. He described in detail the organs of hearing and speech, and wrote two anatomical works, *De vocis auditusque organis historia anatomica* published in 1601 and *Tabulae Anatomicae* published posthumously in 1627.

1553 The first work on forensic medicine, *Constituto Criminalis Cardina*, was published.

1553 A modern work on comparative anatomy was written by Pierre Belon, a French physician from Le Mans.

1554 Anemia in young women, noted during puberty (chlorosis), was first described by Johannes Lange, and was later explained by a lack of iron.

1554 First description of aortic aneurysm was given by French physician, Antoine Sapporta.

1555 Andreas Vesalius made an antemortem diagnosis of aortic aneurysm, confirming this two years later at the autopsy of the same patient.

1556 The suprapubic cystotomy procedure was first performed by French surgeon, Pierre Franco.

1566 *John Woodall* born. A British naval surgeon who was first to suggest that lime juice could prevent and cure scurvy, and who described the circular method for amputation of limbs in 1617.

1560 *Wilhelm Fabry of Hilden (Fabricius Hildanus)* born. The father of German surgery, who recommended amputation above the diseased part of the limb, was the first to amputate through the thigh, and wrote a monograph on gangrene. He illustrated scoliotic spine, and described an operation for it.

1560 *Caspar Bauhin* born. A professor of anatomy from Basel in Switzerland, who wrote important treatises in the field of gynecology, including *Gynaecivorum sive de muliarium affectibus commentari.*

1560 *Peter Chamberlen, the Elder* born. A French-born Huguenot surgeon and obstetrician who emigrated to England as a child and who is credited with the invention of the obstetric forceps (1630), designed to assist childbirth.

1561 *Sanctorius* born. An Italian physician who invented a pulse clock (1602), a clinical thermometer (1612), a trocar and canula for use in tracheotomy, and designed a balance to study body weight in relation to food intake, excretion, perspiration and breathing.

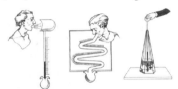

Sanctorius experiments on metabolism

1561 Falloppius' *Observationes Anatomicae* published.

1562 Bartolommeo Eustachio described the passage lined by mucosa connecting the middle ear with the nasopharynx – the Eustachian tube.

1562 Ambroise Paré, the famous French surgeon, carried out a judicial post-mortem, and autopsies became commonplace for members of Parisian high society as a result.

1564 Eustachio's *Opuscula anatomica* (Anatomical Studies) published

which contained one of the earliest illustrations of the structure of the kidneys and the suprarenal glands. A year earlier he described primary and secondary dentition.

1564 Dutch physician, Balduinus Ronsseus, was probably the first to use orange and lemon to prevent scurvy in sailors.

1565 Simon de Vallambert published the first French book on pediatrics.

1565 Hay fever was first described under the name 'summer catarrh' by Leonardo Botallo, an Italian physician. He also gave a description of the ductus arteriosus and the foramen ovale.

1570 The first report of a patient allergic to cats was given by Italian physician, Pietro Mattioli, after keeping the patient in a room where a cat was concealed.

1571 *Hans Lippershey* born. A Dutch spectaclemaker who is credited with inventing the telescope and the first useful compound microscope in 1608. This instrument had limited resolution due to spherical and chromatic aberration.

1574 A detailed account of the ductus venosus and foramen ovale was given by Italian anatomist, Leone Giambatista Carcano.

1575 *Christoph Scheiner* born. A Jesuit astronomer and student of eye refraction who pioneered physiological optics and demonstrated lens changes in accommodation, and images in relation to the retina.

1575   The University of Leiden in The Netherlands was founded by Prince William of Orange. It later gained an international reputation as a center of medical learning, largely due to the teaching of Hermann Boerhaave.

1575   *Zacutus Lucitanus* born. A Jewish physician from Portugal who gave one of the first statements on the falsely conceived contagiousness of cancer.

1576   Closure of penetrating chest wounds by suture was advocated by Felix Wurtz of Switzerland.

1578   Whooping cough was described as 'tussis quintana' by Paris physician, Guillaume de Baillou.

1578   *William Harvey* born. An English physician and anatomist who demonstrated that blood circulated through the body and was pumped by the heart. He discussed his findings in his lectures in 1616

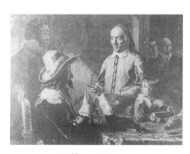

William Harvey

and published them in *Exercitatio Anatomica de Motu Cordis et Sanguinis in Animalibus* (1628). He also published *Exercitationes de Generatione Animalium* (1651), a study in embryology.

1579   *Jan Baptista van Helmont* born. A Dutch physician and founder of biochemistry who coined the term 'gas', described lipemia in diabetes mellitus, and gave a description of seasonal asthma with itching skin eruptions and also of psychosomatic asthma.

1580   *Jean Riolan* born. An early French endocrinologist who introduced the term 'capsulae suprarenalis' for adrenals and described the seminiferous tubules (1626).

1581   *Gaspare Aselli* born. An Italian physician and anatomist who discovered the lymphatic system in 1622 whilst dissecting a dog, and demonstrated the existence of lacteal vessels in 1627, referring to them as milky filaments or white veins.

1583   First excision of the eye in a case of cancer was done by German ophthalmologist, Georg Bartisch.

1584   The first clinical manual on the ear was published by Hieronymus Mercurialis an Italian professor of medicine, who also wrote a text on children's speech.

1584   Falloppius' *Opera omnia*, published posthumously. It included descriptions of abscesses, gangrene, erysipelas, edema, scirrhus, struma and hydrocephalus.

1585   *Caspar Berthelsen Bartholin (Caspar Bartholin the Elder)* born. A Danish physician, theologian and early endocrinologist who described a humor in the cavity of adrenals, that passed to the kidneys and then urine. He wrote *Anatomicae Institutiones Corporis Humani* (1611), one of the most widely read textbooks of anatomy of the time.

1585 *Richard Banister* born. An English ophthalmologist who wrote *Banister's Breviary of the Eyes*, and *A Treatise on One Hundred and Thirteen Diseases of the Eyes and Eye lids*.

1585 The conservative surgical approach by Ambroise Paré of France was extended to cancer in his work *Oevres*, in which he described cancer of the lip and of the breast.

1586 The first complete treatise on cesarean section was written with case histories and illustrations by François Roussette, a French physician to the Duke of Savoy.

1586 A case of gastric ulcer was recorded by Italian physician, Marcello Donati.

1586 The first English monograph on ophthalmology, *A briefe treatise touching the preservation of the eie sight*, was published by Walter Bayley.

1588 *Ole Worm* born. A Danish anatomist who described the Wormian bodies or ossa suturalia of the skull.

1588 An account of ileocecal valve was given by Gaspard Bauhin of Switzerland.

1590 Dutch spectacle maker, Zacharius Jansen, assisted by his father Hans, invented a compound microscope using a simple objective lens and an eyepiece. Hans Lippershey is also credited with the invention.

1591 The first report of an operation for an extrauterine or ectopic pregnancy was made in France.

1591 Italian physician, Sebastianus Petritius, recognized that the discharge from the penis in gonorrhea is pus, and not semen.

1592 The term areola for the pigmented area around the nipple was coined by Swiss naturalist, Gaspard Bauhin.

1592 *Pierre Gassendi* born. A French philosopher and one of the first members of the French Académie de Sciences. He showed the vestigial foramen ovale in the heart, and was one of the first researchers on the atomic theory of matter.

1592 *Jacobius Bontius* born. A physician at Leiden who regarded tropical medicine as a distinct branch of medicine in his works *Medicina Indorum* and *De Medicina Egyptorum*.

1593 Swiss anatomist, Felix Platter, published an accurate description of the anatomy of the eye.

1594 Coraco-brachialis muscle was described by Italian anatomist, Giulio Casserio. It was previously observed around 1571 by Julius Caesar Arantius.

1595 *Johannes Scultetus (Johann Schultes)* born. A German orthopedic surgeon who advocated gradual correction for scoliosis and contracture, and catalogued several surgical instruments, including the use of screw traction.

1596 Arrow poison mentioned by Sir Walter Raleigh in his book *Discovery of the Large, Rich, and Beautiful Empire of Guiana*.

1596 *René Descartes* born. A philosopher, mathematician and scientist who explained the mechanism of vision in his work, La Dioptrique (1637), in which he compared the eye to a camera obscura. Two of his major works were published several years after his death, Tractatus De Homine, a text on physiology (1662) and *L'homme, et un Traité de la Formation du Foetus* (1664).

1597 The first monograph on diseases of the larynx was written by Giovanni Battista Codronchi of Italy.

1597 *Francis Glisson* born. Regius Professor of Physiology at Cambridge, England and a Fellow of the Royal Society, who wrote *De Rachitide* (1650), a classical account of infantile rickets and *Anatomia Hepatis* (1654) in which he gave the first accurate description of the capsule of the liver and the hepatopancreatic sphincter.

1598 *Johann Vesling* born. A professor of anatomy at the University of Padua who described the *linea media scroti* which is named after him.

1600 The term gastrocnemius was used for the calf muscle in the leg by

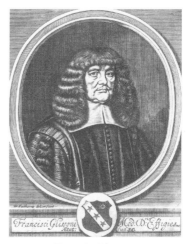

Francis Glisson

Spigelius, professor of anatomy from Padua.

1600 Fabricius ab Aquapendente's *De Formato Foetu* published, in which he described fetal development in animals and man and which contained the first detailed description of the placenta and uterine decidua. He gave an account of the larynx as a vocal organ and was the first to demonstrate that the pupil of the eye changed size in response to light.

1601 *Athanasius Kircher* born. A Jesuit priest and scientist from Geissen in Germany who was the earliest to attempt to view microscopic organisms using his own primitive microscope with which he examined pus or red cells in plague victims.

1603 Fabricius ab Aquapendente's *De Venarum Ostiolis* was published. It contained the first clear description of the semilunar valves of the veins. His findings provided the basis for Harvey's argument for the circulation of blood.

1607 The earliest known classification of burns was made.

1607 *Claude Tardi* born. A French physician who proposed the theoretical basis for blood transfusion from human to human.

1608 *Giovanni Borelli* born. An Italian physiologist, physicist and professor of mathematics who was the first to explain muscular movements and other body functions in terms of mechanical principles in *De Motu Animalium*, published posthumously in 1680. He is considered to be the founder of iatrophysics

1611 In Copenhagen, Denmark, Caspar Bartholin, the Elder, described the functions of the olfactory nerve which he defined as the first cranial nerve

1611 Rheumatism was recognized as an affliction of the joints by French physician Guillaume de Baillou, who was also the first to distinguish between gout and rheumatic fever in his book *Liber de Rheumatismo et Pleuritide Dorsali*.

1611 *Job van Meekeren* born. A Dutch surgeon who gave the first description of torticollis.

1612 Peter Lowe of London classified chest wounds into curable, incurable and mortal.

1614 *Thomas Wharton* born. An English physician who discovered the duct of the submaxillary glands (Wharton duct) and described it in *Adenographia* (1656). He also described the mucoid connective tissue which forms the basic substance of the umbilical cord (1656) and the thyroid gland.

1614 *Konrad Victor Schneider* born. A German anatomist who wrote *De Catarrhis*, a treatise on the membranes of the nose, which led to him naming the mucous membrane of the nasal cavities.

1614 *De Statica Medicina* was published by Sanctorius and provided the first systematic study of basal metabolism.

1615 *Cecilio (Caesilius) Folli* born. A professor of anatomy in Venice after whom the anterior process of the malleus (Folli process) is named. His *Nova auris internae delineatio* was published in 1645.

1616 One of the first books on pediatric surgery for infants was published by Swiss surgeon, Felix Würtz.

1616 *Nicholas Culpeper* born. An English herbalist and astrologer who published a book on herbal remedies, *A Physicall Directory* (1649) which was an unauthorized translation of the College of Physicians' *Pharmacopoeia*. An enlarged version, *The English Physician* (1653) became known as *Culpeper's Herbal* and was one of the most popular works on the subject, running to several editions and in use for three centuries.

1616 *Thomas Bartholin* born. A Danish physician and anatomist who wrote *Vasa Lymphatica et Hepatis Exsequiae* (1653) in which he described the lymphatic system and chyliferous vessels and confirmed the existence of the thoracic duct. He edited one of the earliest medical journals Acta Medica Hofmensia.

1621

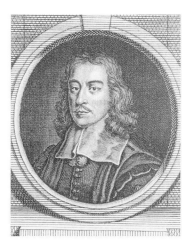

Thomas Willis

Thomas Willis born. An English physician and leader of the English iatrochemists, who made several contributions to medicine. His *Cerebri Anatome, cui accessit Nervorum descriptio et usus* (1664) contained an accurate description of the nervous system, while his *Pathologiae cerebri et nervosi generis specimen* (1667) was a treatise on the nervous origins of convulsive disorders. He coined the term 'neurologie' and is considered to be the founder of neuroanatomy and neurophysiology.

1621 *Moritz Hoffmann* born. A professor of surgery at Aldorf, Germany, who described the pancreatic duct and gave an account of the perineal muscle as 'compressor hemispherius'.

1621 One of the greatest monographs on melancholy, *The Anatomy of Melancholy*, was written by Robert Burton, a pioneer in psychiatry in England.

1621 One of the earliest references to the 'microscope' was made by Cornelius Jacobson Drebble of Holland.

1622 *Jean Pecquet* born. A French anatomist and physician from Montpellier, France, who discovered the receptaculum chyli, a dilated sac at the lower end of the thoracic duct (1647), and developed the concept of its importance in assimilation from the intestines. He clarified the lymphatic system in 1651.

1622 *Richard Wiseman* born. The father of English surgery, who wrote *Treatise of Wounds* (1672), containing graphic accounts of gunshot wounds, and *Several Chirurgical Treatises* (1676), the greatest work on surgery in England to that time, which helped to raise the status of the surgeon. He described scrofula or King's Evil, (cervical tuberculous lymphadenitis) and was one of the first to distinguish between tubercular and gonococcal arthritis.

1622 Hardness of the eyeball in glaucoma was observed by English oculist Richard Banister.

1623 *Johann Sigmund Elsholtz* born. A German physician who pioneered the intravenous injection of chemicals and wrote an early treatise on blood transfusion (1665).

1623 Trichuriasis, caused by an intestinal nematode parasite (trichura), was described by Spanish physician, Alexo de Abreu.

1624 *Thomas Sydenham* born. The English Hippocrates, he relied on careful observation and recording of phenomena of disease. He was one of the first to describe individual diseases including rheumatic fever, smallpox, dysentery, Sydenham chorea and gout, and distinguished between scarlatina and measles. He was one of the

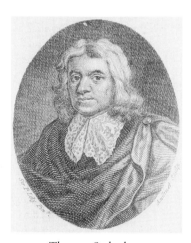

Thomas Sydenham

first to prescribe iron for anemia, and promoted the use of quinine from cinchona bark for treatment of ague or malaria. He devised a tincture of opium in alcohol with saffron, cloves and cinnamon, known as Sydenham's laudanum, that was a popular remedy for many years.

1624 *Francesco Folli* born. An Italian physicist who advocated blood transfusion.

1624 One of the first accounts of malaria was given by Andrein van der Spieghel, professor of anatomy in Venice and Padua.

1625 Use of ipecac in amebic dysentery was described by an English traveler, Samuel Purchas, in his *Pilgrimes*.

1625 One of the first treatises on old age, *A Gerocomice de Senum Conservatione, et Senilum Morborum Curatione*, was published by François Ranchin, professor at Montpellier in France.

1626 Louise Bourgeois, a female midwife in France, published *Observationes Diverses sur la Sterilité*, a book on obstetrics, in addition to texts on female infertility, birth and neonates. As a result of her work, from 1631, Paris midwives began to receive some formal training at the Hôtel Dieu. One of her books was translated as *The Compleat Midwife's Practice Enlarged* (1659).

1626 *Francesco Redi* born. An Italian physician from Arezzo credited with being the first parasitologist who, in 1684, demonstrated that maggots developed from eggs laid by flies, and also described the reproductive process of the roundworm.

1627 Professor of anatomy in Venice and Padua, Andrein van der Spieghel, described the caudate lobe of the liver (the Spieghel lobe).

1627   An early monograph on fever was published by Daniel Sennert, professor of medicine at Wittenberg, Germany.

1627   *De Lactibus*, a classic work by Gaspare Aselli of Milan and published two years after his death, included descriptions of the lymphatic vessels which he discovered.

1627   *Robert Boyle* born. An Anglo-Irish chemist and pioneer in the physiology of respiration, noted for his experiments which proved that air was necessary for life, respiration and combustion. He and Robert Hooke constructed an air pump, a forerunner to the respirator. He wrote *New Experiments Physio-Mechanicall, Touching the Spring of the Air and its Effects* (1660) and reported his work on the relationship between volume and pressure of gas at a constant temperature, Boyle's Law, to the Royal Society in 1661. He wrote a book of remedies including one for urinary calculi.

1628   *Marcello Malpighi* born in Bologna, Italy. The founder of microscopic anatomy who discovered capillary anastomosis and pulmonary alveoli, he was the first to describe the layers of the skin, the lymph nodes of the spleen (Malpighian bodies), the glomeruli of the kidney and red blood cells, and observed the ductus epoöphori longitudinalis.

1628   William Harvey's classic *Exercitatio Anatomica de Motu Cordis et Sanguinis Animalibus* published in which he described circulation,

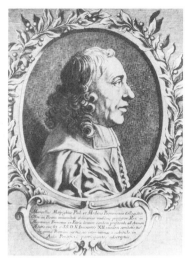

Marcello Malpighi

heart valves, arterial pulse, pulmonary circulation, venous valves and proposed the existence of capillaries.

1629   *Edmund King* born. A London physician to Charles II who published an important paper on dissection of the brain in relation to the pineal gland.

1629   *Johann Heinrich Glaser* born. A professor of anatomy from the University of Basel who described the petrotympanic fissure.

1629   *Nathaniel Hodges* born. A London physician who remained in the city during the plague epidemic and gave a historical account, *Loimologia*, giving symptoms, means of prevention, and treatment.

1630   *Hugh Chamberlen, the Elder* born. A British male midwife who popularized obstetric forceps, invented by his grandfather Peter Chamberlen the Elder.

1630 *Olof Rudbeck* born. A Swedish anatomist and botanist who (as a rival to Caspar Bartholin) claimed to have discovered the lymphatic system whilst working as professor of medicine at Uppsala.

1631 *Richard Lower* born. A physician from Cornwall, England and pioneer of experimental and respiratory physiology, who performed the first blood transfusion between dogs in 1665, and recognized the effect of air on the color of blood.

1632 *Antonie van Leeuwenhoek* born. A pioneer microscopist, protozoologist and bacteriologist from Delft, Holland, who was the first to observe bacteria and protozoa, and whose observations led to the discovery of spermatozoa.

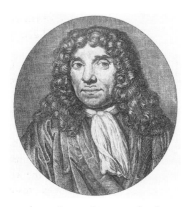

Antonie van Leeuwenhoek

1632 The first illustrated book of surgical pathology was published by Marcus Aurelius Severinus. His *De Recondita Abscessuum Natura*, included descriptions of neoplasms, granulomas and bubos, and provided illustrations of cases such as a probable sarcoma of the right arm.

1633 *Bernadini Ramazzini* born. An Italian physician considered to be the founder of occupational medicine, who wrote the first complete treatise on occupational diseases, *De Morbis Artificum Diatriba* (1700).

1633 *William Croone* born. An English physician and professor of anatomy at the Company of Surgeons, who suggested the reaction of substances passing from nerves in muscle causes contraction.

1634 Two fatal cases of traumatic diaphragmatic hernia were described by Ambroise Paré of France.

1635 An early description of lingual cancer was reported by English surgeon, Alexander Read.

1635 *Robert Hooke* born. An English scientist and pioneer in microscopy, who was Curator of the Royal Society in England. He made improvements to the compound microscope, published *Micrographia* (1665), an outstanding text describing his microscopic observations, and was the first to demonstrate artificial respiration.

1635 Yellow fever was reported in the Antilles by Father J.B. Dutertre.

1637 Vision was first scientifically explained in detail by the French philosopher and scientist, René Descartes in *La Dioptrique*.

1637 *François Mauriceau* born. A French obstetrician who dispensed with the obstetric chair and delivered his patients in bed, and wrote *Des Maladies des Femmes Grosses et de celles qui sont Accouchées* (1668).

1637 *Jan Swammerdam* born. A Dutch naturalist who observed and described red blood cells under the microscope (1658), and discovered the valves in lymphatic vessels.

1638 *Frederik Ruysch* born. A Dutch professor of anatomy who was the first to use the word 'bronchial' to describe arteries and veins around the bronchi (1665), and described the internal circulation of the heart, and the capillaries in the deepest part of the choroid (tunic of Ruysch).

1638 *Nicolaus Steno (Niels Steensen or Stensen)* born. A Danish anatomist from Copenhagen who published *De Musculus et Glandulis Observationum Specimen*, and discovered the duct of the parotid gland which is named after him. He showed that muscle contraction could occur in an isolated muscle, and that its power was the sum of the fibrils.

1639 The French established a hospital, the Hôtel-Dieu du Précieux Sang, in Quebec city, Canada.

1639 A landmark in therapeutics was the introduction of cinchona as treatment for malaria by Spanish physician, Juan del Vego.

1640 *Theodorus Kerckring* born. A German-born anatomist in Amster-dam who described a separate center (Kerckring ossicle) of ossification at the posterior margin of the foramen magnum.

1641 *Regnier de Graaf* born. An eminent Dutch physician who was one of the first to experiment on the pancreas and published a treatise

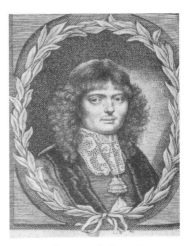

Regnier de Graaf

on pancreatic juice, described the egg-containing follicle (Graafian follicle), and coined the term 'ovary'.

1641 *Raymond de Vieussens* born. A French anatomist who made an antemortem diagnosis of an aortic aneurysm, described the anterior medullary velum, central canal of the cochlea columella, ansa subclavia of the sympathetic nerves, and pathological changes associated with chronic rheumatism.

1642 A description of dry beriberi was published by Jacobus Bontius, a physician from Leiden, in *De Medicina Indorum*.

1642   *John Browne* born. An English surgeon who gave a description of cirrhosis of the liver in the *Philosophical Transactions of the Royal Society*.

1642   *Sir Robert Tabor* born. An English apothecary from Cambridge who became famous through his secret remedy for malaria whose active ingredient, after his death, was found to be the well-known cinchona bark, already in wide use as a cure for malaria.

1642   *Liber de Rheumatismo et Pleuritide Dorsali*, a famous and ground-breaking work on gout, rheumatic fever, acute polyarthritis, gouty arthritis and rheumatoid arthritis (and the differences between them) was published posthumously based on the writings of French physician, Guillaume de Baillou.

1642   First publication on cinchona by Spanish physician, Pedro Barbo.

1642   The pancreatic duct (Wirsung duct) was discovered by Bavarian anatomist, Johann Georg Wirsung, a professor in Padua.

1643   *Lorenz Bellini* born. A great European doctor who described the gross anatomy of the kidney, discovered the renal excretory ducts (Bellini ducts) (1662), and explained fever through the physics of capillary circulation.

1643   *John Mayow* born. An English chemist and physiologist who demonstrated the difference between arterial and venous blood, and observed the process of combustion or burning with a necessary chemical union with a component in the atmosphere, later proving to be oxygen.

1644   *Johannes Nicolaus Pechlin* born. A medical graduate from Leiden, who gave original descriptions of several structures of the alimentary canal.

1644   A hospital built of axe-hewn logs was established on the island of Montreal by Jeanne Mance, a French noblewoman. This became the Hôtel-Dieu de St Joseph, from which the Sisters of St Joseph, the oldest organized nursing group in North America, grew.

1645   *Nova auris internae delineatio* published by Cecilio Folli, a professor of anatomy in Venice. The apparatus of the middle ear, including the cochlea and the semicircular canals, were described in depth.

1645   *Armamentum chirurgicum*, written by Johann Schultes of Ulm, contained many instruments and procedures for cancer, including for mastectomy with recommendation for total slice-removal followed by cauterization.

1645   Use of the microscope in comparative anatomy was initiated by Marcus Aurelius Severinus in his *Zootomia Democritae*.

1645   *Jean Mery* born. A surgeon from Paris who described the Cowper glands of the male urethra, later named after William Cowper who redescribed them.

1646   *Opera*, written by German surgeon Wilhelm Fabry, included clear descriptions of a number of operations for cancer of the breast, and the development of forceps for amputation.

1646   An important treatise on plague was written by Dutch physician, Isbrand van Diemerbrock.

1647   *Denis Papin* born. A French physician and physicist who invented the steam digester with a safety valve, which he used to dissolve bone and other products under pressure.

1648   *James Yonge* born. An English surgeon who described the use of turpentine to arrest hemorrhage, and improved the method of flap operation in amputation.

1648   *Joseph Guichard Duverney* born. A professor of anatomy from Paris who demonstrated the role of the periosteum in the growth and nutrition of the bone, carried out research on the inner ear, and wrote an early treatise in otology.

1648   The first report of tropical dysentery in the East Indies was given by Leiden physician, Jacob de Bontius.

1648   A scientific study of apoplexy, with associated changes in the brain, was published by Johann Jacobus Wepfer, a German physician from Schaffhausen.

1649   *Sir John Floyer* born. An English physician who wrote a treatise on asthma, invented the pulse watch

Floyer's pulse watch

and wrote the first monograph on geriatrics, *Medicina Gerocomica*.

1649   Drainage of the pericardium was first suggested by Jean Riolan, professor of anatomy at Paris.

1650   *John Radcliffe* born. An English physician to King William III, whose estate funded the new Radcliffe Hospital and Radcliffe Library (both in Oxford), and the Radcliffe Observatory.

1650   *Peter Chirac* born. A professor of medicine at Montpellier who wrote several important treatises on wounds, fevers, and the use of iron rust in incubus.

1650   Thomas Willis, an English physician, described the fourth cranial nerve, the trochlear nerve (patheticus oculorum), which causes the downward and outward movement of the eye, and gives an appearance of suffering to the face.

1651 *Hendrick van Deventer* born. A Dutch obstetrician who introduced pelvimetry and defined the oblique diameter of the pelvis and the anteroposterior shortening of the pelvis.

1651 Nathaniel Highmore from Hampshire, England described the maxillary antrum (antrum of Highmore), and suggested that the suprarenals have an absorbent function of exudates from the large vessels. He wrote *Corporis Humani Disquisitio Anatomicae* and several other works.

1651 *Exercitationes de Generatione Animalium*, by William Harvey, was published and contained descriptions of chick and deer embryology.

1652 The thoracic duct and the lymphatic vessels were described by Danish physician, Thomas Bartholin who, a decade later, named the pancreas the 'biliary vesicle of the spleen'

1652 *Augustus Quirinus Rivinus* born. A professor of physiology and botany in Leipzig who described the duct of the sublingual glands (duct of Rivinus).

1653 *Humphrey Ridley* born. An English anatomist and physician who described the cerebral vessels of the brain in *The Anatomy of the Brain* (1695), and has the coronary sinus (Ridley sinus) named after him.

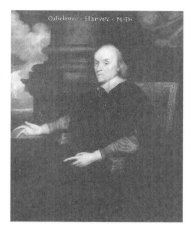

William Harvey

1653 *Johan Conrad Peyer* born. A Swiss anatomist from Schaffhausen who described nodular lymphatic aggregations in the small intestines (Peyer patches).

1653 *Johan Conrad Brunner* born. A Swiss anatomist who conducted the first experiments on endocrinology, demonstrated the symptoms of thirst and polyuria of diabetes, and described the duodenal glands (Brunner glands).

1654 Early blood transfusions were undertaken by Francesco Folli, an Italian physician, who used a silver tube and a bone cannula for transfusion of animal blood.

1654 The first clear description of the blood supply to the liver was given by Francis Glisson, physician, anatomist and Regius professor of physick at Cambridge, in his *De Hepate*.

1654 *Giovanni Maria Lancisi* born. An Italian anatomist, clinician and epidemiologist who is considered a pioneer of public health. He served as physician to three Popes

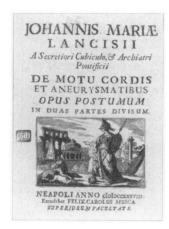

De Motu Cordis by Giovanni Lancisi

and wrote monographs on influenza, malaria and cattle plague. He related the presence of mosquitoes to the prevalence of malaria in swampy districts in his book *De noxiis paludum effluvis* (1717).

1654 Artificial teeth made of ivory and whale-bone and wired together, were mentioned in a treatise on surgery written by Peter Lowe, a surgeon from Glasgow.

1654 The Oddi sphincter, the bile duct at the entrance to the duodenum, was described by English physician and anatomist, Francis Glisson, and later re-described by Italian physician, Ruggero Oddi.

1655 *William Musgrave* born. An English physician who published a series of case studies on pulmo-

nary osteoarthropathy, arthritis with urethral discharge, arthritis with psoriasis, and arthritis with renal colic.

1655 *Caspar Thomasen Bartholin (Caspar Bartholin the Younger)* born. A Danish anatomist and physician from Copenhagen who identified a small lubricating gland adjacent to the vaginal opening in female mammals, the Bartholin gland (1677), described its enlargement (Bartholin cyst), and discovered the sublingual gland and its duct (1684).

1656 Pierre Borel, a French physician, developed the first skin test. He found that blisters occurred on the skin of hypersensitive patients following application of egg. He also recorded that physical weakness, fainting, and asthma occurred in some patients after contact with dogs, cats, mice and horses.

1658 *Francesco Torti* born. An Italian physician who introduced cinchona into Italy and proposed the term 'mal'aria' (bad air) to describe ague in *Therapeutica Specialis ad febres quasdam perniciosa*.

1658 *Johann J. Rau* born. A Dutch anatomist who discovered the long process of the auditory ossicle, anterior to the malleus, the Rau apophysis.

1658 Johann Jacobus Wepfer, a German physician, demonstrated at postmortem that apoplexy (stroke) was caused by hemorrhage from the cerebral blood vessels.

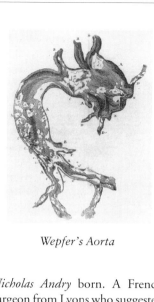

Wepfer's Aorta

1658 *Nicholas Andry* born. A French surgeon from Lyons who suggested the germ theory of disease, coined the term orthopedics, and wrote extensively on the subject.

1659 An early description of an epidemic of typhoid fever was given by English physician, Thomas Willis in his *De febribus*.

1661 A report of cerebrospinal fever (meningitis) was given by English physician, Thomas Willis.

1661 *De pulmonibus* was published by Marcello Malpighi. In it he described the network of tiny blood vessels which connected the venules with the arterioles in a frog's lung, and thus provided confirmation of the circulation of blood.

1662 *Tractatus De Homine*, a text on physiology by René Descartes, was published posthumously, and contained a description of the involuntary response of the nervous system (reflex action).

1662 Nasal catarrh caused by exudation from nasal mucosa was described by German anatomist, Konrad V. Schneider.

1662 John Graunt published his *Natural and Political Observations made upon the Bills of Mortality*. This was the first book on vital statistics and, although there is some dispute regarding authorship, it introduced numeracy into its subject.

1662 Gerhard Blasius, professor of anatomy at Amsterdam, discovered the duct of the parotid gland.

1663 Several cesarian sections were recorded by Dutch surgeon, Hendrik van Roonhuyze.

1663 The beneficial effects of cinchona were published by Italian physician, Sebastiano Bado

1663 *Friedrich Hoffman* born. A German physician who recognized pathology as an aspect of physiology, developed the idea that a vital fluid in the nerves gives 'tonus' to the muscles, and wrote *Systema Medicinae Rationalis and Medicina Consultoria*.

1663 *Guillaume Amontons* born. A French mathematician and instrument maker who invented an air thermometer, conical nautical barometer, folded barometer, and a hygrometer.

1663 An early English treatise on the anatomy of the head, *A Treatise de Merborum Capitis Effentis et Prognosticis*, was published by Englishman, Robert Bayfield. It dealt with cerebral and mental affections and diseases of the head.

1663 The muscular nature of the heart was first described by Danish anatomist, Niels Stenson, in *De Musculis et Glandulis Observationum Specimen*.

1664 *François Parfour du Petit* born, a French pupil of Duverney in Montpellier. He later became a skilful eye surgeon in Paris and wrote several treatises on the comparative anatomy of the eye, and described the Petit canal, encircling the periphery of the lens.

1664 *Cerebri Anatome, cui accessit Nervorum descriptio et usus*, by Thomas Willis, was published. This was the most accurate account of the anatomy of the nervous system to that time, and contained one of the first descriptions of the brain, the arterial supply to the base of the brain (circle of Willis), and the 11th cranial nerve responsible for motor stimulation of the neck muscles. Willis suggested that the cerebellum controlled involuntary movements, and the cerebrum presided over voluntary movements, and described the aortic depressor nerve, a branch of the vagus supplying the aorta, as a wandering nerve.

1665 *Antonio Pacchioni* born. An Italian neurologist who studied the structure and function of the dura mater, and described arachnoidal granulations and depressions in the skull.

1665 Christopher Wren, the English architect, astronomer, and scientist inaugurated intravenous administration of drugs by injecting opium into the veins of dogs using a quill and a bladder.

1665 Marcello Malpighi published three texts. In *De lingua* he distinguished between the outer layer of the tongue and the reticular mucous layer and isolated the taste buds of the tongue. His *De externo tactus organo* contained descriptions of the papillae of the skin, and his *De cerebro* demonstrated that the white matter of the nervous system was made up of bundles of fibers which connected the brain with the spinal cord.

1665 *Micrographia* published by Robert Hooke, an English scientist and microscopist. A classic work on microscopic observations in plants, in which he used the word 'cell' to describe the cavities that he observed in thin slices of cork. He described similar structures in other plants and observed that in some tissues the cells were filled with liquid. He considered that the function of cells was to transport substances within the plant.

1666 *Antonio Maria Valsalva* born. A professor of anatomy at Bologna who described several anatomical structures including the aortic sinuses, anterior ligament of the auricle and the muscle of the tragus (all named after him).

1666 The Académie des Sciences in Paris was established through the influence of John Baptiste Colbert, a French statesman, and was accorded the royal patronage of Louis XIV. It brought together many eminent figures in science.

1666 *William Cowper* born. An English surgeon who wrote *Myotomia Reformata and Anatomy of Human Bodies*, and described the pair of glands (Cowper glands) close to the male urethra.

1666 Eustachio Divini gave an account of his compound microscope to the Royal Society.

1666 *De viscerum structura* was published by Marcello Malpighi. This showed that the liver secreted bile, not the gallbladder, and that the kidneys functioned as sieves. His *De polypo cordis* contained an early description of red blood cells.

1666 *Ippolito Francisco Albertus* born. An Italian physicist from Bologna who advocated bed rest and abstinence from food as treatment for aortic aneurysm.

1666 The sebaceous follicles between the tarsi and the conjunctiva of the eyelids (Meibomian glands), were described by the German anatomist, Heinrich Meibom.

1667 In his *Pathologiae cerebri et nervosi generis specimen*, Thomas Willis suggested the nervous origins of convulsive disorders such as epilepsy, asthma, apoplexy, narcolepsy, and convulsive coughs. He gave an account of whooping cough, described the role of bronchial innervation, and the late-stage effects of syphilis on the brain.

1667 *Daniel Turner* born. An English physician regarded as the founder of dermatology who wrote an important treatise on syphilis.

1667 Robert Hooke, an English scientist and microscopist, gave the first demonstration of artificial respiration, on a dog, by inserting a bellows into the trachea.

1667

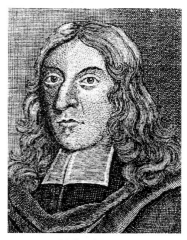

Richard Lower

Richard Lower, an English physician, performed the first successful direct blood transfusion on a human being when he transfused the blood of a lamb into a man.

1667 The effect of blood transfusion in animals was investigated by Jean Baptist Denys from Paris who, following these experiments, transfused 12 ounces of blood from a lamb to a dying man.

1668 *Giorgio Baglivi* born. A founder of the Iatrophysical School of Medicine in Italy who published several significant works including *De*

Praxi Medica and *Opera Omnia Medico Practica et Anatomica.*

1668 Physiology experiments in respiration were carried out by English physiologist and chemist, John Mayow, who demonstrated the difference between arterial and venous blood. He described orthopnea, a state in which a patient can only breathe comfortably when in an erect position, and explained the symptoms and mechanisms of the phenomenon.

1668 *Des Maladies des Femmes Grosses et de celles qui sont Accouchées* published by French obstetrician, François Mauriceau. This introduced the terms 'fourchette' and 'fossa navicularis', and he wrote extensively on female anatomy, providing the first accurate study of the female pelvis. The book was translated into several languages and became a standard text into the 18th century.

1668 *Hermann Boerhaave* born. An eminent physician from Leiden who described rupture of the esophagus (Boerhaave syndrome) in 1723, established the site and nature of pleurisy, and emphasized the chemical factors in functional activity, especially in digestive processes.

1668 The retina's 'blind spot' was discovered by Edmé Mariotte from Burgundy, France.

1668 An early account on the structure of the testicles was given by Dutch physician, Regnier de Graaf.

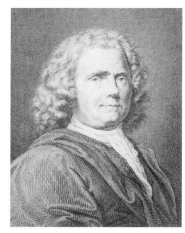

Hermann Boerhaave

1669 *Jacob Benignus Winslow* born. A Danish anatomist who gave his name to the foramen between the greater and lesser sacs of the peritoneum (1732), named the 'grand sympathetic' for the ganglion chain and called the smaller branches 'lesser sympathetic'.

1669 *Tractus de Corde* published by Richard Lower, an English physician. He reported the interaction between air and the blood and determined that respiration added something to the blood since the blood from the lungs was more red than dark venous blood returning to the heart. He gave the earliest description of constrictive pericarditis.

1669 The vessels of the umbilical cord were described as forming valve-like projections by Nicolaas von Hoboken from Utrecht, Holland.

1669 Hennig Sebastian Brandt, a German alchemist, isolated white phosphorus from urine

1670 Thomas Willis noted the presence of sugar in the urine of diabetics and published a treatise on hysteria. A year later he gave first description of myasthenia gravis, and also described puerperal (childbed) fever.

1670 The term epithelium was first used to refer to the skin on the papilla of the lips by Dutch anatomist, Frederik Ruysch.

1671 The first description of Fallot tetralogy was given by Niels Stensen, professor of anatomy in Copenhagen, Denmark.

1671 *Benedict de Spinoza* born. A Dutch philosopher and lensmaker who wrote an important treatise on optics.

1671 *George Cheyne* born. A Scottish physician who wrote *A New Theory of Fevers, An Essay on Method of Treating the Gout,* and *The English Malady*, a treatise on nervous diseases.

1672 *Francis Chicoyneau* born. A French physician who advocated a theory that plague was not contagious in a treatise he wrote after studies carried out during a plague epidemic in Marseilles.

1672 The first account of ovulation on an anatomical, physiological and pathological basis was given by Regnier de Graaf of Holland, who also described the Graafian follicle, a structure or sac which appears on the surface of the ovary,

1672 An early pathological description of the occupational lung disease, silicosis, was given by Isbrand van Diemerbroeck, professor of medicine in Holland.

1673 A description of seasonal rose coryza in Basel was given by Swiss physician, Johannes Binneringus.

1673 Benedicte de Bacquerre published *Senum Medicus.*

1674 *Jean Louis Petit* born. A surgeon from Paris who performed the first mastoidectomy, and defined the inferior lumbar triangle (Petit triangle) bounded by external oblique, latisimus dorsi muscles and the iliac crest.

1674 *On the Respiration of the Foetus* was written by London physician, John Mayow, who carried out some of the first scientific work on respiratory physiology and wrote a second classic in this field, *On Respiration*. He also described mitral stenosis.

1674 Microscopic forms of 'animalcules' from pond and well water, the human mouth and intestine were described by Dutch microscopist, Antonie van Leeuwenhoek. The 'animalcules' were identified as bacteria and protozoa. He described the striped nature of voluntary muscle.

1675 *Martin Naboth* born. A German anatomist and chemist who described cystic distention of the mucous gland (Nabothian gland) of the cervix uteri (Nabothian cyst).

1675 *James Douglas* born. A Scottish physician and midwife who described the rectouterine peritoneal pouch (pouch of Douglas) in *A Description of the Peritoneum.*

1676 The first suggestion that ergotism was due to contamination of rye by biological agents was made by the Paris herbal physician, Denis Dodart.

1677 Binocular lenses were applied to the microscope by French friar, mathematician, and philosopher, Père Le Cherubin.

1677

Stephen Hales

Stephen Hales born. An English clergyman and scientist who is considered to be the father of sphygmomanometry, and was the first person to quantitatively measure blood pressure.

1677 The vulvovaginal gland and its duct were described by Caspar Bartholin the Younger, professor of anatomy at Copenhagen.

1678 *Pierre Fauchard* born. A French dental surgeon who described alviodental periositis (Fauchard disease).

1679 A postmortem description of calcific aortic stenosis was given by Theophile Bonet, a Swiss pathologist. *His Sepulchretum sive Anatomica Practica* included almost 3,000 necropsy protocols.

1680 The first microscopic studies of pollen grains were carried out by American physician, Nehemiah Green.

1680 A special alphabet for deaf mutes was devised by Scottish educator, George Dalgarno.

1681 One of the earliest treatises on comparative anatomy was published by Dutch anatomist, Gerard Blaes.

1681 The Royal College of Physicians of Edinburgh was founded by Sir Robert Sibbald.

1681 *Giovanni Santorini* born. An Italian anatomist and pupil of Malpighi who described the accessory duct of the pancreas (Santorini duct) and several other structures in *Observationes Anatomicae.*

1682 *James Bartholomew Beccaria* born. An Italian physician who wrote treatises on the impurities in air and on the motion of fluids.

1682 The excretory duct (Stensen duct) of the parotid gland and its function were described by Niels Stensen, professor of anatomy at Copenhagen, Denmark.

1682 *Giovanni Battista Morgagni* born. An Italian anatomist, pathologist and professor of anatomy at Padua,

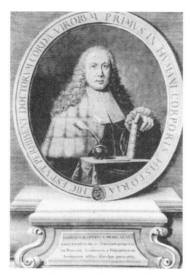

Giovanni Morgagni

who wrote *Adversaria Anatomica* (1706–1719). His work helped to make pathological anatomy an exact science. He studied the anatomical difference between the unhealthy and healthy body and correlated postmortem findings with clinical symptoms. He is considered the founder of pathological anatomy, and several anatomical structures which he identified carry his eponym.

1683 *René Ferchault Réamur* born. A French mathematician and biologist who studied regeneration, movement, formation, growth and digestion of animals and birds, wrote the historic *Memoires pour servir l'histoire des Insectes*, and devised a method of hatching eggs with artificial heat.

1683 *Lorenz Heister* born. The founder of scientific surgery in Germany who introduced the spinal brace, and was the first to describe

appendicitis. As a cancer surgeon, he operated on salivary gland tumors and described thyroid cancer.

1683 The first treatise on the structure, function and disease of the ear was written by Parisian anatomist, Guichard Joseph Duverny.

1683 A classic treatise on gout, *Tractus de Podagra et de Hydrope*, was written by Thomas Sydenham an English physician.

1684 Antonie van Leeuwenhoek extended Malpighi's work on blood capillaries and gave the first accurate description of red blood cells.

1684 An important early text on neurology, *Neurographia*, was written by French neurologist, Raymond de Vieussens, who also studied white matter of the brain, described the cerebellum, and the structure of the ear.

1684 *Jean Astruc* born. A Paris physician who wrote treatises on syphilis, smallpox, women's diseases, skin diseases, the plague, and also wrote extensively on tumors.

1684 *Abraham Vater* born. A professor of anatomy and pathology at Wittenberg who described the duodenal papillae and the ampulla of the bile duct which are named after him, and also the pacinian corpuscles.

1684 Night blindness (nyctalopia) was described by William Briggs, a physician at St Thomas' Hospital, London

1684 The first medical journal in England, *Medicina Curiosa*, was published.

1684 London physician, David Abercromby, first suggested a parasitic cause for syphilis.

1684 The human race was distinguished into five species, on the basis of geographical distribution and physical features, by F. Bernier of France in an essay, *Journal des Scavans*.

1684 The sublingual gland and its duct (Bartholin duct) were described by Danish physician, Caspar Bartholin the Younger.

1685 *Henri François Le Drau* born. An important figure in the development of surgical concepts for the treatment of cancer, he divided it into four categories; of the skin, breast, menstrual products, and produced by abnormal lymph.

1686 Several important treatises including *Histoire de Theriaque and Dissertation sur les Tremblements de Terre, et les Epidemies* were written by French physician, Charles Bagard.

1686 A chronic tropical skin disease found in people of the Malay Archipelago and Southeast Asia (tinea imbricata) was described by English navigator, Sir William Dampier.

1686 A form of chorea accompanied by involuntary irregular jerky movements occurring in children and young adults (St Vitus' dance), was described in *Schedula Monitoria de Nove Febres Ingressu*, written by English physician, Thomas Sydenham.

1686 *Adam Christian Thebesius* born. A German anatomist at Leiden who gave a description of venarum minimarum cordis (Thebesius veins), and the coronary sinus of the heart (Thebesius valve).

1686 The intestinal glands of the simple tubular type (Galeati glands) were described by Italian surgeon, Domenico Gusmano Galeati.

1687 Giovanni Bonomo and Giacento Cestoni of Italy established that the mite *Acarus scabei* caused scabies, the first time a microscopic organism had been established as the cause of a specific disease.

1688 *John Freke* born. A London physician who described myositis ossificans progressiva.

1688 *William Cheselden* born. Chief surgeon at St Thomas' Hospital who published a book on human anatomy, carried out extensive studies in lithotomy, and wrote a treatise on the anatomy of the bones.

1688 The Lieberkühn glands, in the lining of the intestines, were discovered by Marcello Malpighi of Italy.

1688 The symptoms of thirst and polyuria indicative of diabetes were produced in dogs by surgical incision of the pancreas by Johann Conrad Brunner, a Swiss anatomist and pioneer in endocrinology.

1689

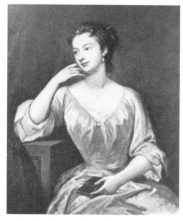

Lady Mary Wortley Montagu

Lady Mary Wortley Montagu born. The wife of the British ambassador in Turkey, she introduced inoculation for smallpox into England and described the procedure for 'ingrafting'.

1690　Pelvic measurement of the mother in relation to childbirth (pelvimetry) was first applied by Henrick van Deventer, a surgeon from Amsterdam, Holland.

1690　The practice of puncturing the amniotic sac to stop hemorrhage in placenta previa was introduced by German midwife, Justine Sigemundin.

1691　*Gaspar Casal* born. A Spanish physician who gave his name to the 'Casal necklace', the pattern of dermatitis involving the neck in pellagra.

1691　The tubule of the peritoneum descending from the uterus into the inguinal canal in young females (Nuck canal) was described by Dutch anatomist, Anton Nuck.

1691　Motor cortex was first suggested by the father of modern chemistry, Robert Boyle, who recorded the case of a man who developed palsy of the arm and leg following a depressed fracture of the skull.

1691　The interconnected spaces in the compact tissues of the bone (Haversian canals) were described by Clopton Havers, an English anatomist and physician, in *Osteologia Nova*, the first complete book on osteology. His study of the physiopathology of bone, and bone growth and repair led to his description of the canals

1691　Marcus Gerbezius, a physician from Slovenia, gave the first report of syncope due to cardiac arrest or heart block.

1691　The corpuscles forming small prominences of arachnoid tissue under the dura mater (Pacchioni bodies) were described by Italian professor of anatomy, Antonio Pacchioni of Rome.

1693　The Achilles tendon, connecting the calf muscle to the heel was first used as an anatomical term by Philippe Verheyen, professor of anatomy at Louvain.

1693　*Jean Baptiste Senac* born. A Paris physician who wrote *On the Structure Action and Diseases of the Heart*, translated Heister's Anatomy, and used quinine in treatment of palpitations.

1693　*Antoine Ferrein* born. A professor of surgery and anatomy from

Montpellier who described the cortical pyramids of the kidney and bile canaliculi, which are unconnected to the lobules.

1694 Use of the trocar and canula for drainage of empyema was undertaken by D.V. Drouin of France.

1694 The accessory lachrymal gland in the orbit was described by Johann Jacob Harder, professor of anatomy at Basel, Switzerland.

1694 Richard Morton, a physician to James II, described patients suffering from the classic symptoms of anorexia nervosa, calling it 'nervous atrophy'.

1695 The first clear written description of ankylosing spondylitis (an inflammatory joint disease of unknown cause) appeared in medical texts.

1696 *Buckhard David Mauchart* born. A professor of surgery at Tübingen who described the Mauchard ligaments, found at the neck of the ocular muscles.

1696 Le Clerc of Paris advocated drainage of empyema in his book *The Compleat Surgeon*.

1697 The term brachial plexus, for nerves in the brachial area, was introduced by French anatomist, Joseph G. Duverney.

1697 Esophageal atresia associated with tracheoesophageal fistula was described in a 2-year-old child by Thomas Gibson, an English physician and grandson of Oliver Cromwell, in *Anatomy of Human Bodies Epitomized*.

1697 *Alexander Monro, Primus*, born. A professor of anatomy in Edinburgh, who played a key role in founding the Edinburgh Royal Infirmary and published work on osteology and comparative anatomy.

1697 *William Smellie* born. A Scottish surgeon and obstetrician who designed practical straight forceps for use in obstetrics, described brachial birth palsy (Erb palsy), and introduced pelvimetry.

1698 Walter Harris, physician to William III, wrote a book on the diseases of children, *A Full View of All the Diseases Incident to Children*.

1698 The earliest pathological account of emphysema of the lung was given in a book by Sir John Floyer, an English physician, in which he described several precipitating causes of asthma, citing dust, tobacco smoke, environmental factors, perfumes, and some types of food as causes. He also described the role of heredity in asthma.

1698 *Henry Baker* born. An English microscopist in London who improved the microscope and wrote *Microscope made Easy*.

1699 Excessive accumulation of fluid causing dilation of the cerebral ventricles (hydroadentitis) was first described by John Friend of Northamptonshire.

1699 *Frank Nicholls* born. A physician to George II who described the dissecting aneurysm of the aorta, and also described its pathogenesis.

1700 The flexible Gooch splint, made of leather for treatment of fractures, was devised by English surgeon, Benjamin Gooch.

1700 *Recherches sur la Nature et la Guerison des Cancer* was published by a French physician from Montpellier, Claude Deshais Gendron.

1700 Giorgio Baglivi of Italy distinguished between smooth and striped muscles.

1700 *De Morbis Artificum Diatriba* was published by Bernadini Ramazzini, a professor of medicine at the University of Modena. It described the health hazards of irritating chemicals, and other agents encountered by workers, gave the earliest description of the symptoms of farmer's lung, miner's lung, baker's asthma, and lead poisoning.

Bernadini Ramazzini

1701 Infection by germs as a cause of disease was proposed by French surgeon, Nicholas Andry.

1701 The first successful operative treatment of an ovarian tumor (ovariotomy) was performed by Robert Houston of Glasgow.

1702 The space within the crista galli of the ethmoid communicating with the frontal and ethmoidal (Palfyn sinus) was described by Jean Palfyn, professor of anatomy at Paris.

1702 *Josias Weitbrecht* born. A German professor of anatomy who described the Weitbrecht fibers, (retinacular fibers of the neck of the femur), and the Weitbrecht foramen (a gap between the capsule of the shoulder joint and glenohumeral ligament).

1703 *De Arthritide Symptomatica Dissertatio*, containing comprehensive case histories and secondary symptoms such as scurvy, asthma, fever and lues venerea, was published by William Musgrave, an English physician.

1704 One of the earliest monographs on the ear, *De Aure Humana*, which included the anatomy and physiology, was published by Italian physician, Antonio Valsalva.

1705 The pathological state of mitral stenosis and aortic insufficiency associated with chronic cases of rheumatism was described by French anatomist, Raymond de Vieussens.

1705 William Cowper from Hampshire noted aortic insufficiency.

1705 The first description of osteomalacia was given by French surgeon, Jean Louis Petit.

1706 French ophthalmologist, Antoine Maitre-Jean, described the nature of the cataract.

1706 *Benjamin Franklin* born. An American scientist and statesman who invented the bifocal lens, pioneered the treatment of nervous diseases using electricity, and wrote on many medical subjects, such as deafness, gout and inoculation for smallpox.

1706 *Edme Gilles Guynon* born. A French scientist who made the first attempt at catheterization of the Eustachian tube via the oral route.

1707 Sir John Floyer introduced his pulse watch that ran for one minute, and published a book on it He attempted to establish a numerical standard for determining abnormality when checking the pulse.

1707 Small retention cysts of the mucous glands of the uterine cervix (Naboth follicle), were described by French surgeon, Guillaume Desnoues, professor of anatomy at Genoa.

1707 *De subitaneis mortibus* was published by Giovanni Maria Lancisi, in which he attributed causes of sudden death to cerebral hemorrhage, cardiac hypertrophy and dilatation, and vegetations on the heart valves.

1708 *Albrecht von Haller* born. A Swiss anatomist who described several anatomical structures, particularly related to the mechanical automatism of heart muscle function.

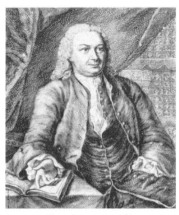

Albrecht von Haller

1708 *Institutiones Medicae* was published by Dutch chemist and physician Hermann Boerhaave, who also gave a classic description of urea and gout.

1710 Alexis Littré of Paris proposed an artificial anus in the colon (colostomy), and advised opening the sigmoid flexure in the iliac region in certain cases of imperforate anus. The operation was first performed successfully by Dinet.

1710 *William Heberden the Elder* born. A London physician who described angina pectoris, acute rheumatic fever, summer catarrh, asthma, the association of renal stones with urinary tract infection, night blindness, and observed the nodes in the fingers of patients with osteoarthritis.

1710 *Sir Fielding Ould* born. An Irish obstetrician from Galway who wrote *Treatise on Midwifery* which included a description of the mechanism of labor and an incision on a rigid peritoneum (episiotomy).

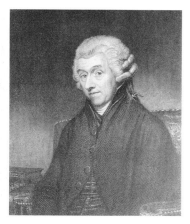

William Heberden

1710   *William Cullen* born. A Scottish physician famed for his innovative teaching methods, who coined the term 'neurology' and wrote *Synopsis Nosologicae Practicae* (1769) in which he initiated a classification of disease (nosology) into fevers, neuroses, cachexiae and local disorders, divided polyarthritis into acute and chronic rheumatism, and described gout.

1710   Femoral hernia was observed by Philippe Verheyen of Belgium.

1710   Empyema was defined as a procedure or surgical incision for draining fluid from the chest by Pierre Dionis of Paris. Others, including H. Bennet (1843) and François Aran (1842), used the term in the same sense.

1711   *William Cadogan* born. An English pediatrician who wrote an early treatise on infant care and feeding, and published an important treatise on gout.

1712   The first surgeon to catheterize the lachrymal duct was Dominique Anel from Toulouse in France.

1712   Madura disease or mycetoma, caused by the fungus *Actinomyces madurae*, was observed by Engelbert Kampfer, a physician from Westphalia in Germany.

1712   *John Fothergill* born. A Quaker physician from Yorkshire England who was the first to record the association between coronary arteriosclerosis and angina pectoris.

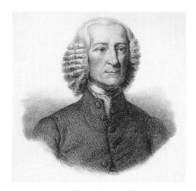

John Fothergill

1712   Use of cinchona for malaria in Italy was introduced by Francesco Torti.

1712   *Thomas Dimsdale* born. An English physician who wrote a treatise on smallpox inoculation, *Thought on General and Partial Inoculation.*

1712   William Penn established one of the first hospitals in Philadelphia.

1713   *Matthew Dobson* born. A British physician and early endocrinologist who wrote *Experiments and*

Observations on the Urine in Diabetes, showed the presence of sugar in urine and the blood, and described hyperglycemia.

1713   The current terminology related to the heart and valves was established by English surgeon William Cheselden, in his *Anatomy of the Human Body*.

1714   Gabriel Fahrenheit invented the mercury in glass thermometer.

1714   Illustrations from *Tabulae Anatomicae* by Italian anatomist Bartolommeo Eustachio were published by Lancisi, 140 years after Eustachio's death. Among them were accurate illustrations of the thoracic duct, facial muscles, the larynx, the kidney, and the sympathetic nervous system.

1714   *Justus Gottfried Gunz* born. A professor of anatomy at Leipzig who discovered the anastomosis between the epigastric and the mammary arteries.

1714   *Robert Whytt* born. A Scottish professor of medicine who described tuberculose meningitis in children in *Observations on Dropsy of the Brain*, and described hydrocephalus due to tuberculose meningitis (Whytt disease).

1714   *Percivall Pott* born. A surgeon at St Bartholomew's Hospital in London who described paralysis caused by caries (tuberculosis) of the spine, the fracture involving the lower end of the tibia and fibula (Pott fracture), and cancer of the scrotum.

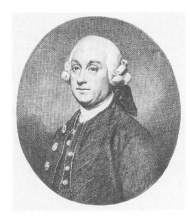

Percivall Pott

1715   *Etienne de Bonnet* born. A contemporary of Jean Jacques Rousseau and a disciple of John Locke who proposed the theory that all knowledge comes from the senses.

1715   *New Treatise on the Structure of the Heart and on the Causes of Spontaneous Heart Beat* was written by the French anatomist, Raymond de Vieussens. It contained a description of the coronary circulation.

1715   *Prudent Hevin* born. A surgeon from Paris who wrote *Pathologie Chirurgica* and a memorandum on strange substances in the esophagus.

1717   In his *Account of the Dissection of a Child*, William Blair-Bell, an British obstetrician, gave a description of congenital hypertrophic pyloric stenosis.

1717   The spiral folds of mucous membrane in the neck of the gall bladder and the cystic duct (Heister valves) were first described by the German surgeon, Lorenz Heister. In 1718 he published *Chirurgie*, which included various suggestions on the treatment of cancer, including the removal of the axillary lymph nodes and the underlying pectoral muscle in breast cancer, and introduced the term tracheotomy.

1717   *Acta Medicorum Berolinensium* was the first medical journal to be published in Germany.

1718   *William Hunter* born. An eminent Scottish anatomist and obstetrician who was a lecturer to the Society of Surgeons, and who built a private theater, dissecting room, and museum at his home in London.

1718   The screw tourniquet, an instrument for stopping the flow of blood into a limb by applying pressure was invented by Jean Louis Petit of France. He performed surgery for mastoiditis in 1720

1719   Determination of the specific gravity of blood was made by English physician, James Jurin.

1719   *Friedrich Wilhelm Hensing* born. A professor of anatomy from the University of Giessen who wrote *De Peritonaeo* and described the phrenico-colic ligament of the spleen.

1719   The Littré glands in the mucous membrane of the spongy part of the urethra were described by Alexis Littré, an anatomist and surgeon from Paris.

1719   *Francis Home* born. An Edinburgh physician who pioneered experimental inoculation against measles and published much of his work and research on measles, croup, diabetes and many other areas in *Medical Facts and Experiments*.

1719   Westminster Hospital in London was founded.

1720   German anatomist, Abraham Vater, described the anatomical abnormality known as a choledochal cyst.

1720   *Bonaventura Corti* born. An Italian anatomist who described the receptor organ for sound, consisting of a complex structure of the basilar membrane, cochlea, hair cells, and other structures, collectively known as the organ of Corti.

1721   *Pierre Brasdor* born. A French surgeon who devised a distal ligation applied to an aneurysm (Brasdor operation).

1721   The infective nature of tuberculosis was shown through microscopy by E. Barry of Dublin.

1721   First use of the word anesthesia in its present sense was given in Bailey's dictionary. It defined anesthesia as 'loss or defect of sense, as in such as have the palsy or are blasted'.

1722   *Théophile de Bordeu* born. A physician who was the first to suggest that the internal secretions of the testis and ovary had a remote and overall effect on the organism.

1722   *Pieter Camper* born. A Dutch orthopedic surgeon who gave a description of the fascia and olecranon bursa, and wrote on shoe-induced deformities.

1722   The Chandos professorship (in medicine and anatomy) at St Andrew's Medical School in Scotland was created by the Duke of Chandos.

1723   Cuneiform cartilage of the larynx (Morgagni cartilage) was described by Giovanni Battista Morgagni, the founder of pathological anatomy.

1723   Drainage of empyema was described by Renatus Garengeot of Paris.

1724   Indirect and direct hernia were differentiated by Lorenz Heister of Germany.

1724   A monograph on the gynecological diseases of spinsters was written by a surgeon and gynecologist from Bavaria, Georg Ernst Stahl.

1724   A much later edition of *De Recondita Abscessuum Natura* by Severinus, divided tumors of the breast into 4 categories; glandular, stromal, scirrhous and cancerous.

1724   *Johann Friedrich Meckel, the Elder* born. A professor of anatomy and gynecology at Berlin who described the sphenopalatine ganglion (Meckel ganglion) and the dural space (Meckel cavity) in which the Gasserian ganglion was lodged.

1724   The duct of the sublingual salivary gland (Walther canal) was named after August Friedrich Walther, professor of pathology from Leipzig, Germany.

1725   Thomas Guy, a bookseller from Southwark, London and a governor at St Thomas' Hospital, founded Guy's Hospital as a hospital for 'incurables'

1725   *Leopold Marco Antonio Caldani* born. A professor of anatomy from Padua who described the coraco-clavicular ligament.

1725   *Pierre Tarin* born. A French anatomist who studied the brain, and described the thickening of the velum medullare at the vermis of the cerebellum (Tarin valve).

1726   English surgeon, Robert Houstoun, 'tapped' a cyst in a case of ovarian dropsy or cystoma.

1726   *William Giffard* born. An English obstetrician who recognized and described a case of extrauterine pregnancy, and documented the first use of obstetric forceps.

1727   *Johann Gottfried Zinn* born. A professor from Göttingen who described the annulus tendineus as the origin of ocular muscles (Zinn ligament), the central artery of the retina (Zinn artery), and completed an anatomical study of the eye.

1727   French surgeon François Parfour du Petit introduced the concept of the action of spinal nerves independent of cerebral influence and described mydriasis, exophthalmos and changes in the orbit of the eye due to irritation of the sympathetic nervous system (Petit syndrome),.

1727 The first report of perforating gastric ulcer was given by English physician, Christopher Rawlinson.

1727 Two feet of gangrenous bowel were resected from a strangulated hernia for the first time (intestinal resection) by Karl A. Ramdohr of Halle.

1728 *John Hunter* born. A leading Scottish surgeon and founder of surgical pathology who made widespread investigations into embryology, venereal disease, and dentistry, and developed a technique for tying off arterial aneurysms.

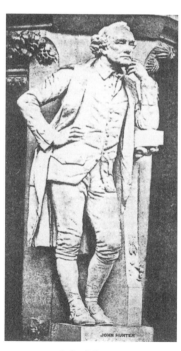

John Hunter

1728 *Joseph Black* born. A Scottish chemist who isolated carbon dioxide in 1754, after its initial discovery by Dutch physician, Jan Baptista van Helmont, and showed its relation to respiration. He presented a famous thesis *De Humore acido a cibis orto, et Magnesia Alba*, which is regarded as a model of philosophical investigation.

1728 The first description of aneurysms of syphilitic origin were published in *De motu cordis et aneurysmatibus* by Giovanni Maria Lancisi. He contributed to knowledge of cardiac pathology with his discussions of the various causes of heart enlargement

1729 *John Leake* born. An eminent English physician who founded the lying-in-hospital at Westminster, published several books on midwifery and gynecology, and introduced a modified delivery bed for women in labor.

1729 One of the earliest modern works on the swollen mass of dilated veins in anal tissue (hemorrhoids), was written by George Ernst Stahl of Bavaria.

1729 The Royal Infirmary in Edinburgh was established.

1729 *William Buchan* born. A Scottish physician who wrote three important works, *Domestic Medicine, Advice to Mothers and Treatise on Venereal Disease*.

1729 *Lazzaro Spallanzani* born. An Italian physiologist who showed

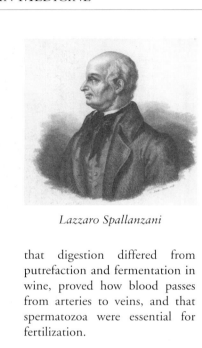

Lazzaro Spallanzani

that digestion differed from putrefaction and fermentation in wine, proved how blood passes from arteries to veins, and that spermatozoa were essential for fertilization.

1730 The first tracheotomy in a case of diphtheria was performed by Scottish physician, George Martin.

1730 One of the first anatomical lectures in the American colonies was given by Thomas Cadwalader, a physician from Philadelphia and a founder of the Pennsylvania Hospital.

1730 *Abbada Felix Ferdinand Gaspar (Felice) Fontana* born. An Italian anatomist who described the Fontana canal, the sinus venosus sclerae, and Fontana's spaces, spaces of the iridocorneal angle, irregular shaped endothelium-lined spaces within the trabecular reticulum.

1730 *Jan Ingenhousz* born. A botanist, chemist and physician from Breda who introduced the concept of the balance between animal and vegetable life, and that green plants in light fix carbon dioxide from air.

1730 The first clinical description of pellagra was made by Gaspar Casal, a Spanish physiologist, who identified the disease among peasants in the Asturias region of Spain and called it Mal de la Rosa.

1730 Stephen Hales carried out pioneering investigations into reflex actions and the spinal cord.

1731 The Royal Academy of Surgery in France was founded.

1732 The Philadelphia General Hospital was established in connection with the Philadelphia Almshouse and was known for several generations as the Blockley Hospital.

1732 German surgeon, Lorenz Heister introduced the expression 'arch of the aorta'.

1732 *Raphael Bienvenu Sabatier* born. A French surgeon from Paris who devised the Sabatier suture, a method of approximation of the intestinal wound using cardboard soaked in turpentine.

1733 An accurate description of all the bones with illustrations was contained in *Osteographia or Anatomy of Human Bones*, published by William Cheselden of St Thomas' Hospital, London.

1733 *Haemastaticks* by Stephen Hales was published. This treatise was the most important contribution to the physiology of blood circulation since that of Harvey and contained a description of Hales measurements of blood pressure in a horse. Hales recorded that arterial pressure was far greater than venous pressure.

1733 Two cases of congenital atresia of the ileum were described by Scottish surgeon, James Calder.

1733 Ichthyosis hystrix, a form of ichthyosis with 'dry and warty knobs', was described by English physician, John Machin.

1733 *Alexander Monro, Secundus* born. A famous Edinburgh anatomist who studied under William Hunter in London, Meckel in Berlin, and Albinus in Leiden, and published important works on the nervous system, eye, ear and general anatomy.

1733 Arsenic and its compounds were investigated by Swedish chemist, Georg Brandt, who published a systematic treatise on the subject.

1733 *Thomas Denman* born. An English obstetrician who first described spontaneous version of transverse presentation in obstetrics, occurring through rotation of the head and shoulder (Denman evolution).

1733 A morbid anxiety about health, leading to hypochondriasis (Cheyne disease), was described by Scottish physician, George Cheyne.

1733 *Caspar Friedrich Wolff* born. A Berlin professor of anatomy who described ren primordialis (Wolffian body), ureter primordialis (Wolffian duct), and proposed the theory of epigenesis.

Caspar Friedrich Wolff

1733 St George's Hospital at Hyde Park Corner, London was founded (now at Blackshaw Road).

1734 *Anselme Louis Bernard Berchillet-Jourdain* born. A French surgeon who described chronic suppurative peridonditis (Jourdain disease).

1734 *Johann Gottlieb Walter* born. A professor of anatomy working in Berlin who gave his name to the smallest branch of the splanchnic nerve passing through the renal plexus (Walter nerve).

1735 Werlhof disease (thrombocytopenic purpura) was described as purpura hemorrhagica in *Opera Omnia* by German physician, Paul Gottlieb Werlhof.

1736 St Phillip's Hospital in Charlestown, Carolina was established.

1736 *Domenico Cotugno* born. A professor of anatomy from Naples, Italy, who described several structures of the labyrinthine apparatus and also gave a classic description of sciatica.

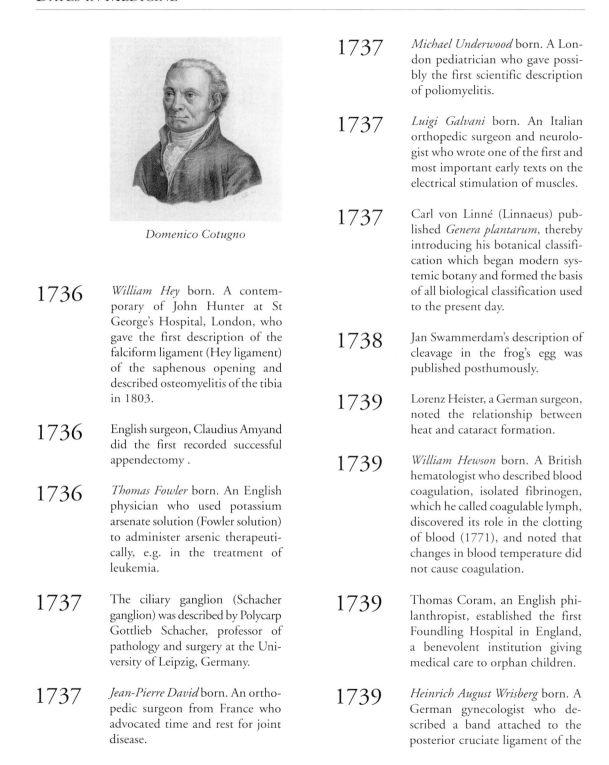

Domenico Cotugno

1736 *William Hey* born. A contemporary of John Hunter at St George's Hospital, London, who gave the first description of the falciform ligament (Hey ligament) of the saphenous opening and described osteomyelitis of the tibia in 1803.

1736 English surgeon, Claudius Amyand did the first recorded successful appendectomy .

1736 *Thomas Fowler* born. An English physician who used potassium arsenate solution (Fowler solution) to administer arsenic therapeutically, e.g. in the treatment of leukemia.

1737 The ciliary ganglion (Schacher ganglion) was described by Polycarp Gottlieb Schacher, professor of pathology and surgery at the University of Leipzig, Germany.

1737 *Jean-Pierre David* born. An orthopedic surgeon from France who advocated time and rest for joint disease.

1737 *Michael Underwood* born. A London pediatrician who gave possibly the first scientific description of poliomyelitis.

1737 *Luigi Galvani* born. An Italian orthopedic surgeon and neurologist who wrote one of the first and most important early texts on the electrical stimulation of muscles.

1737 Carl von Linné (Linnaeus) published *Genera plantarum*, thereby introducing his botanical classification which began modern systemic botany and formed the basis of all biological classification used to the present day.

1738 Jan Swammerdam's description of cleavage in the frog's egg was published posthumously.

1739 Lorenz Heister, a German surgeon, noted the relationship between heat and cataract formation.

1739 *William Hewson* born. A British hematologist who described blood coagulation, isolated fibrinogen, which he called coagulable lymph, discovered its role in the clotting of blood (1771), and noted that changes in blood temperature did not cause coagulation.

1739 Thomas Coram, an English philanthropist, established the first Foundling Hospital in England, a benevolent institution giving medical care to orphan children.

1739 *Heinrich August Wrisberg* born. A German gynecologist who described a band attached to the posterior cruciate ligament of the knee, internal cutaneous nerve to minor brachi, and cuneiform cartilage of the larynx (all named after him).

1739   *John Andrée* born. A physician from Switzerland who settled in London and played a major role in setting up the London Hospital.

1739   An arterial cause for gangrene was published by Parisian surgeon François Quesnay, in *Traité de la Gangrene*.

1740   The role of external and internal intercostal muscles in respiration was explained by George Erhard Hamberger of Germany.

1740   *Johann Ernst Wichmann* born. A German physician who described laryngismus stridulus (Wichmann asthma) and demonstrated the parasitic cause of scabies in 1786.

1740   *John Haygarth* born. An English physician who published the first detailed monograph on acute rheumatism, *A Clinical History of the Acute Rheumatism and Rheumatic Fever and a Clinical History of the Nodosity in the Joints* in 1798. He gave his name to the subcutaneous nodules (Haygarth nodes) of the joints in rheumatoid arthritis.

1740   A hospital, recognized as among the earliest facilities for cancer, was opened with money bequeathed by Jean Godinot, a canon of Rheims Cathedral.

1740   The London Hospital was founded in the East End of the city after a

meeting of philanthropists at the Feathers Tavern, Cheapside.

1740   *Jean André Venel* born. A Swiss orthopedic surgeon and generally regarded as the father of his field, who founded the first orthopedic institute in the world, and stressed the benefits of sunlight in treatment.

1740   Jacob Bigemus Winslow, an anatomist and surgeon from Denmark, used the term basilare to denote the basilar artery.

1741   *William Withering* born. An English physician who demonstrated that the plant foxglove alleviated certain forms of dropsy and thus gave the first clinical description of the effects of digitalis on heart patients.

1741   John Jacob Huber, a professor of anatomy at Göttingen, described the aberrant ganglion on the posterior root of the first cervical nerve.

1741   *Guiseppe Flajani* born. An Italian surgeon who described and gave his name to Flajani disease (exophthalmic goiter).

1742   The Chinese medical text *The Golden Mirror of Medicine* listed four forms of inoculation against smallpox that had been used in China since 1695.

1742   *Nicolas Leblanc* born. A French physician and chemist who developed the process for making soda ash (sodium carbonate) from salt (sodium chloride) and sulfuric acid. The Leblanc process became an important chemical process in the 19th century.

1742 *Johann Ernst Neuberger* born. A German anatomist who described a deep thyroid artery (Neuberger artery).

1742 *Antoine Portal* born. A professor of anatomy at the Jardin du Roi in Paris, who gave original descriptions of several anatomical structures, observed bleeding due to esophageal varices, and published an important work on epilepsy.

1742 *Edouard Sandifort* born. A physician from Holland who described congenital cyanotic heart disease and whose work on pathological anatomy is held equal to that of Giovanni Battista Morgagni.

1742 Permanent grafting of animal tissue was demonstrated in the hydra by Swedish biologist, Abraham Trembley.

1742 A new system of thermometry was described by Anders Celsius of Sweden.

1742 *Carl W. Scheele* born. A Swedish urologist who studied and analyzed urine and made an examination of pulverized bladder calculi from patients with gouty arthritis which led to the discovery of uric acid and calculus acid. He wrote *Chemical Treatise on Air and Fire*, which debunked the phlogiston theory.

1743 Hartwig Wilhelm Ludwig Taube of Germany described a body in the artery, referring to it as 'ganglion minutum' (carotid body).

1743 *Sir William Blizard* born. A founder of the London Hospital Medical School who was famous for tying the superior thyroid artery for goiter.

1743 Curare was brought from the Amazon to Europe by French scientist and explorer, Charles Marie de la Condamine.

1743 Fibrosis and deformity of the penis (Peyronie disease) was described by French surgeon, François de la Peyronie.

1743 Jean Louis Petit, a leading Paris surgeon, made the first suggestion that a distended gallbladder could be relieved by a puncture (cholecystostomy).

1743 Stephen Hales designed a ventilator which enabled fresh air to get into prisons and other enclosed spaces, and consequently the death rate from jail fever was reduced considerably..

1743 *Antoine Lavoisier* born. The French founder of modern chemistry who demonstrated the significance of oxygen in combustion, which he named the acidifying principle (in Greek, oxygine principle, hence the derivation of the word oxygen).

1744 The inferior carotid ganglion, found in the cavernous plexus, was first described by Kasimir Christoph Schmiedel, a professor of anatomy and botany at Erlangen.

1744 *Pierre Joseph Desault*, founder of the Paris surgical clinic, born. A French physician who devised a treatment of aneurysm, better methods of treating fractures and dislocations, and published treatises on venereal disease, and on stones in the bladder and kidneys.

1744 First recorded successful case of mouth-to-mouth respiration or expired air respiration in a coal-miner was given by William Tossak of Edinburgh.

1744 *Henry Park* born. An English surgeon who first described arterio-venous aneurysm which communicates with two veins (Park aneurysm).

1745 *Philippe Pinel* born. A neuropsychiatrist from Paris who was one of the first to follow William Cullen's psychological theory on insanity, and to refer to it as an illness, unchain patients, and treat them humanely.

1745 The English physician, William Heberden, published his *Essay on mithridatium antheriaka*. This pivotal work did much to rid the pharmacopeia of the superstition and irrationality which had previously clouded it and paved the way to modern therapeutics.

1745 *William Cruikshank* born. A surgeon and anatomist from Edinburgh who published Anatomy of the Absorbent Vessels of the Human Body and gave a description of the lymphatics as an absorbing system for blood, and observed that carbon dioxide, salt and other substances are eliminated by the skin, in detailed studies on perspiration. He demonstrated the passage of the impregnated ovum through the fallopian tubes.

1745 French male midwives, or accoucheurs were recognized in the 17th century, but the first recorded American was John Duppy of New York.

1745 *Peter Johann Frank* born. A Bavarian physician who was the first to focus studies on diseases of the spinal cord, the first to describe diabetes insipidus in 1794, and to differentiate it from diabetes mellitus.

1745 *Benjamin Rush* born. Regarded as the first psychiatrist in America, who wrote *Diseases of the Mind*, the first American book on the subject, and introduced occupational therapy in the treatment of mental diseases.

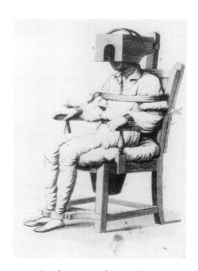

Rush tranquilizing chair

1745 The Middlesex Hospital at Marylebone, London was founded.

1745 *Alessandro Codivalli* born. An Italian orthopedic surgeon and neurologist who differentiated efferent and afferent nerve action in muscles.

1745 The Lieberkühn glands in the lining of the intestines were named after Johann Nathaniel Lieberkühn, an anatomist from Berlin who described them in detail.

1746 Pyorrhea alveolaris or marginal periodontitis was originally described by Pierre Fauchard, and was later named Riggs disease because of a new treatment consisting of tooth scraping developed by US dentist, John Mankey Riggs.

1746 *Recherches sur Glandes* was written by Théophile de Bordeu, a physician at Montpellier. In it he suggested that the ovary secreted internal substance which had a remote and overall effect on the organism.

1746 The discovery of iron in the blood was made by Vincenzo Antonio Menghini, an Italian physician.

1746 *Jean-Louis Baudelocque* born. A French gynecologist who devised a method of removal of the ovum for the treatment of extrauterine pregnancy by making an incision in the posterior vaginal cul-de-sac.

1746 A postmortem account of the emphysematous appearance of the lung in asthma was given by Englishman, Sir William Watson.

1746 John André, a physician at the London Hospital, published *Cases of Epilepsy, Hysteric Fits, and St Vitus Dance, with the Process of Cure*, the first monograph on epilepsy.

1746 *François Chaussier* born. A French anatomist and surgeon who discovered the external circumflex branch of the deep femoral artery which supplied the quadriped muscles.

1747 The concept of impulse and irritability of living tissues was introduced in *Primae Lineae Physiologiae* by Swiss physician, Albrecht von Haller, regarded as one of the greatest physiologists of his century.

1747 The pathological changes related to dysentery were described by Giovanni Battista Morgagni, professor of anatomy at Padua.

1748 *Charles Blagden* born. An English physician who demonstrated the ability of the body to maintain its temperature despite high room temperatures, the cooling effect of water evaporation (1774), and the importance of perspiration in regulating body temperature (diaphoresis) (1775). He also described heat cramp.

1748 *Louis Odier* born. A physician from Geneva who studied at the Universities of Leiden and Edinburgh, is widely credited as being the first to introduce vaccination, and published *A Manual of Practice of Medicine*.

1748 An authoritative description of diphtheria was given by John Fothergill, a Quaker physician, in his *Account of the Putrid Sore Throat.*

1748 *Félix Vicq D'Azyr* born. A French physician and comparative anatomist from Paris who first described the mammilothalamic tract which bears his name.

1748 Osmosis was first discovered by a French abbé, Jean Antoine Nollet, a professor of physics at the College de Navarre in Paris, France. He also invented an electrometer.

1749 French oculist, Jacques Daviel, performed surgical treatment for cataract by excision of the lens (Daviel operation).

1749 *Georgius Prochaska* born. A Moravian professor of anatomy at Prague who demonstrated the integrated functions of the brain in producing movements of the body, and wrote on the heart, and blood circulation.

1749 *David Pitcairn* born. A physician at St Bartholomew's Hospital, London who noted lesions in the heart valves following rheumatic fever, and who introduced the term rheumatic into the description of heart disease in 1788.

1749 Quinine, an alkaloid of cinchona which suppresses the malarial parasite, was used for 'rebellious palpitations of the heart' by French physician, Jean Baptiste Senac.

1749

Edward Jenner

Edward Jenner born. An English physician who introduced vaccination against smallpox and wrote *An Inquiry into the Causes and Effects of the Variola Vaccinae.* He also wrote *Remarks on a disease of the heart following acute rheumatism, illustrated by dissection*, one of the earliest treatises on the subject.

1749 *Benjamin Bell* born. A surgeon at the Royal Edinburgh Infirmary who differentiated between syphilis and gonorrhea in his work *Gonorrhoea Virulenta and Lues Venera* (1793).

1750 The effect of various substances on putrefaction was investigated by Sir John Pringle, the founder of military medicine in England.

1750 *Robert Chessher* born. A British orthopedic surgeon who specialised in the treatment of deformities.

1750 The procedure of staphylorraphy for cleft palate was performed on a child by Parisian dentist, M. le Monnier.

1750   *Peter Middleton* born. An American physician of Scottish origin who performed the first dissection on record in America and founded a medical school in New York.

1750   Straight obstetric forceps were designed by Scottish surgeon, William Smellie.

1750   The first modern surgical description of hematocele was given by London surgeon Percivall Pott.

1751   Pupillary reaction was established as a reflex in *Essay on Vital and Other Involuntary Motions of Animals* by Robert Whytt, a Scottish neurologist.

1751   Curved forceps were designed by French surgeon and obstetrician, André Leveret.

1751   The first establishment in North America devoted to the relief of the sick and suffering, the Pennsylvania Hospital, was chartered by the Assembly of Pennsylvania, through the efforts of Benjamin Franklin, Thomas Bond, a physician from Philadelphia, and Rev Richard Peters.

1752   Gastric juice was isolated from animals by French natural philosopher, René Antoine de Réaumur, who demonstrated its solvent effects on food.

1752   First successful operation for a brain abscess (tempero-sphenoidal abscess following an ear infection)

was performed by French surgeon, Sauveur François Morand.

1752   *Alexander Gordon* born. An obstetrician from Aberdeen who proposed the contagious nature of puerperal fever, and advocated disinfection of clothes of the midwife and doctor attending the mother.

1752   *Paul Mascagni* born. An anatomist from Tuscany, Italy who gave original descriptions of several anatomical structures in his *Historia et Scenographia Vasorum Lymphaticorum corporis humani.*

1752   *Johann Friedrich Blumenbach* born. A German craniologist from Göttingen who studied the variation of skull, face, and skin in different races, in his *Generis Humanis Varietae.*

1752   *Antonio Scarpa* born. An Italian surgeon, anatomist, and ophthalmologist who made several important contributions to surgery including the first comparative study of the organs of hearing, and the discovery of the membranous labyrinth of the ear. He was the first to describe the femoral tri-

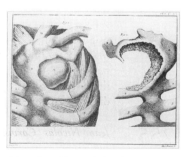

Plate from Scarpa's book on surgery

angle (Scarpa triangle) and wrote *Traité des Hernies*, (1814), one of the first scientific monographs on hernia.

1752 Albrecht von Haller, an eminent Swiss physician, proposed the concept of sensitivity to nerve impulse and resulting irritability of tissues.

1752 An early description of connective tissue disease, scleroderma, was given by Italian, Carlo Crisio.

1754 Bony nodules appearing at the distal joints of the fingers in cases of osteoarthritis were described by English physician, William Heberden (Heberden nodes).

1754 *Benjamin Waterhouse* born. The first professor of medicine at Harvard who introduced inoculation for smallpox into America, and his book, *History of Kinepox*, is a classic on the subject.

1755 *Samuel Thomas Sömmering* born. A German professor of anatomy who described the long pudendal nerve, the suspensory ligament of the lachrymal gland, and several other structures that are named after him.

1755 *Jean Alfred Fournier* born. A professor from Paris who made several important contributions to the study of syphilis, and gave his name to fulminating gangrene of the scrotum and perineum in diabetic patients.

1755 *Jean Nicolas Corvisart* born. A French physician who revived the clinical sign of percussion (de-

Jean Nicolas Corvisart

scribed by Leopold Auenbrugger), and wrote an important treatise, *Diseases of the Heart*.

1755 The first use of electroconvulsive therapy for mental illness was that of French physician, J.B. Le Roy.

1755 *Antoine François Fourcroy* born. A French chemist who gave an account of lumpy tissues in a body on opening a grave in Paris, which he named 'adipocere', and worked with another chemist, Vanquelin, in isolating urea.

1755 *Caleb Hillier Parry* born. An English physician and cardiologist who gave a detailed account of exophthalmic goiter of the thyroid (Parry disease) in *Enlargement of the Thyroid Gland* (1786).

1755 Albrecht von Haller, a Swiss physiologist, adopted the term atheroma to denote fatty degenerative lesions in the arteries.

1755 British surgeon Charles White conducted early studies in anthropometry.

1755   First record of scrapie. A debate took place in the British Parliament regarding the economic effect of a fatal disease in sheep.

1756   Bifocal lenses for spectacles were introduced by American scientist and statesman, Benjamin Franklin.

1756   *Jean Antoine Sassy* born. A French physician who wrote a treatise on diseases of the internal ear.

1756   *William Babbington* born. A physician at Guy's Hospital, London who was a founder of the Hunterian Society and the Geological Society.

1756   *Sir Everard Home* born. A pupil of John Hunter and a surgeon at St George's Hospital who described the median lobe of the prostate (Home lobe) and published *Lectures on Comparative Anatomy, Practical Observations*, and several other works.

1756   *James Currie* born. A Scottish physician, noted for his methods of inducing hypothermia, and was one of the first to employ the thermometer in the management of febrile diseases.

1756   *Joseph Adams* born. A British physician who conducted the first scientific study of hereditary disease, wrote *A Treatise on the Supposed Hereditary Properties of Disease*, and described gout, scrofula and goiter in cretinism.

1757   The ganglion of the trigeminal nerve (Gasser ganglion) was named after Viennese anatomist, Johann Laurentius Gasser.

Joseph Adams

1757   *William Charles Wells* born. An English physician who wrote a treatise on vision, made suggestions on the theory of natural selection, described nodules in acute rheumatism and cardiac complications in rheumatic fever (1810), and demonstrated the presence of albumin and blood in the urine of patients with renal dropsy (1812).

1757   Domenico Maria Gusmano Galeati of Bologna, Italy published a specific account of a case of cardiac aneurysm.

1757   A maximum/minimum thermometer was constructed by English physicist, Charles Cavendish.

1757   *Robert Willan* born. An English physician who wrote *On Cutaneous Diseases* (1796) which categorized cutaneous diseases according to their objective appearance, and contained descriptions of psoriasis, prurigo, pityriasis, and ichthyosis, defined and differentiated sycosis, tinea

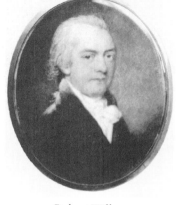

Robert Willan

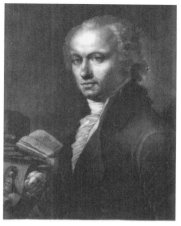

Franz Joseph Gall

versicular, lupus and impeti-go, and classified different kinds of eczema and other skin diseases.

1757 The effects of lemons and oranges in the prevention of scurvy were demonstrated by British physician, James Lind, in his *A Treatise on Scurvy*, after conducting the first controlled trial on record on HMS Salisbury.

1758 The posterior membrane of the cornea (Descemet membrane), was described by Jean Descemet, a professor of anatomy in Paris.

1758 *Franz Joseph Gall* born. A German physician who first proposed the concept of phrenology, the external study of the skull as an indicator of mental powers and moral qualities.

1758 Membrane pupillaris (Wachendorf membrane) was described by Eberhard Jacob, professor of surgery at Utrecht, Holland.

1759 A description of classical symptoms of angina pectoris in his father was provided by Edward Hyde.

1759 The association of amenorrhea with pituitary tumor first suggested by French physician, Anton de Haen.

1759 *Johann Christian Reil* born. A neuroanatomist and physician from Berlin who described the insula of the cerebral cortex, or the lobule of corpus striatum, the island of Reil.

1759 Johann Adam Schmidt born. An oculist from Vienna, Austria who described inflammation of the anterior portion of the uveal tunica or iris due to syphilis, and named it iritis (1801).

1759 Caspar Friedrich Wolff, a professor of anatomy in Berlin, published *Theoria Generationis*, in which he proposed that new structures arise in the course of development, as opposed to the preformation theory. This laid the foundations of modern embryology. Through his anatomical evidence he showed that oxygenated blood from the placenta was brought by the umbilical vein and passed through the heart without mixing, and supplied the head.

1759 Frambesia, later known as yaws, was named by François Boisser de Sauvages, professor of medicine and botany at Montpellier, France.

1759 *Franz Caspar Hesselbach* born. A German surgeon who first described the anatomical area bounded by the inferior epigastric artery, the margin of the rectus abdominis and the inguinal ligament (Hesselbach triangle).

1760 *Matthew Carey* born. An Irish–American physician who gave an accurate account of the yellow fever epidemic that struck Philadelphia at the end of this century.

1760 The nasopalatine nerve was described by Italian anatomist, Domenico Cotugno.

1760 *Peter Rubini* born. An Italian physician from Parma who wrote several treatises on fever.

1760 The posterior round ligaments of the uterus (uterosacral ligaments) were described by Antoine Petit, professor of anatomy in Paris, France.

1760 Scottish physician, William Cullen, gave the first clear account of the skin disease, erysipelas.

1760 *John Barclay* born. A lecturer in anatomy at Edinburgh University who wrote *A New Anatomical Nomenclature, and Muscular Motion*.

1760 *Thomas Beddoes* born. An English physician who founded the Medical Pneumatic Institution in Bristol for the treatment of pulmonary tuberculosis, and to study the role of gas inhalation in the treatment of diseases.

1760 The first British school for the deaf was founded in Edinburgh, Scotland by Thomas Braidwood.

1760 London apothecary, John Hill, published *Caution Against the Immoderate Use of Snuff*. He made some of the first suggestions associating tobacco with cancer and reported polyps showing 'all the frightful symptoms of an open cancer'.

1761 Giovanni Battista Morgagni's *De Sedibus et Causis Morborum per Anatomen Indagatis* was published. The first systematic textbook of morbid anatomy (in 5 volumes), detailing more than 700 case histories and pathological appearances and descriptions of his discoveries. These included cirrhosis of the liver, many forms of tumor, cancers of the breast, stomach, rectum, pancreas and lung, pneumatic consolidation of the lungs, classic descriptions of angina pectoris, myocardial degeneration, and subacute bacterial endocarditis. He was the first to show that cerebral abscess resulted from, rather than caused, suppurative otitis, and the first to connect syphilis with diseases of the cerebral arteries and tumors of the brain. He noted that strokes were caused by changes in the cerebral blood vessels and not from lesions in the brain and that hemiplegia affected the side of the body opposite to the damaged cerebral hemisphere. He described anterior diaphragmatic hernia (Morgagni hernia), atherosclerosis, and aortic coarctation.

1761 Early pathological observations on rheumatoid carditis were made by Lazarus Riverius and Giovanni Battista Morgagni.

1761 John Ulric de Bilguer, a Swiss army surgeon, published *Dissertatio Inauguralis Medico-Chirugica de Membrorum Amputatione Rarissime administranda aur quasi Abroganda.*

1761 *Matthew Baillie* born. An eminent Scottish surgeon who practiced in London and wrote *Morbid Anatomy of the Human Body* and

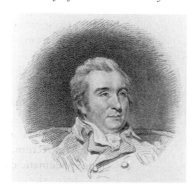

Matthew Baillie

A Series of Engravings to Illustrate the Morbid Anatomy of the Human Body (1797) in which he described dextrocardia with situs inversion viscerum, emphysema of the lung, and associated rheumatic disease with valvular lesions of the heart.

1761 Leopold von Auenbrugger, a physician from Vienna, Austria described percussion, a method of physical examination by striking the surface of the body, and established the regular use of camphor in medicine.

1762 *Eusebius Valli* born. An Italian physician noted for experimenting on himself. He tried the efficacy of plague vaccine on himself and survived, but succumbed to yellow fever whilst visiting Cuba.

1762 The first school of anatomy in North America was opened in Philadelphia by William Shippen.

1762 A book on chiropody was written by Rousselot of Paris.

1762 A method of reducing a shoulder joint which has been dislocated for several months was described by Manchester surgeon, Charles White.

1762 *Nathan Smith* born. A surgeon from Connecticut,, who gave an early account of osteomyelitis, and described the contagious nature of typhoid in *A Practical Essay on Typhus Fever.*

1763 François Boissier de la Croix de Sauvages of France classified arthritis into 14 categories and rheumatism into 10 categories, including rheumatismus arthriticus and gouty rheumatism.

1763 The use of willow in pain relief was first suggested and described by British physician, Edmund Stone.

1763 *Justus Arneman* born. A professor of surgery at Göttingen who did the first clinical studies of ear diseases.

1763 *Whitley Stokes* born. An Irish physician and dermatologist who first described dermatitis gangrenosa infantium, or ecthyma gangrenosum (also called ecthyma terebrans).

1763 *John Bell* born. A Scottish physician and lecturer in anatomy who established the first private anatomy school in Edinburgh in 1790, and wrote the famous *Anatomy of the Human Body* and *The Principles of Surgery*.

1763 *Johann Valentin von Hildenbrand* born. A physician who gave a classic description of typhus (Hildenbrand disease).

1764 A classic description of sciatica was given by Domenico Cotugno, professor of anatomy at Naples, who distinguished two forms: one causing swelling or irritation of the sciatic nerve (Cotugno disease) and the other from inflammation of the hip joint (arthritic sciatica).

1764 *John Abernethy* born. A pupil of John Hunter and later the founder of St Bartholomew's Hospital Medical School, London who ligated the common carotid artery to arrest brain hemorrhage in 1798, and ligated the external artery in cases of aneurysm.

1764 *John Haslam* born. A superintendent at the Bethlem Mental Asylum (Bedlam), London who described general paralysis of the insane (1816), examined the brains of the diseased insane at autopsy, and recorded the changes in the brain due to syphilis.

1764 *Joseph C. Carpue* born. An English surgeon who revived the Indian method of rhinoplasty (Carpue operation).

1764 *John Mason Good* born. An American physician who wrote *A Physiological System of Nosology with a Corrected and Simplified Nomenclature*, an inclusive list for its time of all the synonyms for chronic rheumatism.

1764 First description of a diverticulum of the esophagus was given by Abraham Ludlow in a letter to William Hunter.

1765 The ganglion of the trigeminal nerve (Gasserian ganglion) was named after Viennese anatomist, Johann Laurentius Gasser, by one of his students, Anton Balthasar Raymund.

1765 The term 'croup' was coined by Francis Home of Edinburgh in his *An Inquiry into the Nature, Cause and Cure of Croup*.

1765 *François Ribes* born. An army surgeon from Toulouse who described the uppermost sympathetic ganglion situated on the anterior communicating artery of the circle of Willis, the ganglion of Ribes.

1765   *Thomas Masterman Winterbottom* born. An English physician who described African trypanosomiasis or sleeping sickness which he observed during his travels.

1765   *James Wilson* born. An English surgeon who described the muscle fibers derived from the levator ani surrounding the urethra found above the triangular ligament (Wilson muscles).

1765   John Morgan addressed the College of Philadelphia with *Discourse upon the Institution of Medical Schools in America*. This constituted the formal opening of the first medical school in the country, with Morgan as its first medical professor.

1766   Swiss anatomist Albrecht von Haller, gave a clear, scientific description of cerebrospinal fluid (CSF).

1766   *Dominique Jean Larrey* born. A legendary French military surgeon and one of the first to describe the therapeutic effect of maggots on wounds, a method later revived by American surgeon William Stevenson Baer in treating osteomyelitis.

1766   *William Hyde Wollaston* born. A British chemist who demonstrated the presence of uric acid, calcium, and ammonium in urinary stones (1797), and noted the occurrence of bladder stones in patients with cystinuria (1810).

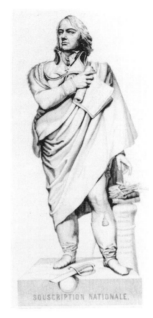

Dominique Larrey

1766   *Thomas Robert Malthus* born. An English physician, clergyman, and pioneering statistician who developed the concept of population control by food supply which had an influential effect on the work of Charles Darwin.

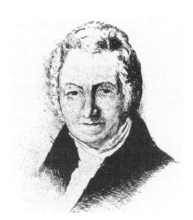

Thomas Robert Malthus

1766   *John Dalton* born. An English chemist who postulated some of the most important laws concerning gases (e.g. partial pressure – Dalton law), determined the atomic weight of many elements, and in 1794 was one of the first to investigate color blindness.

1766   The Wigand maneuver in breech delivery was described by German gynecologist, Justus Heinrich Wigand.

1766   First recorded description of cleidocranial dysostosis was given by French surgeon, Saveur François Morand.

1766   Clinical differentiation between varicella and smallpox was achieved by William Heberden.

1766   First Humane Society for the resuscitation of the apparently drowned was established in Amsterdam.

1767   Nerve generation was first mentioned by Italian anatomist, Felice Fontana, who founded and was the first director of the Natural History Museum in Florence.

1768   *Jean Louis Alibert* born. Considered to be the founder of modern French dermatology, he described mycosis fungoides as piors fungoide and cancroide, keloid, and Aleppo boil.

1768   *Christian Schreger* born. An anatomist from Denmark who described the Schreger line (the bending of dentine tubules near the surface of dentine).

1768   One of the first descriptions of angina was given by French physician, Nicolas F. R. de Magny.

1768   The Great Windmill Street School of Anatomy was founded by William Hunter in London.

1768   *Philip Syng Physick* born. The father of American surgery who introduced many operative techniques, including the use of absorbable sutures, first performed a urethrotomy or internal longitudinal incisidion (1796) and successfully treated gouty arthritis and bladder stones.

Philip Syng Physick

1768   The King's College Medical School in New York, the second medical school in America, was founded.

1768   The first medical society in North America was extablished in Philadelphia.

1768   *Joseph Wenzel* born. A professor of anatomy and physiology from Mainz, Germany who described ventriculus cerebrimus (Wenzel ventricle).

1768   *Sir Astley Paston Cooper* born. An English surgeon and anatomy teacher, who successfully ligated the common carotid artery to treat carotid aneurysm (1805), and the external iliac artery to treat femoral aneurysm (1808).

1768   Robert Whytt, professor of medicine at Edinburgh, wrote a treatise in neurology which concentrated on tuberculose meningitis. He demonstrated that the destruction of the anterior corpora quadrigemina resulted in the abolition of pupillary contraction in reaction to light.

1769   *Georges L.C. Cuvier* born. A French scientist and one of the founders of modern morphology, who discovered the two cardinal ducts, the Cuvier ducts.

1769   Fracture of the lower segment of fibula and malleolus of the tibia with rupture of the internal lateral ligament of the ankle (Pott fracture) was described by London surgeon, Percivall Pott.

1769   An original description of the spasm of the larynx (laryngismus stridulus) was given by Scottish physician, John Millar.

1769   Charles Bonnet of Copenhagen, Denmark described visual hallucinations in old age which were not associated with any mental disorder.

1770   Cancer of the scrotum, the first occupational cancer (chimney sweep's cancer), was described by British surgeon, Percivall Pott.

1770   The association between edema and coagulable substances in urine (nephrotic syndrome) was first observed by Italian anatomist, Domenico Cotugno.

1770   First suggestion of artificial pneumothorax as treatment in tuberculosis was made by M. Bourru of Paris.

1770   *Julien Jean Cesar Legallois* born. A physician and physiologist from Cherneix in France who proposed the concept of maintaining life without need for the heart, by regular injection or supply of blood, and discovered the respiratory center in the medulla oblongata (1812).

1770   *John Stearns* born. The first president of the New York Academy of Medicine who introduced the use of ergot into American obstetrics.

1770   Johann Georg Zimmermann, a physician from Switzerland, published a monograph on bacillary dysentery.

1771   *Karl Asmund Rudolphi* born. A Swiss anatomist and helminthologist who, in 1808, used the term 'echinococcus' to refer to a genus of taeniid tapeworms whose larva form a vesicular hydatid.

1771   An early and detailed description of retroversion of the uterus was given by the British anatomist, William Hunter.

1771   Red cell fragility was noticed by William Hewson, a British hematologist, when he observed that the

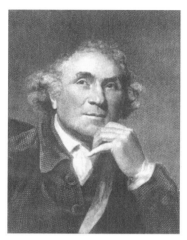

William Hunter

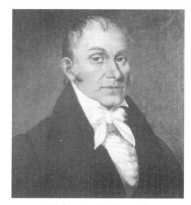

Ephraim McDowell

cells were destroyed in water but remained normal in salt solution.

1771   *Johann Christian Rosenmüller* born. An embryologist and professor of anatomy at Leipzig, Germany who described the pharyngeal recess (Rosenm¸ller fossa).

1771   *Marie François Xavier Bichat* born. A Paris physician and a founder of microscopic anatomy, advocated the study of anatomy on the basis of different tissues in the body, and considered that tumors arose from connective tissue and had a common tissue and structure.

1771   The term reflex to describe the sensory motor reaction was introduced by Johan August Unzer, a physiologist from Halle in Germany.

1771   The New York Hospital received its Royal Charter.

1771   *Ephraim McDowell* born. A pioneer in abdominal surgery from Kentucky who performed the first ovariotomy in 1809, when he successfully removed an ovarian cyst, weighing 22 pounds, without anesthesia.

1771   Samuel Bard, a French Huguenot living in America, introduced the term angina suffocativa for diphtheria.

1771   *Pierre Bretonneau* born. A Paris physician who performed tracheotomy in croup, gave a classical description of typhoid, and demonstrated the characteristics of Peyer patches in the intestines of patients with typhoid.

1771   John Hunter, English anatomist and surgeon who lectured on dentistry, published *The Natural History of the Human Teeth*.

1772   *François Victor Joseph Broussais* born. A French physician who considered irritability of the mucous membrane of the alimentary canal or gastroenteritis as a basis for most diseases.

1772   The membranous labyrinth of the ear, including the semicircular canals, vestibule and cochlea, was discovered by Antonio Scarpa, an Italian anatomist.

1772   *Jacques Matthieu Delpech* born. A surgeon at Montpellier, France who devised a new method of treatment of clubfoot by subcutaneous section of the achilles tendon (subcutaneous tenotomy) in 1816, and recognized that the muscles surrounding the joint give it strength and therefore, that lesions in muscles cause deformities.

1772   *Jean Etienne Dominique Esquirol* born. A French physician, who was a pioneer in mental disease and one of the first to note adult psychiatric illnesses in children and to investigate dementia in senile states.

1772   Nitrogen was obtained from air by Daniel Rutherford, a pupil of Joseph Black, at the University of Edinburgh, Scotland.

1772   *Karl Gustav Himley* born. A professor of ophthalmology at Vienna who designed an operation for irido dialysis, used hyoscyamine to dilate the pupil before the removal of the lens, and established clinical teaching in ophthalmology.

1772   *James Carson* born. An English physician from Liverpool who performed open pneumothorax as treatment for tuberculosis, and suggested that lungs collapsed if the negative pressure was compromised.

1772   William Heberden gave a classic description of angina pectoris and coronary artery disease.

1773   *Thomas Young* born. A physician from Somerset, England, who demonstrated the mechanism of accommodation of the lens in vision, classified diseases in his *Introduction to Medical Literature* and wrote important essays on capillary attraction.

1773   *Luigi Rolando* born. A professor of anatomy in Turin, Italy, who described the sulcus centralis of the brain (Rolando fissure), made a study of the cerebellum, and described several other structures of the brain.

1773   Cancer was considered to be a local process that invaded and generalized through the lymphatics by Bernard Pehrilhe, a Paris surgeon and cancer specialist, who advocated surgical treatment.

1773   *Franz Daniel Reisseisen* born. An anatomist and physician from Strasburg who demonstrated contraction of the smooth muscles in the wall of the smallest bronchial tubes during an asthmatic attack.

1773   John Fothergill, a Quaker physician from England described trigeminal neuralgia as a 'painful affection of the face', Fothergill disease.

1773   Hilaire-Marin Rouelle, a French physician and chemist, isolated urea from urine, conducted the first chemical investigations into blood and discovered sodium carbonate, potassium chloride, and sodium chloride in vertebrate blood.

1773 The Medical Society of London, the oldest of its type in England, was founded by physician and philanthropist, John Coakley Lettsom.

1773 *Abraham Colles* born. An eminent Irish surgeon and professor of anatomy who was one of the first to tie the subclavian artery, and is also thought to have been the first to tie the innominate artery successfully (1811).

1773 *William Stoker* born. An Irish physician who investigated the velocity of sedimentation of blood corpuscles.

1773 *John Bostock* born. A physician at Guy's Hospital who described hayfever in detail in 1817 and included 28 cases of 'estival catarrh' – summer catarrh.

1773 *Robert Brown* born. A Scottish physician and botanist who described the cell nucleus for the first time, explained the process of generation in plants by means of pollen, and discovered Brownian motion.

1773 *John Cunningham Saunders* born. A London surgeon who devised a special cutting needle for cataract operations, and published a treatise on the anatomy of the human ear.

1773 The American Medical Society was founded in Philadelphia by students from different parts of the Union who attended medical lectures there.

1774 One of the most important illustrated gynecology books, *The Anatomy of the Human Gravid Uterus*, was published by William Hunter, a Scottish surgeon.

1774 French surgeon Jean Louis Petit published observations on the removal of not only cancerous axillary nodes, but some of the pectoralis major muscle as well, in breast cancer.

1774 William Hewson a British hematologist and anatomist found that leukocytes arise from the lymphatic glands and the thymus.

1774

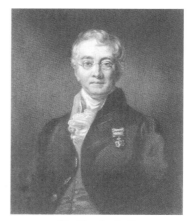

Sir Charles Bell

Sir Charles Bell born. A Scottish anatomist, physiologist, and neurologist who recognized that lesions of the 7th nerve could bring about facial palsy (Bell palsy), and explained the part played by the dorsal root in the sympathetic arc reflex.

1774 *Gaspard Laurent Bayle* born. A French physician from Provence who made important contributions to understanding of the pathology of the lung in tuberculosis.

1774 Porcelain teeth were introduced in France.

1774 *John Conrad Otto* born. A pioneer in the study of hemophilia in America who published his observations on bleeders in families.

1774 The Register of the Royal Humane Society of London, provided evidence of successful cardiac resuscitation using electrostimulation to the thorax in a patient without a pulse.

1774 Uterine curettage (Récamier operation) was devised by French gynecologist, Joseph Récamier.

1774 *Jean Baptiste de Monet Lamarck* born. A French physician and zoologist best known for his theory that acquired traits are inheritable (Lamarckism) which was contradicted later by Darwinian theory. He published *Philosophie Zoologique* (1809) in which he stated that organs were improved with repeated use and weakened by lack of use.

1774 *Jean Marie Gaspard* born. A Parisian otorhinologist who wrote one of the first modern textbooks on the ear and devised a catheter for the Eustachian tube.

1774 Joseph Priestley, an English chemist, isolated oxygen and showed it to be the component in air that made dark venous blood brighter red.

1774 *Pierre Blaud* born. A French physician who prescribed the iron pill (ferrous carbonate or Blaud pill) to treat chlorosis.

1774 French physician, Bernard Pehrilhe, attempted to transmit cancer by injecting material from a human breast cancer into a dog.

1774 The Society for Inoculating the Poor was formed by the physicians of Philadelphia, and was designed to mitigate the horrors of smallpox. This was the first benevolent society to be founded in the Colonies.

1775 *Adam Elias von Siebold* born. A German surgeon who wrote extensively on uterine cancer, believing that the disease was more frequent in women who had had several pregnancies, difficult labor, and leukorrhea.

1775 Oxygen therapy was first suggested for resuscitation by Scottish surgeon, John Hunter.

1775 The concept of internal or endocrine secretion, in which an organ or tissue discharges its secretion directly into the bloodstream to influence other parts of the body, was proposed by Théophile de Bordeu of Paris.

1775 An hereditary allergy to eggs was recorded in *Historia de Materia Medica* by Scottish physician, William Cullen.

1775 British surgeon, Percivall Pott, removed the ovaries of a young woman for the correction of 'ovarian herniae' which stopped menstruation and caused the breasts to shrink.

1776 *René Dutrochet* born. A French physiologist who discovered that green matter in plants absorbs carbon dioxide, identified the role of chlorophyll in photosynthesis, and explained endosmosis.

1776 Italian anatomist, Francesco Gennari, described the structural organisation of the cerebral cortex.

1776 *Charles Frederick Burdach* born. A professor of medicine from Dorpat who described the posterior column of the spinal cord (Burdach column).

1776 *Mauro Rusconi* born. An Italian embryologist and comparative anatomist from Parma who wrote several important treatises on embryology.

1776 The first surgeon to perform cecostomy, the opening of the cecum onto the right iliac region through a peritoneal incision in a patient with carcinoma of the rectum, was H. Pillore of Rouen.

1776 *Conrad Johann Martin Langenbeck* born. A professor of surgery at Göttingen who described the superficial nerve of the scapula (Langenbeck nerve).

1776 *Amedeo Avogadro* born. An Italian physicist who suggested that the molecule was the smallest quantity of a substance, and proposed Avogadro law.

1776 Osteomalacia (bone softness) was described in *A Remarkable Case of Softness of Bones* written by Henry Thomas, a surgeon at the London Hospital.

1777 The first clear description of color blindness was given by English physician, Joseph Huddard, in a letter to Joseph Priestley.

1777 *Louis Jacques Thénard* born. A French organic chemist who carried out a scientific study of the composition of bile, and used the term 'picromel' to denote the sweetish bitter substance in it.

1777 *Treatise on Diseases of the Skin* was written by Anne Charles Lorry. This was the first modern text on dermatology.

1777 The symphysiotomy technique in obstetrics was pioneered by French obstetrician, Jean René Sigault.

1777 *Guillaume Dupuytren* born. A French surgeon who was the first to treat wryneck by subcutaneous section of the sternomastoid, and gave original descriptions of fracture of the lower end of the fibula, and congenital dislocation of the hip.

1777 Antoine Lavoisier renamed Priestley's dephlogisticated air 'oxygen'. He undertook extensive studies on its significance in combustion and respiration and demonstrated that natural organic compounds contained carbon, hydrogen and oxygen.

1777   Bertrand Courtois, a chemist from Dijon, France, serendipitously discovered iodine when he added sulfuric acid to ash of seaweed.

1777   *Johann Georg C.F.M. Lobstein* born. A French pathologist who described osteogenesis imperfecta, a collagen disorder resulting in brittleness of bones and frequent fractures.

1777   *Franz Karl Nägele* born. A German obstetrician who described distorted pelvis in which the conjugate diameter takes an oblique direction (Nägele pelvis).

1777   Maximillian Stoll of Swabia reported carcinoma of the gallbladder.

1778

John Collins Warren

John Collins Warren born. An American surgeon who performed the first operation using ether anesthetic in 1846 when he removed a vascular tumor from just below the mandible in a patient's neck. William Morton administered the anesthetic.

1778   *Thomas Bateman* born. An English dermatologist and surgeon who described lichen urticatus, molluscum contagiosum, and eczema.

1778   *George Ballingall* born. A professor of military surgery from Edinburgh, Scotland who described Madura foot, or Ballingall disease, and clarified the difference between bacillary dysentery and amebic dysentery (1808).

1778   Teeth were first classified into molars, bicuspids, cuspids, and incisors by Scottish surgeon, John Hunter in *A Practical Treatise on the Diseases of the Teeth.*

1778   Spasm of the bronchial muscles (bronchospasm) as a cause of asthma was suggested by Scottish physician, William Cullen.

1779   The first book on public health (in nine volumes), *System of Medical Policing,* was published in Germany by Johann Peter Frank.

1779   Italian physiologist, Lazzaro Spallanzani, proposed that sperm must make physical contact with the egg for fertilization to take place.

1779   *Lars G. Branting* born. A Swedish orthopedic surgeon who developed a system of gymnastics in orthopedic treatment which was adopted by many countries.

1779   *Ludolf Christian Treviranus* born. A German anatomy professor from Bremen who discovered the intercellular spaces in tissues.

1779   Olaus Acrel, a Swedish surgeon who pioneered ophthalmic surgery in Scandinavia, and described the pseudoganglion on the posterior interosseous nerve at the back of the wrist (Acrel ganglion).

1779 *A. Richerand* born. A French professor of surgery and physiology and one of the most skilled in the world, who resected the 5th and 6th ribs.

1779 *Johann C.G. Jörg* born. A German obstetrician who wrote the first orthopedic textbook, and distinguished curvature of scoliosis from spinal tuberculosis.

1779 Deformity and sequelae due to spinal caries (Pott disease) were first described by London surgeon, Percivall Pott, although he failed to recognize the tuberculous nature.

1780 The first clear description of anthrax was given by French veterinarian, Philibert Chabert.

1780 *Philibert Joseph Roux* born. A French surgeon from the Hôtel Dieu in Paris who sutured a ruptured female perineum, pioneered staphylorrhaphy, and the repair of cleft palate.

1780 The first recorded case of suturing after complete division of the intestines (intestinal anastomosis), was achieved by Karl A. Ramdohr of Halle.

1780 The yeast test for the detection of sugar in urine was devised by Edinburgh physician, Francis Home.

1780 Oxygen therapy was suggested in resuscitation of asphyxiated neo-nates by French surgeon, François Chaussier.

1780 *John Abercrombie* born. A surgeon to the Royal Public Dispensary in Edinburgh who wrote *Pathological and Practical Researches on Diseases of the Brain*, the first book on neuropathology.

1780 *Charles Badham* born. A London physician who wrote several important treatises on lung disease, and distinguished acute and chronic bronchitis from pleuro-pneumonia and pleurisy.

1780 Marjolin ulcer, resulting from the breakdown of a cicatrix, was described by French surgeon, Jean Nicolas Marjolin.

1780 One of the first studies on the physiology of digestion was performed by Lazzaro Spallanzani, an Italian physician, who showed that digestion differed from putrefaction and that hydrochloric acid was produced by the stomach.

1781 The boundaries of the infraclavicular fossa (Morenheim space) were first described by Joseph Jacob Morenheim, professor of surgery at St Petersburg, Russia.

1781 *Friedrich Tiedemann* born. A professor of anatomy at Heidelberg, Germany who described the plexus of nerve fibrils around the central artery of the retina arising from the central ciliary nerves (Tiedemann nerve).

1781 Tooth transplantation was introduced into the USA by the French surgeon, Pierre le Mayeur, who offered a fee of two guineas to anybody willing to donate a tooth.

1781 *Laurent Theodore Biett* born. A French physician who gave the first adequate and complete description of lupus erythematosus, also known as Biett disease.

1781 *John Friedrich Meckel the Younger* born. A professor of anatomy at Halle who discovered the diverticulum of the ileum, resulting from the presence of the yolk stalk of the embryo (Meckel diverticulum).

1781 *Réne Théophile Hyacinthe Laënnec* born. A French physician who invented the stethoscope, introduced basic vocabulary to describe heart and lung sounds, coined the

Laënnec Frontispiece

term 'cirrhosis' to describe the appearance of a hard, shrunken liver, and identified bronchospasm as an important component of asthma.

1781 *John Howship* born. A London surgeon who suffered from osteomyelitis of the tibia, studied diseases of the bone, and published *On the Natural and Diseased State of the Bones.*

1781 *Allan Burns* born. A Scottish surgeon and cardiologist who wrote *Observations on Some of the Most Important and Frequent Diseases of the Heart* (1809), in which he described phrenic nerve palsy, a sign of thoracic aortic aneurysm, and suggested that angina was caused by coronary artery obstruction.

1782 Cod liver oil was used for chronic rheumatism in England by Robert Darley, who conveyed his findings to Thomas Percival of Manchester, England.

1782 The laminar structure of the cerebral cortex was shown in the occipital lobe of the brain by Francesco Genneri of Parma, Italy.

1782 The 'yellow spot' or macula lutea on the retina, and the central fovea, were observed and identified by an ophthalmic surgeon from Milan, Francesco Buzzi.

1782 A surgical knife for operating on cataracts, and thus greatly simplifying the procedure, was designed by Baron Wenzel of Austria.

1782 *John Richardson Young* born. An American physiologist who proposed the association between secretions of saliva and gastric juice in digestion, and that the solvent action of gastric juice is due to acids (1803).

1782 The Harvard Medical School was established. The third medical school in America, its founding professors were John Warren, Aaron Dexter and Benjamin Waterhouse.

1783 *François Magendie* born. A pioneer of pharmacology and founder of experimental physiology who described the mechanism of deglutination and vomiting, and the foramen of Magendie (1828), a canal leading to the fourth ventricle.

1783 *Ludwig Levin Jacobson* born. An anatomist and physician from Copenhagen who described the tympanic branch of the glossopharyngeal nerve (canaliculus tympanicus), and the vomeronasal organ, all of which bear his name.

1783 *Benjamin Travers* born. A surgeon at St Thomas' Hospital who described bruit in auscultation of the cranium in a case of caroticocavernous fistula (1809), and performed carotid artery ligation for berry aneurysm.

1783 Alexander Monro, Secundus, of Edinburgh discovered the communication between the lateral ventricles and the third ventricle of the brain (the foramen of Monro).

1783 *Sir Benjamin Collins Brodie* born. A surgeon from St George's Hos-

Sir Benjamin Collins Brodie

pital, London who described a benign serocystic tumor of the breast, performed the first operation for varicose veins, perfected several different surgical instruments, and wrote *Pathological and Surgical Observations and Diseases of the Joints* (1821).

1784 *Bartolommeo Borella* born. An Italian orthopedic surgeon who founded the first orthopedic institute in Italy, and wrote *Cenni d'Ortopedia*.

1784 The hereditary predisposition to asthma was referred to by Scottish physician, William Cullen.

1784 Domenico Cotugno an Italian anatomist, observed and described cerebrospinal fluid (CSF) in fish and turtles, but was unable to detect it in humans.

1784 *John Ball Brown* born. An American orthopedic surgeon who used subcutaneous tenotomy of the Achilles tendon for club foot, and tenotomy for torticollis, scoliosis and other deformities.

1784 The first surgical attempt to correct club foot or talipes was made by the German surgeon, Lorenz Heister.

1784 Swelling of the lower extremities in pregnant women (phlegmasia alba dolens) was thought to be due to the destruction of the maternal lymphatics by Manchester surgeon, Charles White.

1785 Peritonitis was first described by German anatomist, Johann Gottlieb Walter of Berlin.

1785 The presence of collateral circulation of the arteries was discovered by leading Scottish surgeon, John Hunter.

1785 *William Beaumont* born. An American army surgeon who, in 1822, studied human gastric secretion on a patient with a gastric fistula caused by a gunshot wound.

1785 *William Prout* born. An English chemist and physiologist who demonstrated the presence of hydrochloric acid in the stomach (1823).

1785 *Hermann T. Gartner* born. A Danish surgeon who described a benign cyst in the antero-lateral wall of the vagina (Gartner cyst) and the ductus epoöphori longitudinalis (Gartner duct), a rudimentary vestige of the mesonephric duct.

1785 *Jean Charles Athanase Peltier* born. A French physicist from Somme who developed the thermoelectric method of temperature reduction, the Peltier effect.

1785 Auguste Gottlieb Richter, a German surgeon, described Richter hernia, where only part of the lumen protrudes.

1785 English physician William Withering wrote *An Account of the Foxglove, and Some of its Medical Uses, with Practical Remarks on Dropsy, and other Diseases* in which he established a place for digitalis

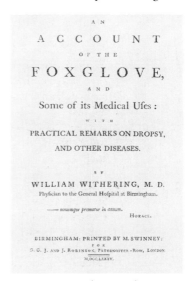

Frontispiece from Withering's book on the foxglove

(foxglove) in the treatment of dropsy. This pharmacological classic is one of the few pivotal volumes that provide the foundation of modern medicine, and can be regarded as the first great monograph devoted to a single medicinal substance.

1785 *Valentine Mott* born. An American surgeon who treated an aneurysm of the subclavian artery by tying it within the scleni muscles (1833), and performed the first successful

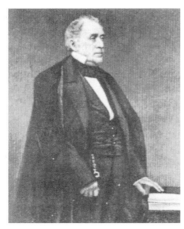

Valentine Mott

amputation at the hip joint in America.

1786   The first excision of the elbow joint was performed by French surgeon, Phillip Brian Moreau. His work was published in 1803.

1786   *Adolph Wilhelm Otto* born. A professor of anatomy at Breslau who gave a clinical description of arthrogryposis multiplex congenita in children and described protrusion of the acetabulum into the pelvic cavity in some cases of osteoarthritis.

1786   John Hunter, a Scottish surgeon and pathologist published *A Treatise on Venereal Disease* in which he described elevated papule in the penis or vulva seen in primary syphilis (Hunter chancre), and gave the first description of lymphogranuloma venereum, a sexually transmitted disease caused by *Chlamydia trachomatis* as a separate disease from syphilis and gonorrhea.

1786   The first modern scientific work on neuroanatomy was written by Félix Vicq d'Azyr of Paris.

1786   Samuel Thomas Sömmering, professor of anatomy at Göttingen, described the optic chiasma, the crossing of fibers within the optic nerve.

1786   *Jean G.A. Lugol* born. A French pathologist whose main interest was scrofula, now known to be a form of tuberculosis, but was then thought to relate to tuberculous necrosis of bone and lymphatic glands.

1786   *Michel-Eugéne Chevreul* born. A French chemist who discovered that fat was composed of fatty acids and glycerol, and isolated oleic, palmitic and stearic acids, the most common fatty acids in fats and oils. He became a professor at the Muséum National d'Histoire Naturelle, Paris, and was also a pioneer in gerontology. He investigated the psychological effects of aging and the psychology of color.

1786   *James O'Beirne* born. An Irish surgeon who described the O'Beirne sphincter, a band at the junction of the colon and the rectum.

1786   Benjamin Rush established The Philadelphia Dispensary for the medical relief of the poor, the first institution of the kind in the United States.

1787   *Carl Ferdinand von Graefe* born. A professor of surgery in Berlin who founded modern plastic surgery and developed rhinoplasty and blepharoplasty. He wrote pioneering works on these subjects and published one of the first books on rhinoplasty in 1818.

1787   *John Lizars* born. A professor of surgery at Edinburgh who described the surgical lines of the buttocks (Lizars line).

1787   *Pierre Charles Alexandre Louis* born. A Parisian physician and expert on tuberculosis and typhoid who described the angle of Louis, between the manubrium and the body of the sternum.

1787   *Johannes E. Purkinje* born. A neurologist from Czechoslovakia who studied aspects of vision, the brain and the heart. He described large nerve cells in the cerebral cortex of the brain, Purkinje cells, and atypical myocardial fibers, Purkinje fibers.

1787   *Samuel Cooper* born. A professor of surgery in London who described spina ventosa, the disease of the bone which discharged its contents through the surface of the skin, and which is essentially chronic osteomyelitis.

1788   *William Gibson* born. An American physician from Baltimore, Maryland who tied the common iliac artery, and devised a bandage for fracture of the lower jaw.

1788   The law relating the volume and temperature of a gas at constant pressure was formulated by J.A.C. Charles of France.

1788   Osteogenesis imperfecta, a congenital disease characterized by brittle bones due to defective ossification was comprehensively described by Swedish physician, Olof Jacob Ekman.

1788   London physician, Charles Kite, described nasal and oral intubation for resuscitating those who had drowned.

1788   Injury to the pancreas as a cause of diabetes was suggested by English physician, Thomas Cawley.

1788   The first description of surgical emphysema associated with ruptured esophagus was given by Dryden, a military surgeon in Jamaica.

1788   An account of pyloric stenosis caused by congenital hypertrophy, in children, was given in America by Hezekiah Beardsley.

1788   Leopold Gmelin, a German chemist and professor of medicine and chemistry at Heidelberg, devised a test for bile pigments, Gmelin test.

1788   A detailed dissertation on artificial teeth was written by French dentist, Nicholas Dubois de Chement.

1788   *Louis François Emmanuel Rousseau* born. A French histologist who described the accessory external lachrymal bone.

1789   *Peter Mere Latham* born. A physician at St Bartholomew's Hospital, London who gave a classical description of the symptoms of coronary thrombosis in 1846, and was one of the first in England to advocate auscultation.

1789   Antonio Scarpa, an Italian anatomist and surgeon, gave one of the earliest and most comprehensive descriptions of the olfactory nerve, and made a comparative study of the organs of hearing in humans and animals.

1789   One of the earliest accounts of congenital heart disease was given by Michael Underwood, a London pediatrician, in his *A Treatise on the Diseases of Children*.

1789   Suturing of the bladder after rupture was first suggested by Benjamin Bell, and then first carried out by Willet of St Bartholomew's Hospital, London.

1789   *Edward Donovan* born. An Irish pharmacist who prepared and marketed Donovan solution, containing iodides of arsenic and mercury, for application to cutaneous and venereal sores.

1789   An important work on cretinism and goiter was written by Italian physician, Michele Vincenzo Giacinto Malacarne.

1789   *Carl Gustav Carus* born. Professor of anatomy and an obstetrician in Montpellier who defined the circle of Carus in his pioneering studies in pelvimetry in 1820.

1789   *Richard Bright* born. A physician at Guy's Hospital, London who differentiated renal dropsy from cardiac dropsy and described

Richard Bright

chronic non-suppurative nephritis (Bright disease) in 1827, one of the earliest studies to focus on renal disease.

1789   Dermoid cysts of the ovaries were described by Scottish physician, Matthew Baillie.

1790   Urological surgery was introduced as a specialty by Pierre Joseph Desault and François Chopart of Paris, France.

1790   Artificial insemination was first performed successfully in a woman by John Hunter, an eminent Scottish surgeon.

1790   *Johann Karl Georg Fricke* born. A German surgeon and pioneer in plastic surgery who described a pedicle graft operation for correcting cicatrical ectropion of the eyelid.

1790   Inflammation of the calcaneal bursa, Swediaur disease, was described by Austrian physician, François X. Swediaur.

80

1790 The first report of central nervous system involvement in mumps was provided by Robert Hamilton of Edinburgh in *An account of distemper in the common people of England vulgarly called the mumps.*

1790 *Jacques Lisfranc* born. A French surgeon who designed an operation for partial removal of the foot, and advocated the extirpation of the rectum as treatment for cancer.

1790 Johannes Ehrenritter, a Viennese anatomist, described the ganglion of the glossopharyngeal nerve.

1790 *Louis Léon Rostan* born. A Paris physician who gave one of the earliest descriptions of cardiac asthma (Rostan asthma), respiratory distress due to cardiac failure.

1790 *Marshall Hall* born. A British neurophysiologist who made the first clear distinction between capillaries and arterioles (1831),

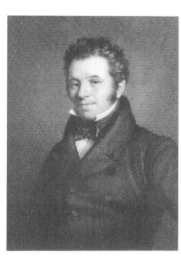

Marshall Hall

pioneered studies on artificial respiration (1855), and studied the nervous system and reflex activity of the medulla and spinal cord.

1790 *Jules Germain Cloquet* born. A professor of anatomy in Paris who described the lymphatic gland in the femoral canal (Cloquet gland), and gave his name to several other anatomical structures.

1790 Luigi Galvani described the electrochemical stimulation of frog muscle, and called it 'animal electricity'.

1791 *John Elliotson* born. A professor of medicine at University College London who described hay fever and asthma, suggested pollen as a precipitating cause (1831), devised pollen counts, and clinical challenge tests.

1791 *Pierre Prosper François Baume* born. A French physician who proposed the theory that a child affected by syphilis will not infect the mother if she has no signs of the disease (Baume law).

1791 *Thomas Calloway* born. A London orthopedic surgeon who devised a test for dislocation of the shoulder (Calloway test).

1791 *Edward Stanley* born. A surgeon at St Bartholomew's Hospital, London who described the retinacular fibers, or reflected capsular fibers on the neck of the femur (Stanley cervical ligaments).

1791 *Joseph Henry Green* born. An English surgeon at St George's Hospital, London and one of the first to perform a thyroidectomy.

1791   *Robert Adams* born. An Irish surgeon who made important advances in understanding chronic arthritis and distinguished rheumatoid arthritis in his treatise on *Rheumatic Gout, or Chronic Rheumatic Arthritis of All the Joints* (1837).

1791   *Charles G. Pravaz* born. An orthopedic surgeon from France who invented a special bed for scoliosis, and appliances for gymnastic corrective exercises.

1791   The first cancer service was established at the Middlesex Hospital in London.

1791   *Jean Cruveilhier* born. A professor of pathology at Montpellier who gave the first description of disseminated sclerosis, or muscular sclerosis, described a form of amyotrophic lateral sclerosis (Cruveilhier disease), and the regional lymph nodes.

1791   The successful removal of a tumor of the maxillary sinus was performed by Plaignaud of Paris.

1791   Luigi Galvani showed that electrical processes are involved in the function of muscles and nerves.

1792   *Carl Ernest von Baer* born. A German scientist and founder of embryology who described germ cell layers and the early processes of embryonic differentiation.

1792   *Gascon Sègalas* born. A French urologist and pioneer in the application of endoscopy to urology, who improved the method initially described by Phillip Bozzoni.

1792   English physician, William Withering, described the medicinal uses of the plant, Cicuta, which was used for centuries in the treatment of cancer and syphilis.

1792   *Charles Delucina Meigs* born. A professor of midwifery at Jefferson Medical College who was the first to recognize embolism as a cause of maternal death (1849).

1792   *John Shaw* born. An orthopedic surgeon from Britain who distinguished between rickets and other curvatures, and advocated exercise in treatment.

1792   François Chopart, professor of surgery in Paris, described astragaloscaphoid and calcaneocuboid articulations (Chopart joints).

1792   *Johan Friedrich Dieffenbach* born. A German surgeon who devised a new method of treatment for strabismus, by severing the tendons of the eye muscles. He also pioneered surgical treatment for vesicovaginal fistula.

1792   The first description of hereditary ectodermal dysplasia with absence of teeth, hair and other ectodermal structures was given by German physician, Ferdinand George Danz.

1793   Modern pediatrics in England was established by Michael Underwood, who described a form of childhood paralysis following a brief illness, thought to be the first scientific account of poliomyelitis.

1793 *Robert Lee* born. A Scottish physician at the Lying-in Hospital in London and lecturer at St George's Hospital, who accurately described the sympathetic ganglion of the cervix uteri (Lee ganglion) in 1841.

1793 *Baron Seutin* born. A Belgian orthopedic surgeon who devised a starch-impregnated linen bandage for fracture that could be incised for inspection and then made rigid again.

1793 Alexander Monro, Secundus, a Scottish anatomist, proposed that arterial supply to the brain was fixed or limited as it was enclosed within a fixed cavity.

1793 *Pierre François Olive Rayer* born. A physician from Paris and an authority on kidney diseases who described pyelonephritis in pregnant women (1841), and was the first to draw the distinction between chronic and acute eczema.

1793 *Sir James Ronald Martin* born. A Scottish surgeon who published an early treatise on tropical diseases, *Influence of Tropical Climates on European Constitutions.*

1793 Manuel Louis Antonio Gimbernat, a Spanish surgeon from Barcelona, described an operation for strangulated femoral hernia, and the ligamentum lacunare.

1793 Matthew Baillie of St George's Hospital, London wrote *Morbid Anatomy of Some of the Most Important Parts of the Human Body*, the first book to treat pathology systematically. It contained descriptions of the symptoms and morbid anatomy of gastric ulcer, cancer of the stomach, bladder, esophagus and testes, and is generally regarded as reaching new heights of clarity in the history and classification of oncology.

1793 The first British physician to give a specific account of heart block was Thomas Spence, in his paper, *History of a Case in Which There Took Place a Remarkable Slowness of the Pulse.*

1793 *Eugéne Soubeiran* born. A French chemist who discovered chloroform, independently of Justus von Liebig.

1793 *William Elmonds Horner* born. An American anatomist who described the small muscles at the internal commisure of the eyelids (muscle of Horner), and prepared the first treatise in America on pathological anatomy.

1793 *Thomas Addison* born. An English physician at Guy's Hospital, London who described a disorder resulting from the destruction of the renal glands (Addison disease), xanthoma diabeticorum, and first described circumscribed scleroderma.

1793 *Charles Aston Key* born. A British surgeon who performed successful ligations for aneurysms of the subclavian artery and external iliac artery, and described a surgical method for relieving strangulated inguinal hernia.

1793 *Johann Lucas Schönlein* born. A German professor of pathological anatomy at Würzberg who introduced the terms hemophilia and tuberculosis, and described peliosis rheumatica (Schönlein disease or purpura rheumatica) (1837).

1794 *John Rhea Barton* born. An American orthopedic surgeon, famed for being ambidextrous, who perfomed arthroplasty and osteotomy, and successfully performed subtrochanteric osteotomy of the femur for deformity.

1794 *John Davidson Godman* born. An American physician from Maryland who described the continuation of the pretracheal fascia into the thorax.

1794 *On the Morbid Effect of Carbonic Acid Gas on Healthy Animals* was published by English physiologist, William Bache.

1794 An outstanding study on inflammation, fundamental to pathology, was recorded by British surgeon, John Hunter in his *A Treatise on blood, inflammation and gun-shot wounds*.

1794 *Guy Benjamin Babbington* born. An English surgeon who invented a laryngoscope, described hereditary epistaxis, and designed a glottiscope.

1794 *Marie Jean Pierre Flourens* born. A French physiologist who was the first to perform extirpation of

different parts of animal brains and later identified the respiratory center in the medulla oblongata.

1794 *Robert Liston* born. An orthopedic surgeon from Scotland who developed a lateral splint for femoral fractures.

1794 *John Conolly* born. A physician from the Middlesex Asylum in Hanwell who was the first to advocate removal of all forms of mechanical restraints for mental patients.

1794 British physician, John B. Davidge, theorized that the ovaries excited the vessels of the womb to menstruate.

1794 James Russell published *A Practical Essay on Certain Disease of the Bones Termed Necrosis*.

1795 A comparative study of the measurements of human and animal bones (osteometry), was founded by English surgeon, Charles White, who also studied the relationship of the humerus to the forearm.

1795 *Ernst Heinrich Weber* born. A German physiologist who showed that digestive juices are products of glands and initiated research in this area.

1795 *Moritz Heinrich Romberg* born. A German professor of neurology who wrote the first formal treatise on nervous diseases, *Lehrbuch der Nervenkrankheiten* (1840), and described the pathognomonic sign in truncal sensory ataxia (Romberg sign).

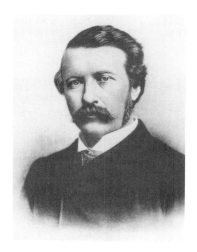

Moritz Romberg

1795 *Thomas Wakley* born. British physician who undertook research into food analysis which led to the Adulteration of Food and Drink Act, and was the founder of *The Lancet* (1823).

1795 The Abernethian Society was first inaugurated at St Bartholomew's Hospital, London.

1795 *Roderick MacLeod* born. A Scottish physician who described a syndrome of effusion into the synovial capsules, bursae, and sheaths in rheumatoid arthritis, and recorded his findings in *On Rheumatism*.

1795 The risk and urgency of treatment of tension pneumothorax was pointed out by James Latta of Edinburgh.

1795 Pipe smoke was identified as an environmental carcinogen by Samuel von Sömmering, professor of anatomy at Göttingen, who described carcinoma of the lip.

1795 Facial paralysis was described by German physician, Nikolaus Friedrich.

1795 *Alfred Armand Louis Marie Velpeau* born. A professor of clinical surgery in Paris after whom several anatomical structures are named: the inguinal canal, ischiorectal fossa, and tela subserosa around the kidney.

1795 Lime and lemon juice were introduced into British navy rations to control scurvy.

1796 *Anders Adolf Retzius* born. A Swedish anatomist and anthropologist who described the ligament of Retzius attached to the extensor retinaculum which acts as a sling to the extensor tendons.

1796 *William Marsden* born. A London surgeon who founded the Royal Free and Royal Marsden Hospitals (formerly the London Cancer Hospital).

1796 *Paul Briquet* born. A French physician who wrote a monograph on hysteria (Briquet syndrome), and described pulmonary gangrene in bronchiectasis (1841).

1796 The first successful ligation of the femoral artery in America was performed by Wright Post of Long Island, New York.

1796 *George McClellan* born. An American surgeon who founded the Jefferson Medical School where he was appointed the first professor of surgery.

1796 *Robert James Graves* born. An Irish physician who gave an accurate account of exophthalmic goiter, Graves disease, and published *Clinical Lectures on the Practice of Medicine.*

1796 *Jean Baptiste Bouillaud* born. A French physician who correlated carditis with acute rheumatic fever (Bouillaud syndrome), described acute rheumatic polyarthritis and localized the area of speech to the temporal lobe.

1796 Edward Jenner, a English country physician, performed the first inoculation when he scratched a child's skin with a needle contaminated with cowpox pus from a milkmaid to protect the child from smallpox. In 1798 he published *An Inquiry into the Causes and Effects of the Variolae Vaccinae, a Disease Known by the Name of Cow Pox*, and described accelerated secondary local inflammatory response in a smallpox immune patient.

1797 *Jean Baptiste Hippolyte Dance* born. A French physician who described the empty right iliac fossa found in children with intussusception (Dance sign), and carried out important work on uterine phlebitis and cholera.

1797 *Nathan Ryno Smith* born. An American surgeon who described an anterior suspensory apparatus for fractures of the lower extremities.

1797 French surgeon, Jean Antoine Rigal, devised the Rigal suture which utilized rubber rings instead of thread to close wounds.

1797 *William Fetherston Montgomery* born. An Irish obstetrician from Dublin who described the sebaceous glands of the areola of the nipple (Montgomery glands).

1797 A description of the Venturi tube was given by Giovanni Battista Venturi of Modena, Italy.

1797 *Emil Huschke* born. A professor of anatomy at the University of Jena who described the prominent lower margin (Huschke valve) of the lachrymal duct at its junction with the lachrymal sac.

1797 *Marc Jean Bourgery* born. A Paris surgeon who described the posterior ligament of the knee joint.

1797 The complex organic substance in blood contributing to color and containing heme (hematin) was described by William Charles Wells, a physician at St Thomas' Hospital, London.

1797 *Camille Melchior Gibert* born. A French dermatologist who gave a complete description of pityriasis versicolor and pityriasis rosea (1834)

1797 *Jacob Schroeder van der Kolk* born. A physician from Utrecht who made microscopic studies of the medulla of the brain, and whose name is associated with the fibers of the reticular formation of the medulla.

1797 *Gabriel Andral* born. A French physician who described the Andral sign (the characteristic posture in pleurisy) whereby the patient assumes a supine position, resting on the healthy side.

1797 Affusion therapy, the application of hot or cold water for treatment of disease, was pioneered by Scottish physician James Currie and recorded in his treatise on the subject.

1798 Thomas Robert Malthus published *An Essay on the Principle of Populations*, a work which influenced Darwin and Wallace and suggested the idea of 'survival of the fittest'.

1798 *Marie Devergie* born. A French dermatologist who was the first to recognize and demonstrate the fungal cause of tinea cruris, an epidermomycosis affecting the inguinocrural region (eczema marginatum).

1798 *Thomas Hodgkin* born. An English pathologist who introduced the stethoscope to England, described the neoplastic disease (Hodgkin

Thomas Hodgkin

disease), and gave an account of aortic valve insufficiency.

1798 *Louis Florentine Calmiel* born. A French physician who demonstrated the pathological lesions in the brain of patients with general pathesis, during a period when general knowledge on the cause of syphilis was unknown.

1798 *Hans Karl Leopold Barkow* born. A professor of anatomy at Breslau who described several of the ligaments attached to the carpels and tarsals.

1798 The first clinical description of strangulated hiatus hernia was given by Sir Astley Paston Cooper of London.

1798 Robert Willan, a physician and dermatologist from Yorkshire, England, described psoriasis diffusa (baker itch), an occupational disease affecting the hands and arms of bakers.

1798 Pneumatic medicine, the science which treats disease with gases, was established by English physician from Bristol, Thomas Beddoes.

1798 *Gustav Adolf Michaelis* born. An obstetrician from Kiel who described the diamond-shaped area over the aspect of the pelvis bounded by the dimples of the posterior iliac spines.

1798 *John Kearsley Mitchell* born. An American surgeon who wrote extensively on rheumatism, osmosis, ligature, mesmerism and neurology, and gave an original description of neurotic spinal arthropathies.

1799   *John Scott* born. A Scottish surgeon well respected for his skill in the treatment of diseased joints, who performed some of the first jaw removals in England, and published *Chronic Inflammations and Diseases of the Joints* which described ways to treat inflamed joints.

1799   George Washington succumbed to excessive 'bloodletting' by his physicians, causing some to question the practice.

1799   *Sauveur H.V. Bouvier* born. An orthopedic surgeon from France who wrote on bone deformities, the corset in history, and was the first to use the term 'locomotor apparatus'.

1799   *Karl Adolph von Basedow* born. A German physician who described the Merseberg triad, consisting of exophthalmos, goiter and palpitations in hyperthyroidism, Basedow syndrome (myeloneuropathy in thyrotoxicosis), and Basedow disease (thyrotoxicosis).

1799   *Sir Charles Locock* born. A British physician who suggested crowded teeth, onanism and menstruation as causes of epilepsy, for which he suggested treatment with potassium bromide.

1799   *James Syme* born. A British surgeon who performed several surgical procedures for the first time in Britain, such as amputation at the hip joint, and excision of the lower jaw for sarcoma.

1799   *Antoine Laurent Jessie Bayle* born. A Paris physician who studied pathological lesions of the brain and described general paresis.

1799   *Phillipe Ricord* born. An American pioneer in venereology who demonstrated the different etiology of syphilis and gonorrhea, and described the three stages of syphilis.

1799   *Jean Poiseuille* born. A French physiologist who invented a mercury hemodynamometer for the measurement of blood pressure (showing changes in respiration), and described the speed of current in a capillary tube as being proportional to the square of the diameter of the tube (Poiseuille law).

1799   The Royal College of Surgeons of England was given a Royal Charter by George III.

1800   James Gardette from Philadelphia used reduced atmospheric pressure to fix dentures to the jaw.

1800   The first eye infirmary in the United States was opened in New London, by Elisha North of Goshen, Connecticut.

1800   *Valentine Flood* born. An Irish anatomist who discovered the superior glenohumeral ligament of the shoulder joint which now bears his name.

1800   The contagious nature of trachoma was first noted by French military surgeon, Dominique Larrey.

1800   The contagiousness of erysipelas was first recognized by English physician, William Charles Wells.

1800   *Jacob von Heine* born. A German orthopedist and one of the first to describe infantile paralysis or poliomyelitis (1840).

1800   A doctoral thesis on rheumatoid arthritis, based on detailed clinical studies of the female occupants of the SalpÍtrÉrie Hospital in France, was presented by Augustin-Jacob Landré Beauvais.

1800   *Francis Kiernan* born. A London surgeon who described the interlobular spaces (Kiernan spaces) of the liver.

1800   Samuel von Sömmering, a professor of anatomy at Göttingen, identified a crescent-shaped grayish black nuclear material lying in the midbrain between the pedunculi and tegmentum and named it the substantia nigra.

1800   Chlorine was used to purify water by Edinburgh surgeon and anatomist, William Cruikshank.

1800   Infrared radiation was discovered by Sir Frederick William Herschel, who passed light though a prism and set up thermometers beyond the red end of the spectrum to demonstrate the heating effect of infrared light.

1800   *Willard Parker* born. A New York surgeon who described an incision parallel with the Poupart ligament over the area of maximum dullness due to appendicular abscess (Parker incision), and performed appendectomy in America.

1800   Gray matter was first interpreted as the active and functioning part of the brain by German physician, Franz Joseph Gall.

1800   A complete course of anatomy, surgery and medicine started at The Great Windmill Street School in London.

1800   Skin grafting was first carried out by Italian surgeon, Guiseppe Baronio, who demonstrated the fundamental principle that an autograft from the same animal would take, while an allograft from another animal was rejected.

1800   *Hermann Friedrich Kilian* born. A German gynecologist who described the level of promontory of the sacrum (Kilian line), and demonstrated the importance of spondylolisthetic pelvis in pregnancy.

1800   *Alfred Wilhelm Volkmann* born. A German professor of physiology and anatomy who described the Volkmann canal found in the bones which carry blood vessels from the periosteum.

Volkmann's spoon

1800   *Friedrich Wöhler* born. A German chemist and pioneer in the chemical interpretation of living phenomena, who synthesized urea for the first time from potassium cyanate and ammonium sulfate (1829), which signaled the beginnings of organic chemistry.

1800 The earliest histopathological study of the tissues was carried out without the benefit of a microscope, by Marie François Xavier Bichat of Paris.

1800 Alessandro Volta investigated the effects of electricity on muscles.

1800 The first use of bougies to dilate esophageal stricture was undertaken by Alexis Boyer of France.

1800 Common cardinal veins were described by French naturalist, Geroges L.C.F. Cuvier.

1801 *Johannes Peter Müller* born. A German physiologist who gave the first demonstration of the electrical nature of the heart, described the primordial female genital tract (Müller duct), and proved that the embryo respired by examining changes in blood color entering and leaving it.

1801 *Francis Henry Ramsbotham* born. A lecturer in obstetrics and the first obstetrics physician to the London Hospital. He opposed the use of chloroform and published the famous *Principles and Practice of Obstetric Medicine and Surgery* (1841).

1801 *Armand Trousseau* born. An eminent French physician who performed the first tracheotomy in France (1865), was a pioneer of intubation, described the Trousseau sign for hypocalcemia, and received the prize of the Academy of Medicine for his treatise on laryngeal phthisis.

Armand Trousseau

1801 *César Alphonse Robert* born. A French surgeon who described the fascicle of fibers arising from the posterior cruciate ligament to the lateral meniscus of the knee (Robert ligament).

1801 Carl Johann Christian Grapengiesser of Berlin first used galvanic current therapeutically.

1801 *George Rainey* born. A demonstrator at St Thomas' Hospital, London who described ectopic calcifications in tissues (Rainey tubes).

1801 In *Mechanisms of the Eye*, published by English physician Thomas Young, astigmatism was described.

1801 *Richard Dugard Grainger* born. A British neurologist who demonstrated the role of gray matter in the spinal cord in reflex activity.

1801 Dublin physician John Cheyne published his first book, *Essays on the Diseases of Children*.

1801 Inflammation of the anterior portion of the uveal tunica or iris due to syphilis was named 'iritis' by Johann Adam Schmidt of Vienna. He founded the first journal of ophthalmology, *Ophthalmologische Bibliothek.*

1801 *Sir Thomas Pridgin Teale* born. An English surgeon from Leeds who wrote a monograph on abdominal hernia (1846), and published treatises on plastic surgery and amputation.

1801 The Institute for Investigating the Nature and Cure of Cancer was formed in England by Thomas Denman, and has had such notables as Matthew Baillie and John Abernethy among its members.

1801 *James Hope* born. An English cardiologist who wrote an important monograph on cardiac disease and morbid anatomy, and is best known for *A Treatise on the Diseases of the Heart and Great Vessels*, in which he described the Hope murmer.

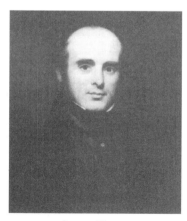

James Hope

1801 *Jules Guérin* born. An orthopedic surgeon from France who used tenotomy and myotomy for scoliosis and congenital hip displacement, and advocated plaster bandages for club foot.

1801 *Friedrich Wilhelm Theile* born. A German anatomist who described the space formed by the reflection of the pericardium on the aorta and the pulmonary artery (Theile canal).

1801 *Alfred Donné* born. An anatomist from Montpellier who pioneered the microscopic study of blood fluids and secretions, described *Trichomonas vaginalis*, and made the first observations of platelets in the blood (erroneously considering them to be fat globules).

1801 Extract of opium was crystallized and morphine obtained by Adam Friedrich Wilhelm Sertürner, a German chemist.

1802 *Alexander Friedrich Hueck* born. A professor of anatomy at the University of Dorpat who described ligamentum pectinatum iridis (1841).

1802 *Horace Green* born. An laryngologist from Vermont who wrote one of the earliest treatises in America on chronic laryngitis and bronchitis (1846).

1802 *Sir Dominic John Corrigan* born. A physician from Dublin who described the Corrigan or water-hammer pulse, famine fever, and the Corrigan button.

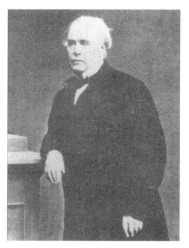

Dominic Corrigan

1802   *William Sharpey* born. A professor of anatomy and physiology at the University of London who discovered and named the Sharpey fibers, connective tissue fibers found between the periosteum and the bone. He was the first specialist in physiology in England.

1802   *Antoine Jerome Balard* born. A French chemist who discovered that iodine turned blue in the presence of starch, an important finding which formed the basis of testing for starch.

1802   *Alexander Bryson* born. An English physician who described reduced expansion of thoracic movement seen in exophthalmic goiter (Bryson sign).

1802   The first description of the fat or sucking pad of the cheeks was given by French anatomist, Marie François Xavier Bichat.

1802   *Auguste Berard* born. A Paris surgeon who described the suspensory ligament of the pericardium (Berard ligament).

1802   *Heinrich Gustav Magnus* born. A German physician who made the first analysis of blood gases, demonstrating relative amounts of carbon dioxide and oxygen in venous and arterial blood, respectively.

1803   *Joseph Stoltz* born. A French gynecologist who designed the Stoltz operation for cystocele, by denuding a patch on the anterior abdominal wall and running a purse-string suture around the edge.

1803   *Louis Daniel Beauperthuy* born. A West Indian pioneer in tropical medicine who investigated the virulent epidemics of yellow fever in Venezuela, and noted the causal relationship between mosquitoes and marshes.

1803   Seishu Hanaoka of Hirayama, Japan used a mixture of alkaloids, mainly scopolamine and atropine (tsusensan), to give pain relief to sufferers of breast removal due to cancer.

1803   *Friedrich Arnold* born. A professor of anatomy from Heidelberg who described the otic ganglion of the 5th cranial nerve (Arnold ganglion).

1803   *Auguste Theodore Vidal de Cassis* born. A French surgeon who devised a method of subcutaneous ligation of veins for varicocele.

1803   The first excision of the elbow joint was performed by French surgeon, P.F. Moreau from Nancy.

1803   *Arnold Adolphe Berthold* born. A German physiologist who proved the existence of internal secretions (hormones) when he transplanted the testes of a cock to another bird that had been castrated, preventing the sequelae of castration in the second bird.

1803

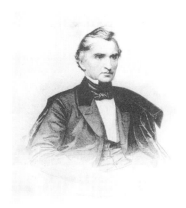

Justus von Liebig

Justus von Liebig born. A German chemist and the father of industrial chemistry, who discovered chloroform, studied nutrition and the degradation of proteins to purines, urea, and uric acid, and wrote *Orgnic Chemistry in its Application to Physiology and Pathology.*

1803   Noscapine (narcotine), an alkaloid of opium with antipyretic properties and without narcotic effects, was isolated by Charles Louis Derosne of France.

1803   British naval surgeon, David Fleming, performed a successful ligation of the carotid artery following trauma.

1803   Instability of the knee joint due to injury to the medial semilunar cartilage was described by English surgeon, William Hey. He gave the first description of the falciform ligament (Hey ligament).

1803   An account of strictures of the urethra and esophagus was published by Sir Everard Home. He gave the first description of the esophageal web in his *Practical Observations on the Treatment of Strictures in the Urethra and in the Esophagus.*

1804   The first accurate account of the symptomatology of a lower esophageal diverticulum was given by Dèguise of Paris.

1804   Philipp Bozzini invented a cystoscope for the bladder.

1804   *Matthias Schleiden* born. A German botanist who studied the role of the nucleus in cell division and tissue formation, and developed the concept of the cell as the essential building block of all living things in his *Grundzuge der wissenschaftlichen Botanik.*

1804   *Karl Freiherr von Rokitansky* born. A Czech professor of pathology in Vienna and founder of modern pathological anatomy who gave many original descriptions, especially of the stomach, liver and heart.

1804   *John Hilton* born. An English surgeon who performed the first operation for internal strangulation of the small intestines, described the nematode *Trichinella spiralis*, suggested its involvement in trichinosis, and its parasitic nature. In 1863 he published *On the Influence of Mechanical and Phyiological Rest on the Treatment of Accidents and Surgical Diseases.*

1804   *George Philip Cammann* born. A New York physician who devised one of the first binaural stethoscopes (Cammann stethoscope).

1804   The infectious nature of the saliva of a dog suffering from rabies was noted by George Gottfried Zinke of Jena.

1804   *Joseph Dietl* born. A Polish physician who described symptoms of acute pain in the costavertebral angle due to partial obstruction caused by kinking of the ureter in a floating kidney (Dietl crisis).

1804   *William Stokes* born. An Irish physician who gave a description of paroxysmal tachycardia, heart block associated with syncopal attacks, and described Cheyne–Stokes breathing in apoplexy. He wrote *A Treatise on the Diagnosis*

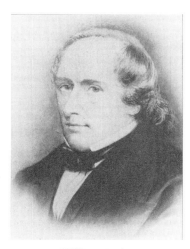

William Stokes

and Treatment of the Diseases of the Chest.

1804   *Pierre Charles Huguier* born. A French gynecologist who invented one of the first uterine sounds, described lymphogranuloma venereum, leiomyoma (Hugier disease), and gave his name to the canal from which the cauda tymphani emerges in the petrotymphanic fissure.

1804   *John Dalrymple* born. An English ophthalmologist who published many classic texts including *Anatomy of the Human Eye and Pathology of the Eye*, and described abnormal widening of the palpebral fissure in exophthalmic goiter (Dalrymple sign).

1804   *Louis Theodore Helie* born. A Paris professor of anatomy and gynecologist who described the superficial musculature of the uterus and founded the famous anatomical museum in Paris.

1804   *Izaak Abrahamzoon van Deen* born. A Dutch physiologist who devised a test for blood in gastric juices, using guaiac and glacial acetic acid as reagents (van Deen test).

1804   *George Ludwig Kobelt* born. A German anatomist who gave his name to the Kobelt venous plexus, formed by the veins of the bulb of the vestibule below the clitoris.

1805   *Antoine Mathijsen* born. A Belgian surgeon who introduced plaster-of-Paris into surgery and pioneered the use of galvano-cautery.

1805   *Joseph Pancoast* born. A New Jersey professor of anatomy and surgery who performed a section of the trigeminal nerve at the foramen ovale as treatment for trigeminal neuralgia, and published *A Treatise on Operative Surgery* (1844).

1805   *Observations on Cancer* was published, a collection of cases representing the state of knowledge regarding cancer that existed among post-Hunterian surgeons.

1805   *Manuel Patricio Rodriguez* born. A Spanish physician who invented the laryngoscope, consisting of two mirrors.

1805   *Marie Edouard Chassaignac* born. A Paris surgeon who described the space between the pectoralis major and the mammary gland (Chassaignac space), and a carotid tubercle on the transverse process of the 6th vertebra (Chassaignac tubercle).

1805   The radial fibers of the ciliary muscles were described by Sir Philip Crampton, a surgeon from the Meath Hospital, Dublin.

1805   Friedrich W. Sertürner published his work on the isolation of morphine. This followed the 1802 publication *Sur l'opium* by Charles L. Derosne reporting the isolation of alkaloids from opium. These works marked important milestones in the extraction of pure substances and the development of the modern pharmacopoeia.

1805   *Charles Williams* born. An English physician who described dull tymphanitic resonance over the second intercostal space in cases of large pleural effusion (Williams sign), and developed the popular trumpet-shaped stethoscope.

1805   The first journal of psychiatry *Magazin für psychische Heilkunde* was founded by Johann Christian Reil.

1805   *François Lucien Gaillard* born. A French surgeon who described a surgical method for the treatment of ectropion.

1805   The first recorded colostomy for intestinal obstruction was performed by Pierre Fine.

1805   *James Yearsley* born. The first physician to practice otorhinology as a specialty in London, who pointed out that deafness may arise from diseases of the nose and throat, developed the artificial tympanum, and founded the Metropolitan Ear and Throat Hospital in 1838 and the *Medical Directory* in 1845.

1805   *Edward Cock* born. A surgeon at Guy's Hospital who gave his name to the ulceration of a sebaceous cyst giving it an appearance of epithelioma (Cock peculiar tumor), and performed the first pharyngectomy.

1805   *Samuel David Gross* born. An American surgeon who introduced laparotomy for ruptured bladder, suprapubic incision for the prostate, distinguished prostatic hypertrophy from bladder disease, and wrote *Elements of Pathological Anatomy and The Anatomy, Physi-*

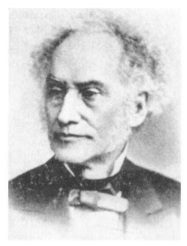

Samuel Gross

ology, and Diseases of the Bones and Joints.

1805   *Josef Skoda* born. An Austrian physician who popularized the use of Laënnec's stethoscope in clinical medicine, and described many auscultatory sounds in the chest (e.g. Skoda resonance).

1806   *Guillaume Benjamin Amand Duchenne* born. A physician from Paris who was one of the earliest workers on the electrophysiology

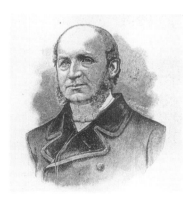

Guillaume Duchenne

of muscles. He described Duchenne muscular dystrophy occurring in early childhood, different forms of lead palsy, and distinguished rheumatic and lachrymal forms of facial paralysis from brain or nerve lesions.

1806   *Simon Joseph Honore Beau* born. A French cardiologist who described cardiac insufficiency and cardiac asystole, sometimes known as Beau syndrome, and Beau lines seen as transverse grooves on the fingernails in cases of serious illness.

1806   Walter Brashear of Maryland was the first to perform a successful amputation of the hip in the United States.

1806   Jean-Pierre Robiquet and Louis Nicholas Vanquelin obtained the first amino acid, asparagine, from asparagus.

1806   *Louis Alexander Dugas* born. An American surgeon who devised the Dugas test for dislocation of the shoulder, and published an important paper, *New Diagnosis in Shoulder Dislocations.*

1806   *Joseph François Malgaigne* born. A professor of surgery from Paris who described the superior carotid triangle, and was the first to use ether for anesthesia in France.

1806   *Appollinaire Bouchardat* born. A French endocrinologist who first used polariscopic and chemical methods to detect diabetes, developed diets, and invented gluten bread.

1806   *Henry G. Davis* born. An American orthopedic surgeon and a pioneer in sanatoria for tuberculosis, who carried out open evacuation of suppurative arthritis, washed out with chlorine and water.

1806   *Luther V. Bell* born. An American physician who described mania resulting from acute periencephalitis (Bell disease).

1807   *John Watson* born. A New York surgeon who performed esophagotomy for esophageal stricture.

1807   *Alonzo Clark* born. A New York physician who described the obliteration of liver dullness due to distension in peritonitis (Clark sign), and introduced large doses of opium for peritonitis, monitoring the respiratory rate as an indicator of the opium level.

1807   *François Louis Valleix* born. A French physician who first described the tender points in a nerve that cause neuralgia (Valleix points).

1807   *Eduard Zeis* born. A professor of surgery at Marburg who described the sebaceous glands in the eyelids (Zeis glands).

1807   *Robert William Smith* born. A professor of surgery at Trinity College, Dublin who first described the hand fracture (Smith fracture, a reversed Colles fracture). He published the first treatise on neurofibromatosis in 1849, *Treatise on the Pathology, Diagnosis, and Treatment of Neuroma*.

1807   *Louis Ripault* born. A French physician who described a method of applying pressure to the eye ball; if the distortion was permanent the patient was declared dead (Ripault sign).

1807   *Auguste Nélaton* born. A French surgeon from Paris who introduced a rubber urethral catheter and electrocautery into surgery, and described the Nélaton line in congenital dislocation of the hip: extending from the anterior superior iliac spine to the ischial tubercles.

1807   *Gurdon Buck* born. A New York surgeon who established traction through a system of weights and pulleys for the treatment of thigh fractures, and described the fascial sheath of the penis in 1848.

1807   *Ernest Pierre Antoine Bazin* born. A French dermatologist who described symmetrical purple nodules due to vasculitis of the calf, which break down to form ulcers and leave pigmented scars (Bazin disease), and proposed a parasitic cause for ringworm.

1808   *Washington Lemuel Atlee* born. A surgeon from Pennsylvania who pioneered the surgical treatment of uterine fibroids in America, and performed over 400 ovariotomies.

1808   *Charles Pierre Denonvilliers* born. A professor of surgery in Paris who described the plastic correction of a defective ala nasi by transferring a triangular flap from the side of the nose (Denonvilliers operation), and prostoperitoneal aponeurosis.

1808 *The Radical Cure of Empyema* was published by M.F.M. Audouard.

1808 A pioneer in rheumatology, British physician David Dundas, concentrated his studies on the heart and published *An Account of Peculiar Diseases of the Heart*, in which he described rheumatic heart disease.

1808 Inflammation of the cornea with many differing causes (keratitis) was first described by James Wardrop, a surgeon from Edinburgh. He resected the lower jaw and advocated distal ligation of an artery for aneurysm (Wardrop operation).

1808 *Sir William Fergusson* born. A Scottish surgeon who wrote *System of Practical Surgery*, devised several surgical instruments (vaginal speculum, mouth gag, lion forceps), and excised the head of the femur for incurable diseases of the hip.

1808 *Senses and the Intellect and Emotions and the Will* were published by Alexander Bain of Aberdeen, who is considered a founder of modern systematic psychology.

1808 An account of wet beriberi was given by C. Rogers in *De Hydrope Asmatico Ceylonia*.

1808 *William Ludwig Detmold* born. An American orthopedic surgeon who established a public clinic for the treatment of crippled children, and carried out the first subcutaneous tenotomy in the United States.

1808 The contraction of the smooth muscles in the wall of the smallest bronchial tubes during an asthma attack was described by anatomist and physician, Franz Daniel Reisseisen of Strasburg.

1808 Bronchiectasis was first noted by French physician René Laënnec who differentiated it from similar conditions such as pleurisy and empysema, and recognized this as an important component of asthma.

1808 *George Budd* born. A professor at King's College London who described Budd–Chiari syndrome of hepatic vein occlusion resulting in hepatosplenomegaly, jaundice, ascites and portal hypertension, and cirrhosis of the liver due to the nematode, *Fasciolopsis*.

1809 *John Reid* born. An Edinburgh surgeon who promoted the study of pathology, differentiated between typhoid and typhus fever, and published several treatises on pathology, anatomy and epidemic fevers of Scotland.

1809 *Francesco Rizzoli* born. An Italian orthopedic surgeon who invented an instrument used to break the bone in orthopedic surgery (osteoclast), to fracture a normal femur to compensate for shortening, and founded the Rizzoli Institute.

1809 *Louis Braille* born. He attended the first blind school in Paris and devised an alphabet for the blind by using varying combinations of embossed dots on the page that (with modifications) is still in use today.

1809 *Bartholemy Alphonse Bardinet* born. A professor of medicine at Limoges who described the humero-olecranon ligament of the posterior part of the capsule of the elbow joint (Bardinet ligament) in 1869.

1809 *Charles Robert Darwin* born. The most influential biologist of the 19th century who developed the concept of evolutionary adaptation of organisms to their environment which he described in *On the Origin of Species by Means of Natural Selection* (1859).

1809 *Allen Thompson* born. A Scottish physician from Edinburgh who described the yellow fibers covering the inner half of the external abdominal ring (Thompson fascia).

1809 *Thomas Wilkinson Kingsley* born. An American dentist and pioneer in maxillofacial surgery who designed several devices for use in fracture of the upper jaw (Kingsley oral bars) and fractured maxilla (Kingsley splint).

1809 *William Wood Gerhard* born. An American physician who gave an early, clear clinicopathological description of typhoid (1837), and made an accurate study of tuberculous meningitis (1834).

1809 *Henri Louis Roger* born. A French physician who wrote extensively on disorders of the liver, heart and gastrointestinal tract. He described excessive salivation caused by obstruction or blockage of the esophagus by tumors (Roger reflex or syndrome), and Maladie de Roger caused by a defect in the interventricular septum of the heart.

1809 *Friedrich Gustave Jacob Henle* born. A German anatomist who discovered the smooth muscle in the middle coat of smaller arteries, the external sphincter of the bladder, the looped portion of the uriniferous tubule (loop of Henle), and described the columnar and ciliated epithelial cells.

1809 *John Stough Bobb* born. An American surgeon who developed cholecystotomy for removal of gallstones.

1809 *Jules Gabriel François Baillarger* born. A French psychiatrist who described the internal and external lines of Baillarger in the cerebral cortex, and the bipolar illness with alternating states of depression and hypermania, now referred to as manic depressive psychosis.

1809 *Andrew Christian Conradi* born. A Norwegian physician who defined the Conradi line, drawn from the base of the xiphisternum to the cardiac apex, to denote the upper limit of normal dullness of the left lobe of the liver.

1810 *Daniel Noble* born. An English physician who took charge of disease control during a typhus epidemic in Manchester, and published *Influence of Manufactures upon Health and Life and The Human Mind in its Relationship with the Brain and Nervous System.*

1810 The Zeller operation, used in the treatment of webbed fingers, was devised by Viennese surgeon, Simon Zeller.

1810 *Theodor Schwann* born. A German physiologist famous for his classic cell theory, who also described the neurolemma (sheath of Schwann), the striped muscle in the upper part of the esophagus, showed that air is needed for putrefaction, and that the tension of a muscle varies with its length.

1810 The amino acid, cystine, was isolated from urinary calculi by an English physician and chemist, William Hyde MacArthur.

1810 *James Knight* born. An American orthopedic surgeon who specialized in braces and trusses, used electrotherapy, rejected plaster castes, and tried to avoid surgery wherever possible.

1810 *Henry Savage* born. A founder and gynecologist at the Samaritan Hospital in London who described the perineal body between the anus and the vulva (Savage perineal body).

1810 *Bernhard Rudolf Konrad von Langenbeck* born. A professor of surgery in Berlin who first observed candidosis, operated on cleft palate, and described the Langenbeck triangle, an area over the head of the femur between the pyriformis and the gluteus medius.

1810 *Nathan Strong* born. An American physician who gave one of the first and most important descriptions of cerebrospinal meningitis (1810).

1810 Dislocation of the hip joint, where the head of the femur is displaced toward the anterior superior iliac spine (Monteggia dislocation), was described by Italian surgeon, Giovanni Battista Monteggia.

1810 *Nicolai Ivanovitch Pirogoff* born. A professor of surgery at Moscow and noted military surgeon who defined the Pirogoff triangle, bounded by the intermediate tendon of the digastric muscle, posterior border of the myelohyloid muscle and the hypoglossal.

1810 *William John Little* born. A British orthopedic surgeon who pioneered the use of intravenous saline in treatment of cholera, performed the first tenotomy and subcutaneous heel tetonomy for club foot, and described a form of cerebral palsy (Little disease).

1810 An apparatus for automatically regulating steam under pressure (autoclave) for sterilization was first used by French confectioner, Nicolas Appert.

1810 *Ludwig Türck* born. A Viennese neurologist and laryngologist who devised a laryngoscope, described the micropathology of the spinal cord in tabes dorsalis, the direct pyramidal tracts (Türck column), and an abnormal leukocyte (Türck cell).

1810 *James Jackson Jr* born. A Boston physician who wrote a treatise on cholera, described the prolonged expiratory sound in tuberculosis, and the difference between the apex heart rate and the radial pulse in cases of atrial fibrillation.

1810 *Louis Auguste Desmarres* born. A Paris ophthalmologist who designed an operation (Desmarres operation) for pterigium, and gave his name to a curved lid retractor for examining the eyes.

1810   *William Henderson* born. A pathologist from Edinburgh, who wrote a treatise on the skin disease, molluscum contagiosum, in which he described the inclusion bodies (1841), and was one of the first to differentiate typhus from relapsing fever (1844).

1810   The first operative treatment on the heart was performed by French military surgeon, Dominique Jean Larrey, when he drained the pericardium following a stab wound.

1810   French physician, Gaspard Laurent Bayle, described carcinoma of the lung and the pathological nature of a tubercule.

1811   Maintenance of artificial respiration in curarized animals was shown by Sir Benjamin Collins Brody.

1811   *William Budd* born. An English physician who proposed excreta as a source of typhoid, and wrote *Typhoid Fever: Its Nature Mode of Spreading and Prevention.*

1811   *Thomas Blizard Curling* born. A London surgeon who gave an accurate clinical description of cretinism, acute duodenal ulceration associated with burns (Curling ulcer), and published *Diseases of the Testis and Diseases of the Rectum.*

1811   *Andrea Verga* born. An Italian neurologist from Milan who

Thomas Blizard Curling

described a small tunnel in the petrous temporal bone, between the corpus callosum and the body of Fornix, which now bears his name.

1811   *John Hutchinson* born. A British respiratory physiologist who developed the spirometer for estimating the vital capacity of the lungs, and carried out research into the respiratory system.

1811   *Idea of a New Anatomy of the Brain*, one of the earliest significant contributions to neurology was written by Scottish anatomist and neurologist, Sir Charles Bell, who differentiated spinal nerves into sensory and motor components.

1811   *Carlo Matteucci* born. An Italian physiologist who showed that current can be made to flow from the cut end of an isolated muscle to its uncut surface, if these points are connected by a galvanometer.

1811   *Louis Philippe Alfred Hardy* born. A physician in France who described the sign of aphonia in early stages of gangrene of the lung.

1811   *Arthur Farre* born. A professor of midwifery at King's College London who gave his name to the line of attachment of the mesovarium to the ovary.

1811   *Sir James Young Simpson* born. A Scottish obstetrician and professor of midwifery at Edinburgh who first used ether as an inhalational anesthetic (1840), introduced chloroform (1847), and acupressure (1864).

1811   The sacroiliac joint was first described by French physician, Joseph Capuron.

1811   *Jean Nicholas Demarquay* born. A French surgeon who described the fixation of the lower end of the larynx during phonation and deglutition as a sign of syphilis of the trachea (Demarquay sign).

1811   *Eugéne Joseph Woillez* born. A French physician who described a form of acute idiopathic congestion of the lung (Woillez disease).

1812   *Edward Selleck Hare* born. An English surgeon who gave an early description of signs due to a cervical sympathetic lesion (Horner syndrome).

1812   Perforated appendix was recognized as a cause of death by London physician, John William Keys Parkinson.

1812   *Anton Wintrich* born. A German physician who described a change in pitch of the percussion note when the mouth is opened or closed in cases of pulmonary cavity (Wintrich sign).

1812   *Casimir Joseph Davaine* born. A French physician from Paris and an originator of the germ theory of disease (before Pasteur), who identified the anthrax bacillus in the blood of animals.

1812   *William Stevens* born. A surgeon at Santa Cruz who successfully tied the internal iliac artery in a case of aneurysm.

1812   *Thomas Bevill Peacock* born. A physician at St Thomas' Hospital in London who wrote an important treatise on the malformation of the heart.

1812   *John Hughes Bennett* born. A professor of physiology in Edinburgh who recognized the impotance of the microscope in determining disease, described leukocythemia, illustrated the microscopic blood picture in leukemia, and wrote on use of cod liver oil, treatment of rheumatism, and physiology.

1812   *Austin Flint* born. A New York specialist in clinical medicine and auscultation who described several physical signs including the eponymous apical mid-diastolic or presystolic functional murmur originating from the mitral valve in patients with aortic stenosis.

1812   The reflecting microscope, consisting of a reflecting mirror instead of an objective lens, was invented by Giovanni Battista Amici of Northern Italy.

1812 *Henry Louis Bayard* born. A French physician who described capillary hemorrhages seen in the pleura and pericardium of babies who attempted to breathe prematurely in utero, Bayard ecchymoses.

1812 Lower segment cesarean section was introduced by German surgeon, Friedrich Benjamin Osiander.

1812 Pierre Hubert, a physician from Liége in Belgium, described the spread of rigor mortis from the face to the feet.

1813 Elective drainage of a lung abscess was performed by Jaymes of Paris.

1813 *James Marion Sims* born. An eminent American gynecologist who was helped to establish gynecology as a specialty, pioneered surgery in the treatment of vesico-vaginal fistula, and designed the Sims duck-billed vaginal speculum.

1813 Delirium tremens, associated with alcoholism was described by Thomas Sutton of London.

1813 *Claude Bernard* born. A celebrated French physiologist who discovered glycogen and its metabolic pathway, established the mechanism of vasomotor reflex responses, and introduced the concept of the internal environment of the body.

1813 *Frank Hastings Hamilton* born. An American army physician who practiced skin grafting for ulcers, published *Deformities after Fractures* (1855), and wrote an important treatise on fractures and dislocations (1860).

1813 *George Owen Rees* born. An English physician who devised the Rees test for detection of albumin in urine, with tannic acid in an alcoholic solution as reagent.

1813 Thomas Baynton of London introduced horizontal posture and modern orthopedic treatment in cases of spinal caries.

1813 *Johan Florenze Heller* born. An Austrian physician who devised the nitric acid test for detecting protein in urine, and wrote an important work on urinary calculi (1860).

1813 *William Benjamin Carpenter* born. A British physiologist and professor of forensic medicine who proposed the concept of the subconscious mind.

1813 *John Snow* born. An anesthetist and epidemiologist from England who virtually put an end to objections to the use of chloroform in obstetrics by administering the agent to Queen Victoria during the birth of one of her children, invented the ether inhaler, and experimented with endotracheal

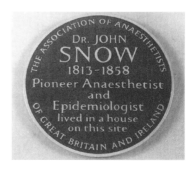

Memorial plaque on Snow's house in London

anesthesia. He implicated sewage in the River Thames as a cause of cholera.

1813 *François Magarite Barrier* born. A French physician who described peribronchitic abscesses (Barrier vacuoles).

1813 *Gaspard Adolphe Chatin* born. A French physician and endocrinologist who showed that cretinism was directly related to iodine deficiency, and calculated the necessary preventative amount.

1813 *Quinton Gibbon* born. An American surgeon who described a large inguinal hernia associated with hydocele (Gibbon hernia).

1813 Myotonic pupils and absent tendon reflexes, Adie syndrome, was described by London surgeon and ophthalmologist, James Ware.

1813 John Blackall, one of the first physicians to demonstrate albuminuria in dropsy, published his findings in *Observations on the Nature and Cure of Dropsies.*

1813 The area between the two tendons of the origin of the sternomastoid in the supraclavicular fossa (Zang space) was described by German professor of clinical surgery, Christoph Bonifacius Zang.

1814 *Louis Bauer* born. An American orthopedic surgeon who wrote the first American handbook on orthopedics (*Lectures in Orthopedic Surgery*), and famously advocated the importance of rest and immobilisation for spinal injury.

1814 The first English monograph on congenital diseases of the heart was written by London physician and cardiologist, John Richard Farre.

1814

Golding Bird

Golding Bird born. A British physician who wrote a monograph on urinary deposits, described oxaluria (Bird disease), and wrote *Elements of Natural Philosophy.*

1814 An important treatise, *Diseases of the Heart*, was published by French physician, Jean Nicolas Corvisart.

1814 Colchicine was extracted from the meadow saffron, and was the only real treatment for gout until the development of anti-inflammatory agents.

1814 *Heinrich L.F. Robert* born. A German gynecologist who described the rudimentary sacrum with marked narrowing of the transverse and oblique diameters (Robert pelvis).

1814 *Francis Sibson* born. A professor of medicine at St Mary's Hospital in

London who described the Sibson fascia, a septum covering the apical pleura attached to the first rib (1846).

1814 English physician, Sir Charles Manfield Clarke, described ulcer at the neck of the uterus in a case of vaginal discharge.

1814 *Edward Mott Moore* born. An American surgeon who described fracture of the lower end of the radius with dislocation of the head of the ulna, and entrapment of the styloid process within the annular ligaments (Moore fracture).

1814 *Anton Nuhn* born. A German anatomist who described and named the anterior linguinal glands (Nuhn glands).

1814 *Sir James Paget* born. A British physician who discovered the parasite, *Trichinella spiralis* and gave an original description of eczema of the nipple and mammary cancer

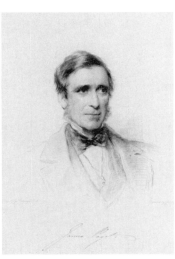

Sir James Paget

(Paget disease), and first described osteitis deformans (ankylosing spondylitis).

1814 *Adolph Hanover* born. A German anatomist from Berlin who published an early classic thesis on the eye, *On the Anatomy, Physiology and Pathology of the Eye*.

1815 *Carl Conrad Theodor Litzmann* born. A German professor of obstetrics at Kiel who published a paper on the surgical treatment of ectopic pregnancy and several other works, including a textbook on obstetrics.

1815 *Sir William Robert Wills Wilde* born. An Irish surgeon and father of Oscar Wilde (the author) who described the optical appearance on the external aspect of the membrana tymphani (Wilde cone).

1815 *Joseph Toynbee* born. An aural surgeon to St Mary's Hospital, London who described the corneal corpuscles (Toynbee corpuscles), and explained the role of the eustachian tubes during swallowing.

1815 *Robert Remak* born. A German professor of neurology who noted that the gray matter of the brain contained cellular tissue, described the unmyelinated nerve fibers (Remak fibers), cardiac ganglia (Remak ganglia), and classified the embryonic germ layers.

1815 Pericardiocentesis was first performed successfully by Spanish surgeon from Barcelona, Francisco Romero.

1815   *Daniel Cornelius Danielssen* born. A Norwegian physician who described Danielssen disease, a form of anesthetic polyneuritis in leprosy.

1815   *Louis Auguste Fredericq* born. A Belgian physician who described a red line in the gums occurring in the presence of pulmonary tuberculosis (Fredericq sign).

1815   *Philip Gustav Passavant* born. A German surgeon who described the Passavant cushion, a ridge projecting from the posterior and lateral walls of the nasopharynx at the level of the free margin of the soft palate in atrophic rhinitis, and the Passavant bar, a ridge on the posterior wall of the pharynx.

1815   *James Archibald Jacques* born. He was the production manager of a London rubber mill who produced the first soft urethral catheter (Jacques catheter).

1815   *Horace Wells* born. An American dentist who introduced nitrous oxide as an anesthetic.

1815   *Carl Reinhold August Wunderlich* born. A professor of medicine at Leipzig who pioneered the application of thermometry to clinical medicine in his *Das Verhalten der Eigenwarme in Krankeiten* (1868).

1816   Thomas Jeremiah Armiger, a demonstrator in anatomy at the London Hospital, wrote *The Rudiments of the Anatomy and Physiology of the Human Body*.

1816   *Ferdinand Ritter von Hebra* born. A Viennese dermatologist who

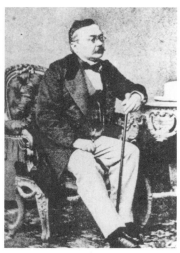

Ferdinand Ritter von Hebra

founded the histological approach to dermatology with his classification of skin diseases, Atlas of Skin Diseases (1845).

1816   John King, a surgeon from South Carolina, saved both mother and child when he performed a complex operation for an abdominal pregnancy, and later published an important work on ectopic pregnancy.

1816   *Augustus Volney Waller* born. An English physiologist who demonstrated that the axis cylinder, if cut off from the nerve cell, will undergo degeneration while the stump will remain viable for a longer time (law of Wallerian degeneration).

1816   *Alois Bednar* born. An Austrian pediatrician who wrote a treatise on diseases affecting infants (1850–1853), and described lesions of the palate in the newborn as a result of sucking foreign objects (Bednar aphthae).

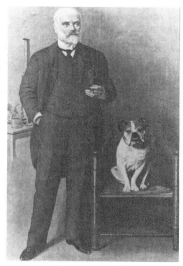

Augustus Waller

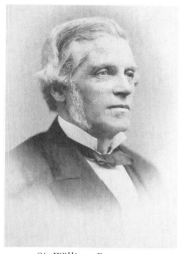

Sir William Bowman

1816 *Louis Alfred Richet* born. A professor of clinical surgery in Paris who described the canal for the umbilical vein in the anterior wall of the umbilical canal (1855).

1816 *James Henry Bennett* born. An English obstetrician who differentiated between benign and malignant tumors of the uterus (1845).

1816 *Ludwig Moritz Hirschfeld* born. A Polish professor of anatomy who described the lingual branch of the facial nerve (Hirschfeld nerve) and the posterior renal sympathetic ganglion (1866).

1816 *Sir William Bowman* born. An English anatomist who developed the concept of glomerular filtration and tubular secretion (1842), described the capsules in the kidneys that filter blood (Bowman capsule), the Bowman membrane which separates the corneal epithelium from the sub-

stantia propria of the cornea (1849), perfected irridectomy and removal of cataracts.

1816 *Ludwig von Buhl* born. A German pathologist who described icterus neonatorum (Buhl disease).

1816 *Edward Sieveking* born. A British physician who produced a paper in 1857 on epilepsy in *The Lancet*, including 15 tested remedies.

1816 *Henry Jacob Bigelow* born. A Boston surgeon who wrote what is regarded as the first American text on the subject, *A Manual of Orthopedic Surgery*, and described the Y-shaped iliofemoral ligament of the hip joint (Bigelow ligament).

1816 The Tenon capsule (fascia bulbi) was named after French army surgeon and professor of pathology, Jacques René Tenon, who specialized in ophthalmology.

1816 The point of emergence of the descending palatine nerve from the palato-maxillary canal (Méglin point) was described by French physician, J.A.M. Méglin, an anatomist at Sultz.

1816 *Alexander Ecker* born. A Swiss anatomist who provided an original description of several convolutions of the occipital lobe, and published works on the movement of the brain and spinal cord (1843), and the structure of the suprarenal glands (1846).

1816 *Karl Friedrich Wilhelm Ludwig* born. A German experimental physiologist who made several important contributions to the understanding of blood pressure and heart activity, including the invention of the kymograph (1846), the mercurial blood pump (1859), and a method of perfusion for isolated organs (1865).

1816 *Adolph Krukenberg* born. A German professor of anatomy who described the central vein (Krukenberg vein) of the hepatic lobule.

1816 *Sir Richard Quain* born. An Irish physician at the Brompton Chest Hospital in London who described a form of fatty degeneration of the heart (Quain fatty degeneration), and compiled a two-volume dictionary of medicine (1882).

1816 *Charles Pajot* born. A Paris obstetrician who designed a decapitating hook, and described a method of using obstetric forceps to exert a tangential force giving a resultant force in the direction of the birth canal during delivery.

1816 Early recognition of the dangers of application of medical knowledge by laymen was noted by French physician Adolphe Pierre Piorry in *On the Danger of Reading Medical Textbooks by the Laity*.

1816 A mechanism for the development of esophageal diverticulum was given by Charles Bell.

1817 The first record of an investigation into the causes of abdominal or ventral hernia was given by Jules Germain Cloquet, professor of anatomy at Paris.

1817 *Johann Baptiste Chiari* born. An Austrian gynecologist who discovered the Chiari–Frommel syndrome (1882) of galactorrhea and atrophy of the uterus associated with low levels of follicle stimulating hormone.

1817 *Charles Edouard Brown-Séquard* born. A French neurophysiologist who demonstrated the importance of the suprarenal capsule, and described hemiplegia associated with crossed anesthesia (Brown-Séquard syndrome, 1850).

1817 The cavernous ganglion around the portion of the carotid artery within the cavernous sinus was described by Russian surgeon, August Carl Bock.

1817 Lithium was discovered by Johann August Arfvedson of Stockholm, Sweden, and was isolated a year later by Jöns Jacob Berzelius.

1817 *John Murray Carnochan* born. A New York surgeon who designed an operation for trigeminal neuralgia, published a treatise on congenital dislocation of the hip which was the first comprehensive view of the subject in America, several years before Bigelow's monograph.

1817   Parkinson disease, characterized by mask-like facies, tremor and slowness of movements, was first described by London physician, James Parkinson.

1817   *Robert Barnes* born. An English obstetrician who designed the Barnes dilator, a rubber bag for dilating the os and cervix uteri.

1817   *Wilhelm Roser* born. A German professor of surgery at Marburg who defined surface marking from the anterior superior iliac spine to the ischial tubercles (Roser line).

1817   *Arthur Hill Hassall* born. An English physician who described the concentric corpuscles of the thymus (Hassall corpuscles), and published the first English textbook on microscopic anatomy, *The Microscopical Anatomy of the Human Body in Health and Disease* (1846).

1817   The first clear account of chronic subdural hematoma was given by M. Houssard of Paris, although the condition had been observed at postmortem for several centuries.

1817   *Jacob Augustus Clarke* born. An eminent London neurologist who described the nucleus dorsalis of the spinal cord (Clarke column), and the pigmented cells of the nucleus dorsalis (Clarke cells, 1851).

1817   *Ludwig Thiry* born. A Belgian physician who induced an experimental intestinal fistula (Thiry fistula) in a dog to obtain intestinal secretions for research.

1817   *George Critchett* born. A London ophthalmologist who described several operations for the eyes, including one for squint.

1817   The thickening of the Descemet membrane of the cornea was described by German professor, Johann Ignas Josef Dollinger.

1817   *Etienne Jules Bergeron* born. A French physician who described hysterical chorea (Bergeron disease).

1817   Lumbar colostomy through a vertical incision in the loin was performed by Danish surgeon, Adolph Callisen of Copenhagen.

1817   *Karl Vogt* born. A German neurophysiologist who defined the Vogt angle, found between the nasobasilar and alveolonasal lines.

1817   Nerve cells in the subthalamic nucleus (Pander cells) were described by German embryologist and anatomist, Christian Heinrich Pander. He coined the term 'blastoderm'.

1817   *Rudolf Albert von Kölliker* born. A Swiss anatomist, embryologist and pioneer histologist who described the structure of tissues and cells, the cellular structure of nerves and smooth muscle, and wrote *Manual of Human Histology*.

1817   Catgut was used in surgery by English surgeon at Guy's Hospital, Sir Astley Paston Cooper.

1817   Xanthine was isolated by Alexander John Gaspard Macet, a physician and chemist from Geneva.

1817   *Alphonse François Marie Guérin* born. A professor of surgery at the Hôtel Dieu, Paris who described the terminal portion of the male urethra (1849).

1817   *Wilhelm Griesinger* born. A physician from Germany and prolific writer who gave his name to the syndrome of pseudohypertrophic infantile muscular dystrophy. He founded the Society of Medical Psychology.

1818   Fetal heart sounds were first heard in a pregnant woman in her fifth month of pregnancy by Geneva surgeon, François Mayor.

1818   *Jean Antoine Eugéne Bouchut* born. A Paris physician who recognized the state of nervous exhaustion and asthenia (nervosisme), described a form of breathing seen in children with bronchopneumonia, and developed tubes for intubation of the larynx.

1818   *An Analysis of the subject of Extra-uterine Foetation, and of the retroversion of the Gravid Uterus*, was written by John King of Edisto Island, South Carolina.

1818   *Ludwig Traube* born. A German pathologist who worked on the pathology of fever and the effects of drugs on muscular activity, used digitalis in the management of

Ludwig Traube

heart disease, gave a clear description of pulsus bigeminus in 1872, and described rhythmic variations of the vasoconstrictor center.

1818   *Eduard Jaeger von Jastthal* born. A Viennese ophthalmologist who devised the Jaeger test for near vision (1854), designed operations for cataract, entropion and ecropion, and published an atlas of ophthalmology (1869).

1818   An instrument to measure cardiac output, the ballistocardiograph, was demonstrated by J.W. Gordon.

1818   *David Hayes Agnew* born. A Philadelphia surgeon who devised the Agnew splint for fracture of the patella.

1818   *Sir Thomas Spencer Wells* born. A British gynecologist who performed hysterectomy for myoma (1861), splenectomy (1865), a complete ovariotomy (1858), and devised forceps for forcipressure, a method of crushing blood vessels by forceps to arrest bleeding.

1818   *Edmé Joules Maumené* born. A French chemist who devised the Maumené test to detect sugar in urine, by adding stannous chloride to give a distinct brown color.

1818   *Auguste Ambroise Tardieu* born. A French physician who described ecchymosis seen on the pleura following suffocation (Tardieu spots).

1818   *Frederick Oldfield Ward* born. An English physician who published *Outlines of Human Osteology*, and gave his name to the triangular area which intervenes amongst the trabeculae of the cancellous tissue of the neck of the femur.

1818   Jean Zuléma Amussat conducted experiments on catheterization.

1818   *Emil Du Bois Reymond* born. A professor of physiology at the University of Berlin who demonstrated that the electrical state of the nerve altered when a current was passed through it, and described the injury potential of the muscle (1840).

1818   *Ignaz Phillipp Semmelweis* born. A Hungarian obstetrician and advocate of asepsis for prevention of puerperal sepsis, and who demonstrated that mortality due to puerperal fever could be reduced if doctors washed their hands (1847).

1818   *Franciscus Cornelis Donders* born. A Dutch ophthalmologist and physiologist who introduced prismatic and cylindrical lenses in spectacles, and whose book, *The*

Anomalies of Refraction and Accommodation (1864), formed the basis for fitting eyeglasses for myopia, strabismus, hypermetropia and other conditions.

1818   *The American Journal of Science* was founded.

1818   *Max Joseph von Pettenkofer* born. A German biochemist who studied the formation of bile and bile salts, respiratory quotients, the metabolism of fat, and pioneered public health and hygiene by taking responsibility for the purification of Munich's water supply. He was director of the first Institute of Hygiene in the world (1879).

1818   *Karl Vierordt* born. A German clinician who made many contributions to medicine including the discovery of a method of calculating the circulation time of blood (1842), and the invention of the hemacytometer (1852) and the sphygmograph (1854).

1818   *John Marshall* born. A professor of surgery at University College London who described the vena cava and associated structures (1850).

1818   A procedure for elective drainage of a lung abscess by resecting the 5th and 6th ribs was described by A. LeClerk Richerand of Paris.

1819   Alternation of generations was proposed by German botanist and poet, Ludwig Adelbert von Chamisso.

1819   *Joseph Ritter von Artha Hasner* born. An ophthalmologist from

Prague who described the valve at the lower end of the naso-lachrymal duct (1850).

1819 *Carl Sigmund Franz Crede* born. A professor of obstetrics and gynecology in Leipzig who described a method of expulsion of the placenta (Crede maneuver) by applying pressure on the uterine fundus through the abdominal wall.

1819 A procedure for opening an obstructed bowel above the site of obstruction and allowing its contents to escape (enterotomy) was first suggested by Mannoury.

1819 *William Holme van Buren* born. An American surgeon who first described hardening of the corpora cavernosa (van Buren disease).

1819 Auscultation, a method of examining the chest, was developed by French physician, René Theophile Laënnec, who published a treatise on his early stethoscope, gave the first description of lupus verrucosus, and a classic description of the physical signs and pathological changes in lobar pneumonia.

1819 The layer of the retina containing rods and cones (Jacob membrane) was described by Irish ophthalmic surgeon, Arthur Jacob.

1819 *Augustin Marie Morvan* born. A French physician who described a form of syringomyelia with trophic changes in the extremities (Morvan disease).

1819 *Ernst Wilhelm von Ritter Brücke* born. One of Europe's leading physiologists who pioneered the functional study of phonetics, described the luminosity of the eye by illuminating the fundus with artificial light, and described the radial fibres of the ciliary muscles (1844).

1819 *Wenzel Treitz* born. A professor of pathological anatomy at Prague who described retroperitoneal hernia through the duodenojejunal recess (Treitz hernia), and the suspensory ligament of the duodenum (Treitz ligament, 1853).

1819 French surgeon Alexis Boyer described the causes and treatment of anal fissure.

1819 *Sir Alfred Baring Garrod* born. A consulting physician from King's College London who discovered the excess uric acid in the blood of patients with gout, introduced the thread test for uric acid, and coined the term 'rheumatoid arthritis'.

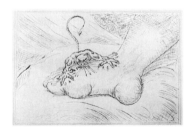

Cartoon of the effects of gout

1819 *Karl Wilhelm Ludwig Bruch* born. A German anatomist who described the lamina vitrea, a transparent membrane next to the retina separating it from the capillaries in the choroid (Bruch membrane, 1844).

1819   *Friedrich Rudolf Voltolini* born. An otorhinolaryngologist from Breslau who described acute purulent inflammation of the internal ear leading to violent pain, delirium, and unconsciousness (Voltolini disease).

1819   *Buckminster Brown* born. An American orthopedic surgeon and a skilled operator on the knee, hip and foot, who was the first to cure bilateral congenital dislocation of the hip.

1820

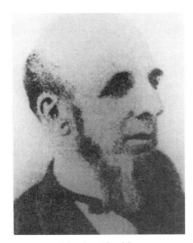

Charles Blackley

Charles Harrison Blackley born. A physician from Manchester who demonstrated the application of grass pollen to the eyes as a cause of hay fever, devised pollen counts and clinical challenge tests, and wrote *Experimental Researches on the Causes and Nature of Catarrhus Aestivus* (1873).

1820   A case of epilepsy associated with a remarkable slowness of the pulse, and one of the first descriptions of heart block, was made by English physician, William Burnett.

1820   The Académie Royal de Médicin of Paris was founded by incorporating the old Académie Royal de Chirurgie and was divided into medicine, surgery and pharmacy.

1820   The importance of the elastic recoil property of the lung in respiration, the effect of venous return of the blood to the heart, and the production of a negative pleural pressure were noted by Liverpool physician, James Carson. He induced pneumothorax as treatment for pulmonary tuberculosis.

1820   *Peter Ludwig Panum* born. A Danish physician who gave the first scientific explanation of how a disease spreads from person to person, and from place to place. He also studied the pathology of embolism (1868), embryonic malformations (1860), and poisonous alkaloids (1856).

1820   The immunity of females to hemophilia despite their ability to transmit the disease (Nasse law) was proposed by Christian Friedrich Nasse of Germany.

1820   *Otto Eduard Heinrich Wucherer* born. A German physician who observed the embryonic form of the filarial worm (*Wuchereria bancrofti*) in 1868, later shown to be the cause of elephantiasis.

1820   The alkaloids cinchona and quinine were extracted from Peruvian cinchona bark, by Pierre Joseph Pelletier and Jean B. Caventou of Paris.

1820   *Lewis Albert Sayre* born. An American orthopedic surgeon from New

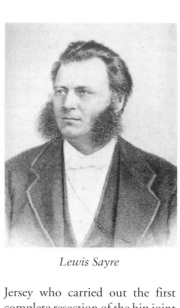

Lewis Sayre

Jersey who carried out the first complete resection of the hip joint and creation of an artificial joint (1863).

1820   The first official United States pharmacopoiea was published in Boston.

1820   *Heinrich Müller* born. A professor of anatomy at Würzberg who described several anatomical structures that have been named after him, including a muscle and a fiber.

1820   German chemist, Friedlieb Ferdinand Runge, obtained an alkaloid from the seeds of *Coffea arabica* (coffee), and distilled phenol from coal tar (1834).

1820   *Sir Henry Thompson* born. An English surgeon who described the surgical treatment of urinary bladder tumors and wrote extensively on prostate cancer. He was also the founder and first president of the Cremation Society.

1820   *Florence Nightingale* born. A British nurse whose dedication and service during the Crimean War led to a dramatic reduction in deaths, and who organized a fund to establish a training institute for nurses at St Thomas' Hospital, London.

1820   *Sir George Murray Humphry* born. A physician from England who founded the *Journal of Anatomy and Physiology*, wrote on the skeleton, coagulation of blood, myology, and on old age. He described the posterior cruciate ligament of the knee joint (Humphry ligament) in 1858.

1820   *Gottfried Ritter von Rittershaim* born. An German dermatologist in Vienna who described dermatitis exfoliativa infantum (Ritter disease), or staphylococcal scalded skin syndrome.

1820   *John Laws Milton* born. A London dermatologist who described angioneurotic edema (Milton disease) as 'giant urticaria'.

1820   Two monographs on botulism, giving detailed descriptions, were published by German physician, Justinus Kerner.

1820   *Richard Payne Cotton* born. A London physician who studied tuberculosis in depth, published *Phthiasis and the Stethoscope* (1852), and gave a description of paroxysmal tachycardia (1869).

1820   *Peter Redfern* born. An Irish orthopedic surgeon and pathologist who described the microscopic structure of the cartilage.

1820   An early form of the galvanometer to measure electric current, the rheometer, was invented by a professor from the école Polytechnique de Paris, André Marie Ampére.

1820   Systematic psychology in Britain was founded by Scottish physician, Thomas Brown, who published *Lectures on the Philosophy of the Human Mind*.

1820   The relation of gastric hemorrhage secondary to portal hypertension was noted by Peter Johann Frank, a physician from Bavaria.

1820   The amino acid glycine was isolated from a hydrolysate of gelatin by Henri Braconnot, who named it 'sugar of gelatin'.

1820   Diphtheria was originally known as croup until it was given its present name by Pierre Bretonneau of France. He also gave a classic description of typhoid, including Peyer patches in the intestine.

1820   *Joseph Gerlach* born. A professor of anatomy at Erlangen who described the lymphatic follicles in the mucous membrane of the eustachian tube, and the mucosal fold near the orifice of the appendix (Gerlach valve).

1820   The first description of cancer due to arsenic was given by John Ayrton, a physician from Penzance.

1820   Iodine-induced thyrotoxicosis was first observed by Jean François Coindet, a physician at Geneva.

1820   An operation for cleft palate was devised by Carl Ferdinand von Graefe.

1821   The first recorded excision of the head of the femur in disease of the hip joint was given by English surgeon, Anthony White.

1821

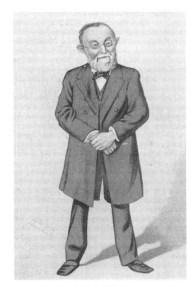

Rudolph Virchow

Rudolph Ludwig Karl Virchow born. An outstanding German pathological anatomist who established cellular pathology, coined the terms leucocytosis (1858), leukemia (1845), neuroglia (1854), thrombosis (1848), and amyloid (1854), and distinguished rheumatic gout (arthritis deformans) from familial gouty arthritis.

1821   *Samuel Haughton* born. A British physiologist who pioneered studies on the function and mechanism of the erect penis, and developed the concept of function with 'least action' in the analysis of muscular mechanism.

1821   Facial palsy arising from nuclear and infranuclear lesions of the facial nerve (Bell palsy) was described by Scottish neurologist, Sir Charles Bell, after original descriptions of the canal of the facial nerve by Gabriele Falloppio.

1821   The triangular ligament or the fascia of origin of the penile musculature was described by Maurice Carcassone, a professor of anatomy from Montpellier.

1821   The ophthalmoscope, an instrument to visualize the fundus of the eye, was designed by Charles Babbage.

1821   *Charles Hewitt Moore* born. An English surgeon who described a method of treating aneurysm by introducing a wire in order to produced coagulation (1864).

1821   *Charles Filippe Robin* born. A professor of histology at the Faculty of Medicine in Paris who described the lymphatic spaces around the arteries (Robin spaces, 1868), and the osteoclastic cells of the bone.

1821   *Richard James MacKenzie* born. An anatomist and surgeon from Scotland whose original contributions to surgery include: *A Successful Ligation of Subclavian Artery, Excision of the Knee Joint*, and *Amputation at the Ankle by an Internal Flap.*

1821   Interstitial cells of the testis (Leydig cells) were first described by Franz von Leydig, a professor of histology and comparative anatomy at Würzberg.

1821

Hermann von Helmholtz

Hermann Ludwig Ferdinand von Helmholtz born. A German surgeon who developed a method of obtaining electromyograms of the muscles (1851), carried out pioneering work on muscle energy, invented an ophthalmoscope (1851), and explained the mechanism of accommodation of the eye and perception of color.

1821   *Elizabeth Blackwell* born. The first woman graduate in America (1849) who later became professor of obstetrics and gynecology at the London School of Medicine.

1821   *Samuel Fenwick* born. An English physician who described atrophy of the stomach occurring in association with pernicious anemia (Fenwick disease), and made excellent observations on perforation of the appendix and abscess formation.

1821   *Henry Willard Williams* born. An American ophthalmologist who designed a special lantern to test color vision, and introduced the method of suturing the flap after cataract excision (1864).

1822 An early treatise on cod liver oil, *Experiences of the Great Curative Powers of Cod liver Oil*, was published by Johann Heinrich Schenckl, a physician from Siegen.

1822 *Hermann Welcker* born. An Austrian physician who described the angle of the basicranial axis (Welcker angle, 1882), was the first to determine total blood volume in mammals, and the relative volumes of plasma and blood cells.

1822 *Louis Pasteur* born. A French chemist and father of modern bacteriology and pasteurization who showed the presence of living cells in fermentation, postulated the germ theory of disease, and first administered the rabies vaccine (1885).

1822 The first successful vaginal hysterectomy was performed by Sauter of Constance.

1822 *Friedrich Matthias Cladius* born. A professor of anatomy at Kiel who described the supporting cells on the floor of the cochlear canal (1858).

1822 *Karl Thiersch* born. A German professor of surgery who described a method of operative treatment for epispadias (1869), and devised the Thiersch method of skin grafting where long broad strips of skin of one half its full thickness are used.

1822 Army surgeon, James Mann, provided the first record in the United States of excision of the elbow joint.

1822 The first clear desciption of the functions of the facial nerve was given by English physician, Herbert Mayo.

1822 Auscultation of fetal heart sounds as a diagnostic procedure was firmly established by French obstetrician, Jean Alexander Lejumeau.

1822 *Heinrich Frey* born. A professor from Zurich who described the crypts at the bottom of the gastric glands (Frey gastric follicles, 1859).

1822 *Alfred Henry McClintock* born. An Irish physician who described pulse rate over 100, indicative of post partum hemorrhage (McClintock sign).

1822 Progressive paralysis of the insane, Bayle disease, was described by French physician, Antoine Laurent Bayle.

1822 *George William Balfour* born. A cardiologist from Edinburgh who wrote several important treatises including *Hematophobia* and *Clinical Lectures on the Diseases of the Heart and Aorta*.

1822 *Friedrich Wilhelm von Bärensprung* born. A German physician who described Bärensprung disease, a chronic contagious skin infection, mainly affecting the scrotum, perineum, and axilla, due to microsporon species (*Tinea cruris*).

1822   *Adolf Kussmaul* born. A German professor of surgery at Heidelberg who made the first attempt at gastroesophagoscopy (1869), described cases of ascending neuropathy (1859), periarteritis nodosa (1866), progressive bulbar palsy (1873), and pulsus paradoxus (1873).

1822   *Jean Charles Eugéne Foltz* born. A French professor of anatomy who described the valvular constrictions at the entry of lachrymal ducts (1862).

1822   The method of bruising the urinary stone with surgical instruments (lithotrity) was first practiced by M. Leroy Etiolles.

1822   *Gregor Johann Mendel* born. The founder of genetics from Moravia who worked on the hybridization of pea plants, artificially fertilizing them to produce specific characteristics, and later published his laws of segregation and independent assortment (1865).

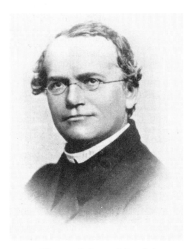

Gregor Johann Mendel

1822   Scottish physician, James Scarth Combe's account, *A Case of Anaemia*, presented before the Medico-Chirurgical Society of Edinburgh, was later recognized as the first on pernicious anemia.

1822   Scottish physician Andrew Buchanan was among the first to investigate blood coagulation.

1823   The first excision of the parotid gland was carried out by Pierre Augustin Béclard, a professor of anatomy at Paris. In 1824 he described the Beclard triangle, the area bounded by the posterior border of the hyoglossus, the posterior belly of the digastric, and the greater cornu of the hyoid bone.

1823   *Bruno Jacques Beraud* born. A Paris surgeon who described the valve located at the junction of the lachrymal duct and its sac (1854), the Beraud valve.

1823   *Carl von Carion Stellwag* born. An Austrian ophthalmologist who described the infrequency of blinking and widening of palpebral fissure seen in exophthalmic goiter (Stellwag sign).

1823   The first American treatise on ophthalmology in America, *A Treatise on Diseases of the Eye*, was published by George Frick of Maryland, the first American to specialize in this field.

1823   *Carl Braun von Fernwald* born. A German physician who described asymmetrical enlargement of the uterus with the appearance of a longitudinal furrow.

1823

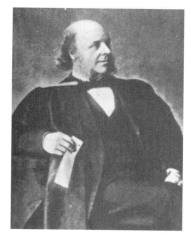

John Braxton Hicks

John Braxton Hicks born. An obstetrician at Guy's Hospital and a pioneer in midwifery who described a combined method of internal and external podalic version (1860), and intermittent contraction occurring after the third month of pregnancy (Braxton Hicks sign).

1823 By successfully tying both carotid arteries, William D. Macgill became the first American to perform carotid artery ligation.

1823 *Aristide August Stanislaus Verneuil* born. A French surgeon who described the syphilitic involvement of the bursae (Verneuil disease), founded the *Revue de Chirurgerie*, and introduced iodoform as treatment for cold.

1823 *Johann Friedrich August von Esmarch* born. A German military surgeon who designed the Esmarch bandage, made of rubber and used for application to the limbs, especially to reduce blood loss.

1823 French surgeon, François Anthime Eugéne Follin born. He described small bodies (Follin grains) consisting of isolated portions of Wolffian tubules in the paravarium (1850).

1823 *William Brinton* born. An English physician who described linus plastica of the stomach (Brinton disease) in his *Diseases of the Stomach* (1859), and studied 7000 postmortem cases of peptic ulcer disease (1857).

1823 *Moritz Schiff* born. A German physiologist who defined the pathways for touch and pain sensations in the spinal cord, and described the Schiff cycle where bile salts secreted into the intestine are re-absorbed and returned to the liver.

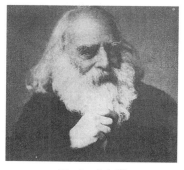

Moritz Schiff

1823 *Trumann Hoffman Squire* born. An American surgeon who wrote a treatise on the stricture of the urethra (1867) and designed a catheter.

1823 *James Donaldson Gillespie* born. A surgeon at the Edinburgh School of Medicine and Surgery who designed an operation for excision of the wrist.

1823 *William Kitchen Parker* born. A London physician who described part of the developing skull which completes the occipital portion of the primitive cranium in lower animals (Parker arch, 1870).

1823 *Heinrich Daniel Ruhmkorf* born. A German mechanic from Hannover who lived in Paris and built the first induction coil which formed the basis for the development of the Geissler tube.

1823 The retroperitoneal passage of the external iliac artery was described by French anatomist, Annet-Jean Bogros.

1824 *Paul Broca* born. A French surgeon and anthropologist who located the motor area of speech in the third frontal convolution of the brain (1861), and founded anthropometry with his inventions of 27 craniometric and cranioscopic instruments.

1824 *Sir Samuel Wilks* born. An English physician who gave a definittive account of myasthenia gravis (Wilks syndrome, 1877), the relationship between renal conditions and nephrotic syndrome (1853), the causes of pyemia and septicemia (1861) and an account of alcoholic paraplegia (1868).

1824 Prostatoperitoneal aponeurosis (Tyrell fascia) was described by Frederick Tyrell, a surgeon at St Thomas' Hospital and nephew of Sir Astley Paston Cooper.

1824 The area bounded by the posterior belly of the digastric, the greater cornu of the hyoid bone and the posterior border of the hyoglossus (Beclard triangle) was described by French anatomist, Pierre Augustine Beclard.

1824 The inhalational effects of carbon dioxide for inducing anesthesia were studied by Henry Hill Hickman.

1824 *Simon Gustav* born. A professor of surgery in Germany who wrote monographs on vesicovaginal fistula, splenectomy, and plastic surgery.

1824 René Joseph Hyacinthe Bertin's classic treatise on the heart, *Traité des Maladies du Coeur et des gros Vaisseaux*, was published.

1824 *John Reissberg Wolfe* born. A German-born ophthalmologist who worked in Australia where he first described the use of a full thickness skin graft (taken from behind the ear) to correct ectropion and other eyelid deformities caused by loss of skin (Wolfe graft).

1824 'Absence', a term describing a minor form of epilepsy, was coined by French physician, Louis Florentine Calmiel. He showed pathological lesions in the brain of patients with general paresis before the cause of syphilis was known.

1824 Intracranial infection as a result of head injury was recognized by Sir Astley Paston Cooper, surgeon to George IV.

1824 *William Tennant Gairdner* born. A professor of medicine at Glasgow

University who wrote an important treatise on cardiac murmurs (1861), and differentiated between postoperative pneumonia and pulmonary collapse (1854).

1824   *Richard Ladislaus Heschel* born. A professor of anatomy at Olmutz who described the transverse gyri of the temporal lobes.

1824   The Massachusetts Eye and Ear Infirmary was founded, one of the first specialist hospitals in the United States.

1824   The first transfusion of human blood was given to a bleeding woman in childbirth by James Blundell.

1824   Compounds with identical chemical composition but different structure and properties (isomers) were first observed by Justus von Liebig.

1824   Epigastric pain preceding pre-eclampsia was described by French surgeon, François Chaussier.

1824   *Bernhard Johannes Gudden* born. A neuroanatomist from Munich who described the tract connecting the medial geniculate bodies and inferior corpora quadrigemina of the opposite side (1870), and pioneered physiological studies of the thalamus.

1824   Characteristic striping of the heart found during postmortem in patients with severe anemia (tabby cat appearance) was described by James Scarth Combe, a physician in Edinburgh in his paper, *A Case of Anaemia*.

1824   The islands of epithelium present in the gums of infants (Serres gland), and the metafacial angle of anthropmetry (Serres angle) were described by Antoine Etienne Renaud Augustin Serres, a professor of anatomy and natural history at the Jardin des Plantes, Paris.

1824   Hippuric acid was discovered by Friedrich Wohler of Germany, a landmark in the study of metabolism.

1824   German physician, Dietrich Schütte, was the first to use cod liver oil in treating rickets.

1825   The first attempt at ovariotomy in Britain was made by Scottish surgeon, John Lizars, but was unsuccessful.

1825   The term lithotrite was coined by French physician, Jean Civiale.

1825   A description of a classic experiment where a curarized animal is maintained on artificial respiration with a bellows through tracheostomy, was given by Charles Waterton.

1825   *Carl Joseph Eberth* born. A bacteriologist from Würzberg who discovered *Salmonella* and showed it was the causative organism of typhoid (1880), and described the broken-line appearance of cardiac muscles under the microscope (1866).

1825   *Jean Baptiste Emil Vidal* born. A French dermatologist who described neurodermatitis (Vidal disease).

1825 *Thomas Henry Huxley* born. An English physician from Middlesex who discovered the inner layer of the root sheath of the hair follicle (Huxley layer).

1825 *Timothy Holmes* born. A London surgeon who described an operation for excision of the calcaneum (Holmes operation).

1825 *Nikolaus Friedrich* born. A German physician who wrote a significant treatise on progressive muscular atrophy, and described a hereditary spinocerebellar degenerative disease (Friedrich ataxia, 1863).

1825 *Luigi Vella* born. An Italian physiologist who described artificial fistula created by dividing the intestine in two places and fixing both pieces to the abdominal wall (Vella fistula).

1825 *Ernst Felix Emanuel Hoppe-Seyler* born. A German physiological chemist who obtained hemoglobin in a crystalline form (1864), named hemoglobin, and quantified the volume of oxygen bound to hemoglobin. He founded the first biochemical journal, *Zeitschrift für physiologische chemie*, in 1877.

1825 *Luigi Maria Concato* born. An Italian physician who originally described tuberculosis as the etiological agent of Concato disease (polyserositis), where today the eponym is applied to all forms of polyserositis.

1825 *Charles Felix Michel Peter* born. A French physician in Paris who described atheroma of the blood vessels in his treatise on the heart and blood vessels of 1883.

1825 *Frederick James Gant* born. A London surgeon who performed subtrochanteric osteotomy (Gant operation) for ankylosis of the hip joint.

1825 *Nathan Bozemann* born. An American surgeon who designed a double-channeled urethral catheter (Bozemann catheter).

1825 *Friedrich Albert Zenker* born. A German professor of pathological anatomy who described necrosis and hyaline degeneration of striated muscle (Zenker degeneration), and the diverticulum of the upper esophagus (Zenker diverticulum).

1825 *Louis Henri Felix Féréol* born. A French physician who described periarticular subcutaneous nodes in acute rheumatism (Féréol node).

1825 *Fessenden Nott Otis* born. An American urologist who designed a method for internal urethrotomy and introduced the use of local anesthesia in urology (1884).

1825 *Pierre Carl Eduard Potain* born. A French cardiologist who explained the mechanism and physiology of heart sounds (1866), the mechanism of the gallop rhythm (1875), and the opening snap of mitral stenosis (Potain sign).

1825 *Jean-Martin Charcot* born. An eminent French neurologist who contributed to work on biliary passages, the liver and kidneys, studied crystals in the sputum of asthmatics, and described tabetic arthropathies (Charcot joints), Charcot triad in mutiple sclerosis, and osteoarthritis attributed to syphilis.

1825 The first amputation of the knee joint in America was performed by Nathan Smith, a surgeon from Connecticut.

1825 The first American textbook on pediatrics, *A Treatise on Physical and Medical Treatment of Children*, was written by William Potts Dewees of Philadelphia.

1825 *Max Johann Sigismund Schultze* born. A German zoologist who described the olfactory mucous membranes and cells (Schultze membrane and cells), defined the cell as the building block of an organism, and introduced osmic acid as a stain for nervous tissue.

1825 Congenital lymphatic cyst of the neck (cervical hydrocele or Maunoir hydrocele) was described by Swiss surgeon, Jean Pierre Maunoir.

1826 Bromine was discovered in seawater by French chemist, Jérome Antoine Balard.

1826 *John Thompson Hodgen* born. A surgeon from St Louis, Missouri who designed the Hodgen splint, made of metal and used for treatment of fracture of the femoral shaft.

1826 *Carl Gegenbaur* born. A German comparative anatomist who demonstrated the unicellular nature of

the ovum in vertebrates (1861), and described osteoblasts (1885).

1826 The first splenectomy was performed by Carl Friedrich Quittenbaum of Germany, although the operation was not successful.

1826 The pretracheal fascia (Porter fascia), and tracheal tug as a sign of thoracic aneurysm (Porter sign) were originally described and named by William Henry Porter, professor of surgery at Trinity College, Dublin.

1826 *Alphonso Dumontpallier* born. A French physician who devised the Dumontpallier test, for detection of bile pigments, using iodine as a reagent.

1826 *Emily Blackwell* born. An American obstetrician who established the New York Infirmary for Indigent Women and Children and became professor of obstetrics at the Women's Medical College (1869).

1826 *Richard Barwell* born. A London surgeon who described the correction of genu valgum by osteotomy of the tibia (Barwell operation).

1826 *Edmé Felix Alfred Vulpian* born. A physician from Paris, who demonstrated the presence of an active vital substance in the adrenal glands (1856), later named epinephrine, and described Vulpian atrophy in progressive muscular dystrophy.

1826 The first description of adenoma sebaceum was given by a physician from Paris, Pierre François Olive Rayer.

1827 Chronic appendicitis was described as a clinical entity by French physician, Francois Mèlier.

1827 Pericardial drainage by aspiration in a 14-year-old girl was performed by Jowett in Nottingham, England.

1827 The term hyperemia was introduced by French physician, Gabriel Andral.

1827 *Auguste Chauveau* born. A French physiologist who pioneered the direct recording of cardiac impulses and the thermodynamics of muscular function.

1827 *Julius Nessler* born. A German chemist from Karlsruhe who prepared Nessler reagent, a test for ammonia used in the analysis of blood, urea and plasma proteins.

1827 *Charles Fayette Taylor* born. An American orthopedic surgeon who introduced remedial exercises, advocated them for many conditions, and perfected a steel brace for Pott disease.

1827 *Lord Joseph Lister* born. A British surgeon and founder of the antiseptic system of surgery who advocated the use of carbolic acid for the prevention of infection during surgery, and used catgut treated with carbolic acid to promote asepsis (1869).

1827 The first surgical removal of the uterus was carried out by Italian surgeon, Augosto Bozzi Granville,

Joseph Lister

but without success. He was a founder of the Obstetrical Society.

1827 *Henry Gray* born. A fellow of the Royal College of Surgeons, he published the famous anatomical work, *Anatomy, Descriptive and Surgical* (1858), popularly known as Gray's Anatomy.

1827 *Bernhard Sigismund Schultze* born. A German gynecologist who demonstrated the remains of the yolk sac are normally incorporated into the placenta, and described the Schultze method which revives the asphyxiated neonate by inverting and swinging the infant.

1827 *Marcellin Pierre Eugéne Berthelot* born. A French physician who produced benzene and napthalene (1851), discovered the enzyme invertin in yeast, named acetylene and succeeded Louis Pasteur as secretary of the French Academy of Sciences in 1889.

1827   *E. Isambert* born. A French physician who described tuberculous ulceration of the larynx and pharynx (Isambert disease).

1827   Trepanning as a treatment for bone necrosis was described in an account written by Nathan Smith, a surgeon from Connecticut.

1827   Observations respecting 'an ulcer of peculiar character which attacks the eyelids and other parts of the face' were made by Irish ophthalmologist, Arthur Jacob, and later named Jacob ulcer.

1827   *James Hinton* born. The first aural surgeon to be appointed to Guy's Hospital in London who performed the first operation for mastoiditis in England (1868), and wrote *The Mystery of Pain* and *The Questions of Aural Surgery* (1874).

1827   The first cesarean section in America was performed by John Lambert Richmond.

1828   *Sir Benjamin Ward Richardson* born. A British physician who invented the ether spray and modified the chloroform inhaler, researched poisons, and described the Richardson sign of death.

1828   *The Medical, Surgical and Medicine Reporter*, a forerunner of the *British Medical Journal* (BMJ), and the British Medical Association (1832) were founded by Sir Charles Hastings.

1828   *Friedrich Wilhelm Ernst Albrecht von Graefe* born. An eye surgeon from Berlin who founded the *Archiv für Ophthalmologie* (1854), introduced modern surgical ophthalmology, and designed operations for squint, glaucoma, cataract, conical cornea, and described the von Graefe sign of eyelid lag in thyrotoxicosis.

1828   *Thomas Bryant* born. An English surgeon who described the iliofemoral triangle (Bryant triangle, 1861), used for surface marking in the diagnosis of fracture of the neck of the femur.

1828

William Alexander Hammond

William Alexander Hammond born. An American neurologist who wrote the first monograph on neurology in America, *Diseases of the Nervous System* (1871), described athetosis, carried out research on snake venom and arrow poisons, and was a founder of the American and New York Neurological Associations.

1828   *J. M. Rodriguez* born. A Mexican obstetrician and pioneer in the diagnosis of pregnancy by palpation and auscultation.

1828   *Lionel Smith Beale* born. An English microscopist who identified malignant cells in sputum (1860), illustrated and described cells of the cardiac ganglion (1863), and wrote the influential book, *The Microscope and its Application to Clinical Medicine*.

1828   *Ulysses Trelat* born. A French surgeon who described small yellowish spots near tuberculous ulcers of the mouth (Trelat sign).

1828   *Jules Bernard Luys* born. A Paris neurologist who carried out research on hypnosis, hysteria and insanity, and described hemiballismus caused by lesions in the subthalamic body or the medial nucleus of the thalamus (nucleus of Luys, 1865).

1828   *Julius Jacobson* born. A German ophthalmologist from Königsberg who used a scleral flap incision for cataract operations, and described syphilitic retinopathy.

1828   John Abernethy of St Bartholomew's Hospital, London, described the Abernethy fascia covering the external iliac artery which bears his name.

1828   A flat instrument applied to the surface of the body to mediate percussion (pleximeter) was invented by French physician, Adolphe Pierre Piorry, who wrote *Traité sur la percussion mediate* in which he described its use.

1828   *Sir Jonathan Hutchinson* born. An English physician who described the peg-shaped incisor teeth in congenital syphilis (Hutchinson teeth, 1861), prepared an *Atlas of*

Sir Jonathan Hutchinson

Skin Diseases which contains a description of Hutchinson–Boeck disease, a 10-volume *Archives of Surgery*, and founded the New Sydenham Society.

1828   A description and illustration of the lesions in multiple sclerosis was given by London pathologist, Robert Hooper in *The Morbid Anatomy of the Human Brain*.

1828   French surgeon, Jacques Mathieu Delpech, first observed the tuberculous nature of spinal caries.

1828   *Robert Battey* born. A Georgia surgeon who performed oophorectomy and excision of uterine appendages for non-uterine conditions such as painful menstruation and neurosis (Battey operation, 1872), used later in the treatment of other pelvic conditions.

1828   *John Scott Burdon Sanderson* born. A professor of medicine at Oxford who pioneeered electrophysiology, devised an improved rheotome to study the action currents of the heart.

1828   *Otto Heinrich Enoch Becker* born. A German oculist who observed pulsation of the retinal arteries in exophthalmic goiter (Becker phenomenon).

1828   *James Hobson Aveling* born. A London obstetrician who designed a repositor (Aveling repositor) which reduced inversion of the uterus.

1828   *Edmund Leser* born. A German surgeon who described the sudden onset of seborrheic dermatosis (senile warts) with malignant tumors, most commonly of the gastrointestinal tract.

1828   *Etienne Stéphane Tarnier* born. A French obstetrician who designed axis traction forceps for applying traction along the line of the pelvic axis (Tarnier forceps, 1860).

1828   *Rocco Gritti* born. An Italian surgeon in Milan who described a method of supracondylar amputation of the femur while retaining the patella (1857).

1828   *Eugene Koeberlé* born. A French surgeon and gynecologist who introduced ovariotomy in France, and modified the artery forceps including a locking device (Koeberlé forceps, 1865).

1828   A mercury manometer to measure blood pressure was devised by Jean Léonard Poiseuille (Poiseuille hemodynameter).

1828   *Alexander Pagenstecher* born. A German ophthalmologist who prepared a secret remedy consisting of yellow oxide of mercury (Pagenstecher ointment), and defined a method of surface marking the origin of attachment of any movable abdominal tumor.

1828   *Johann Nepomuk Czermak* born. A German professor of comparative anatomy at Jena who studied the minute anatomy of the teeth, and improved and popularized the laryngoscope invented by Manuel Patricio Rodriguez.

1828   A study of 28 hay fever cases was provided in *Of the catarrhus aestivus, or country catarrh*, written by English physician, John Bostock.

1828   *John Langdon Haydon Down* born. An important English figure in mental health who published a blueprint for treatment and education of the mentally retarded, *Observations of Ethnic Classification of Idiots* (1866), and is remembered for Down syndrome.

1828   *William Murray Dobie* born. A physician at the Chester Royal Infirmary, England who gave several original descriptions of the histological appearance of muscle fibers.

1828   The first adequate description of lupus erythematosus was given by Laurent Theodore Biett, a physician in Paris.

1828 Probably the first description of a neuroma was given by Scottish physician, William Wood.

1829 English physician, James Lomax Bardsley, was the first to use emetine for amebiosis.

1829 The term metastasis, for spread of a cancer, was introduced by French gynecologist, Joseph Claude Anselme Rècamier.

1829 The earliest record of an abscess in the right iliac fossa (Dupuytren abscess) was given by Guillaume Dupuytren of Paris.

1829 *Benjamin George McDowell* born. A Dublin surgeon who was the first to describe the suspensory ligament of the pectoralis major tendon which is named after him.

1829 *Frederick William Pavy* born. An English worker on carbohydrate metabolism and diabetes who correlated hyperglycemia and glycosuria, described cyclic or recurrent albuminuria (Pavy disease), and the involvement of the joints in typhoid.

1829 *Friedrich August Kekule von Stradonitz* born. A German physician and organic chemist who discovered the benzene ring structure, and proposed that molecules consist of linked atoms, bonded according to valence.

1829 *William Goodell* born. An American gynecologist who described the softening of the cervix occurring as a sign of pregnancy (Goodell sign).

1829 *Ernst Leberecht Wagner* born. A German physician who wrote a treatise on uterine cancer (1858), the path of metastases of cancer of the cervix, and described dermatomyositis (1863).

1829 Cutaneous leishmaniasis, or Baghdad sore, was first observed by the father of dermatology in France, Jean Louis Alibert.

1829 *Anton Friedrich von Tröltsch* born. A German aural surgeon who described the Tröltsch space between the two pouches of the mucous membrane in the upper part of the middle ear, and invented the modern otoscope (1860).

1829 *Theodor Billroth* born. A professor of surgery in Zurich and Vienna who performed the first successful resection of the esophagus (1871), carried out a distal partial gastrectomy (1881), performed a resection of the larynx (1883), and gave his name to the Billroth operations.

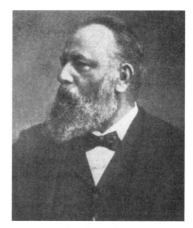

Theodor Billroth

128

1829   *Jules Marie Parrot* born. A French physician who described the Parrot nodes on the parietal and frontal bones of the skull of infants with congenital syphilis, and the Parrot sign, characterized by dilatation of the pupils induced by pinching the skin of the neck of patients with meningitis.

1829   *George Harley* born. A Scottish physician who studied intermittent hematuria, later known as paroxysmal nocturnal hematuria (Harley disease), showed that curare was an antidote to strychnine, and that respired oxygen forms a complex in the blood (hemoglobin).

1829   *Ivan Sechenov* born. A Russian physiologist at St Petersburg and Moscow who gave a description of cerebral inhibition of spinal reflexes, and laid the foundations for future Russian physiology.

1829   A laryngoscope was invented by Guy Benjamin Babington.

1829   *Emiline Horton Cleveland* born. A professor of obstetrics at the Women's Hospital in Philadelphia and the first woman in America to perform major abdominal surgery and ovariotomy.

1829   *Eduard Pflüger* born. A German physiologist who carried out detailed studies of nerve stimulation, respiratory function, and discovered Pflüger cords (made of a linear arrangement of sex cells during the developing ovary).

1829   The first successful excision of the cervix in America was performed by John B. Strachan (cervicectomy).

1829   *John Lewis William Thudichum* born. A German biochemist practicing in London who pioneered studies in phospholipids, and devised the Thudichum test for creatinine, using ferric chloride as a reagent.

1829   *Friedrich Goll* born. A neuroanatomist from Zurich who described fasciculus gracilis of the posterior column of the spinal cord (1868), and wrote a paper on *Minute Anatomy of the Spinal Cord of Man* in 1870.

1829   *Hugo Wilhelm von Ziemssen* born. A Munich physician who advocated treatment for anemia using subcutaneous injections of defibrinated human blood (Ziemssen treatment).

1830   *Richard von Volkmann* born. A surgeon from Germany who described contracture in fingers and wrists following ischemia and secondary to injury to the elbow (Volkmann contracture, 1881), and advocated the excision of tuberculous joints rather than amputation of the limb.

1830   *Henri Ferdinand Dolbeau* born. A Paris surgeon who described the Dolbeau operation for lithotomy, in which the stone is crushed in the bladder through a median incision in the urethra.

1830   *Sigismond Jaccoud* born. A professor of internal pathology from Geneva who described a form of arthritis of the hands and fingers occurring in patients with rheumatic fever (Jaccoud disease), the prominence of the aorta in the suprasternal notch (Jaccoud sign) in aortic dilation, and febrile meningitis in patients with tuberculous meningitis (Jaccoud dissociated fever).

1830   *Silas Weir Mitchell* born. A neurologist from Philadelphia who described a condition associated with painful feet, erythromelalgia (1872), demonstrated knee jerk reflex (1886), and investigated the psychotic properties of mescaline (1896).

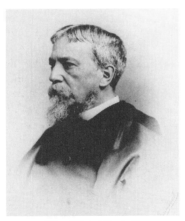

Silas Weir Mitchell

1830   *Etienne-Jules Marey* born. A French physiologist who obtained the first tracing of the impulse of the heart in the radial artery during the cardiac cycle with the invention of the sphygmograph in 1863.

1830   The canal at the junction of the cornea and sclera (canal of Schlemm) was described by German anatomist, Friedrich Schlemm.

1830   Alexander Ziegler, a Scottish obstetrician, invented obstetric forceps in which the Smellie lock was replaced by splitting the shank of one of the shoulder blades to allow passage for the other blade.

1830   *Otto Spiegelberg* born. A German gynecologist who accurately described the paraovarian cysts, performed curettage of the uterus for retained tissues, and wrote *Das Compendium der Geburtshilfe*, a popular textbook of obstetrics.

1830   *William Basil Neftel* born. An American physician who described a hysterical disease in which the patient is unable to sit, stand or walk without pain, but can perform any movement lying down (Neftel disease).

1830   *Jean Baptiste Vincent Laborde* born. A Paris physiologist who described a form of artificial respiration with intermittent traction of the tongue in 1897.

1830   *Jules Émile Pean* born. A French surgeon who (unsuccessfully) resected the stomach in carcinoma of the stomach, and also designed clamp forceps for hematosis.

1830   Thomas Southwood Smith, an English Unitarian minister, observed epidemics of fever at the London Fever Hospital and published *A Treatise on Fever*.

1830   *Edward Clapton* born. London physician who described the green line at the base of the teeth in cases of poisoning due to copper (Clapton line).

1830   *George William Callender* born. A London surgeon who devised maxillary clips (Callender clips) for the treatment of overgrowth of the incisor process of the maxilla.

1830   Salicin in willow bark as a form of pain relief was described by French physician, Henri Leroux.

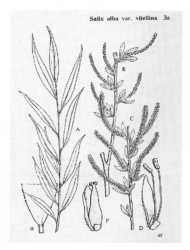

Salix alba var. vitellina 3a

Willow

1830   *Sir William Roberts* born. An English physician who devised the Roberts test for detection of albumin in urine, using a solution of magnesium sulfate and sulfuric acid as reagents.

1830   American social reformer, Robert Dale Owen, published the first book on birth control in America, *Moral Physiology*.

1830   The association between intraocular pressure and glaucoma was pointed out by Scottish ophthalmologist, William Mackenzie.

1830   Venesection was condemned in America by Benjamin Rush in the *Baltimore Monthly Journal*.

1831   A combined dilator and lacerator for esophageal stricture was devised by R. Fletcher of London.

1831   *Henry Vandyke Carter* born. A physician in the Indian Medical Service who described Madura foot, scrotal elephantiasis, and several other diseases.

1831   Intermittent claudication was first described by J. Bouley who gave a description of lameness due to arterial disease in a horse after exercise.

1831   An original description of the fracture of the lower end of the fibula was given by French surgeon, Guillaume Dupuytren, followed by a detailed account of Dupuytren contracture, describing the fibrous thickening of the palmar fascia leading to contractures of the hand.

1831   A classical description of delirium tremens was given by John Ware, professor of medicine at Harvard University.

1831   *Jakob August Estlander* born. An Icelandic surgeon who described an operation for harelip, and resected the ribs lying over empyema (Estlander operation).

1831   *Paul Claude Hyacinthe Meynet* born. A French physician who described the Meynet nodes in the capsules of joints or tendons, found in rheumatic conditions and especially in children.

1831 *Jean Casimir Felix Guynon* born. A professor of surgical pathology in Paris who described the internal os of the uterus and the canal formed by its prolongation (1858).

1831 *Pietro Loreta* born. A professor of surgery at Bologna who described a method for opening the stomach and performing either a digital or instrument dilatation of the pyloric or cardiac orifice (Loreta operation).

1831 *Thomas Murray Drysdale* born. A New York gynecologist who described the Drysdale corpuscles, transparent microscopic cells seen in the fluid of ovarian cysts.

1831 *Wilhelm His Sr* born. A professor of anatomy and embryologist at Basel and Leipzig who promoted developmental mechanics, described the special formative cells of the blood vessels (1868), developed the microtome for cutting thin sections of tissue (1866), and wrote *On the Tissues and Spaces of the Body*.

1831 Chloroform was discovered independently by von Liebig in Germany, Guthrie in New York and Soubeiran in France.

1831 *Theodore Gaillard Thomas* born. A New York gynecologist who published an important treatise on the diseases of women (1868), and performed the first vaginal ovariotomy (1870).

1831 *Karl von Voit* born. A German physiologist who described the cerebellar nucleus accessory to the corpus dentatum (Voit nucleus).

1831 Potassium iodide was used as a treatment for secondary syphilis by Robert Williams of St Thomas' Hospital, London.

1831 *Alarik Frithiof Holmgren* born. A physiologist from Sweden who pioneered the application of electrophysiology to study visual systems, was the first to demonstrate retinal action currents, and developed the Holmgren test for color blindness.

1831 *Carl Friedrich Wilhelm Frommann* born. A professor of histology at Jena who demonstrated the striations in the axis cylinders of the nerve cell (Frommann striae, 1876), using silver nitrate stain.

1831 *Ernest Besnier* born. A French dermatologist who described flexural pruritis amongst infants (1892), later named Besnier prurigo, Besnier–Boeck disease, and a treatise on rheumatism describing chronic arthrosynovitis (Besnier rheumatism, 1876).

1832 Paris professor, Jean *Alfred Fournier*, born. He made several contributions to the study of syphilis and gave his name to fulminating gangrene of the scrotum and perineum in diabetic patients.

1832 *Léon Labbé* born. A Paris surgeon who developed the practice of pre-anesthetic medication (1872), gave his name to the Labbé triangle between the inferior border of the liver and lower border of the 9th costal cartilage, and the Labbé vein.

1832   *Pierre Mauriac* born. A French physician who first described erythema nodosum syphiliticum (Mauriac disease), and a syndrome of growth retardation, obesity and hepatomegaly in juvenile diabetes.

1832   *Ernst Victor von Leyden* born. A German physician who worked on tabes and poliomyelitis, established sanatoria for treatment of tuberculosis, was the first to describe fatty infiltration of the heart (1882), gave a concise account of heart disease (1884), and described a form of muscular dystrophy (Leyden paralysis).

1832   *Cesare Frederici* born. An Italian physician who first described heart sounds ausculated in the abdominal cavity in cases of intestinal perforation, with gas in the peritoneal cavity (Frederici sign).

1832   The membrana flaccida of the membrana tymphani (Sharpnell membrane) was described by Henry Jones Sharpnell, an English military surgeon.

1832   The waterhammer pulse, or Corrigan pulse, characterized by a sudden impact and rapid fall in aortic insufficiency, was described by Dublin physician, Sir Dominic John Corrigan.

1832   *Wilhelm Max Wundt* born. An experimental psychologist from Germany who introduced the concept in his work *Beiträge zur Theorie der Sinneswahrnehmung*, which highlighted studies on voluntary reactions, reflex actions, and sensory perception.

1832   *Monographie des Dermatoses*, a classification of skin diseases, was written by the founder of the modern school of dermatology in Paris, Jean Louis Alibert. He introduced the word 'dermatolysis' in the same year.

1832   *August Breisky* born. A German gynecologist who described kraurosis vulvae (Breisky disease).

1832   German chemist, Justus von Liebig, discovered chloral hydrate, by passing alcohol through chlorine.

1832   *Franz König* born. A German orthopedic surgeon who identified the relationship between hemophilia and hemophilic arthropathy, and three stages in this disease.

1832   *Jacob Gottstein* born. An otorhinologist from Breslau who described the protoplasmic projections of the lateral cells of the cochlear canal (1872).

1832   *Ernst Axle Henrik Key* born. A Swedish professor of pathological anatomy who was one of the first to describe the sensory nerve endings (Key bulb).

1832   *John Parkin* born. An English surgeon who described the use of charcoal filters to purify water and so prevent the spread of cholera.

1832   The Boston Lying-in Hospital, one of the first specialist hospitals in the United States, was founded.

1832   *Nicolaus Rudinger* born. A professor of anatomy at Munich who described the muscles internal to the circular fibers of the rectum (Rudinger muscle, 1879).

1832 *Francesco Fede* born. An Italian pediatrician who (with Antonio Rega) described sublingual fibroma caused by the lower teeth when infants are still suckling (Fede–Rega disease).

1832 *Dioscoride Vitali* born. An Italian physician who devised the Vitali test for detecting alkaloids, with the reagents potassium hydroxide and sulfuric acid.

1832 Intravenous saline was first used as treatment for circulatory collapse following cholera, by Thomas Aitchison Latta.

1832 Codeine, a base alkaloid of opium, was isolated by Jean-Pierre Robiquet.

1832 *Sir William Turner* born. A British surgeon who described the interparietal sulcus of the brain (Turner sulcus), and the subzonal membrane of the amnion in the chorionic vesicle (1872).

1832 *Hermann Arnold Jakob Knapp* born. A leading German ophthalmologist working in New York who designed several operations for squint, pterygium, and cataract, wrote a treatise on curvature of the cornea (1859, and founded the *Archives of Ophthalmology and Otology* in 1869.

1832 Isolation of creatinine from muscle, cholesterol (1815), and glucose from diabetic urine was done by French chemist, Michel Chevreul.

1833 Liver puncture biopsy was performed by English surgeon, Edward Stanley.

1833 The first accurate description of tuberculous meningitis was given by American physician, William Wood Gerhard.

1833 Isolation of atropine was carried out by German pharmacologist, Philipp L. Geiger.

1833 *Paul Bert* born. A French physiologist who experimented on the effect of anoxemia and high altitudes on blood and the circulation using pressure chambers.

1833 The accessory ganglion of the great sympathetic system in connection with the solar plexus (Lobstein ganglion), and osteogenesis imperfecta (Lobstein syndrome) were described by Johann Georg Christian Martin Lobstein, professor of pathology in Strasburg.

1833 *Eduard von Wahl* born. A German surgeon who described distension of the proximal portion of obstructed bowel (Wahl sign), and the systolic murmur over an injured artery (1885).

1833 *Wilhelm Johann Friedrich Krause* born. A professor of anatomy at Göttingen in Germany who described the septa which divide the sarcomeres within muscles (Krause membrane), and several other structures which bear his name.

1833 *William Leishman* born. A professor of midwifery at Glasgow and editor of the *Glasgow Medical*

Journal who published *A System of Midwifery* (1870), which remained a standard textbook into its fourth edition.

1833 *Constantin Charles Theodore Paul* born. A French physician who described feeble apex beat with forcible impulse over the rest of the heart in cases of pericardial adhesions (Paul sign).

1833 The Mayer ligament, a suspensory ligament of the carotid body, was first described by an anatomy professor at Bonn, Germany, M.F. Mayer.

1833 *Sir Thomas Smith* born. A London surgeon who described loss of the femoral head due to acute inflammation in infancy, and gave a description of cranio-hypophysial xanthomatosis (Hand–Schülter–Christian disease).

1833 *James Clark White* born. A Boston dermatologist who described White disease (keratosis follicularis).

1833 *Abel Henry Bouchard* born. A French physician who described miliary aneurysms and associated them with cerebral hemorrhage.

1833 The King's College Medical Society in London which took its name from the King's College Medical and Scientific Society, was founded.

1833 *Edwin Theodor Saemisch* born. An ophthalmologist from Bonn who described serpiginous ulcer of the cornea (Saemisch ulcer) and its treatment.

1833 *Carlos Juan Finlay* born. A Cuban physician who proved that the *Aedes aegypti* species of mosquito was the carrier of arbor virus which causes yellow fever.

1833 *Carl Friedrich Otto Westphal* born. A German neuropsychiatrist who described agoraphobia, demonstrated the absence of knee jerk reflex in tabes dorsalis, and described the third cranial nerve (Edinger–Westphal nucleus).

1833 William Wallace, an Irish physician, was said to have been the first to describe lymphogranuloma venereum.

1833 *Friedrich von Recklinghausen* born. A German pathologist who described a familial disease marked by pedunculated soft tumors over the body (neurofibromatosis, and multiple neuroma, or von Recklinghausen disease).

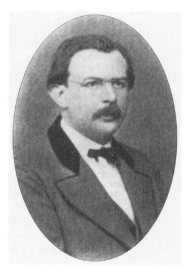

Friedrich von Recklinghausen

1833   *Wilhelm Alexander Freund* born. A German surgeon who introduced abdominal hysterectomy as treatment for cancer of the uterus.

1833   *Carl Jacob Christian Adolf Gerhardt* born. A professor from Germany who was a pioneer in pediatrics and laryngology, described bilateral adductor paralysis of the larynx (Gerhardt syndrome, 1863), and devised the Gerhardt test for detection of ketones.

1833   *Wilhelm Manz* born. A professor of ophthalmology at Freiburg who described epithelial utricles found on the cornea (Manz utricular glands) in 1859.

1834   *Rudolph Peter Heinrich Heidenhain* born. A German professor of physiology and histology who described the parietal and central cells of the gastric secretory glands (1888), and gave his name to the Heidenhain cells.

1834   *Hugh Owen Thomas* born. The father of modern orthopedics in Britain who devised various devices for the treatment of deformities and fractures, and invented the Thomas splint (1876) which caused a drastic fall in mortality in compound fractures of the femur.

1834   *Friedrich Leopold Goltz* born. A German physiologist who pioneered work on vestibular disturbances and vertigo (1870), vagal reflex inhibition in relation to the heart, and showed the difference between cortical and subcortical functions.

1834   *August Friedrich Leopold Weismann* born. A German zoologist who proposed the chromosome theory of heredity in 1892.

1834   *Walther Hermann Heineke* born. A surgeon from Erlangen who devised an operation for pyloroplasty (Heineke–Mikulicz operation) involving a longitudinal incision of the pylorus followed by a transverse suture.

1834   *Hugo Schiff* born. A German chemist who worked in Florence, Italy where he devised the Schiff test to detect carbohydrates in urine, using sulfuric acid, glacial acetic acid and alcohol.

1834   *Alexander Rollet* born. An Austrian professor of histology at the University of Graz who described the colorless stroma of erythrocytes (Rollet stroma) in 1880.

1834   *Fritz Waldemar Rasmussen* born. A Danish physician who described a branch of the pulmonary artery affected by tuberculosis (Rasmussen aneurysm).

1834   *Ernst Haeckel* born. A German zoologist, regarded as the founder of modern morphology, who published *General Morphology* (1866), *Natural History of Creation* (1868), and *Anthropogeny or the Evolution of Man* (1874) on human embryology, and coined the terms 'ontogeny', 'phylogeny' and 'ecology'.

1834   Tuberculous spondylitis of the cervical vertebrae (Rust disease) was described by German surgeon, Johann Nepomak Rust.

1834 *A. Clara Swaine* born. An American medical missionary who graduated from the Woman's Medical College, Pennsylvania in 1869, and went to India where she opened the first medical hospital for women in India (1874).

1834 *Salvatore Tommaselli* born. An Italian physician who described pyrexia and hematuria due to excess use of quinine (Tommaselli disease).

1834 *Arthur Edward Durham* born. An English surgeon who devised the joint tracheotomy tube (Durham tube).

1834 *Karl Ewald Konstantin Hering* born. A German physiologist who (with Joseph Breuer) described the Hering–Breuer neurogenic reflex controlling rate and depth of respiration via the vagal nerve.

1834 *Heinrich Hoyer* born. A Polish professor of embryology who described the communications between small arteries and small veins without the intervention of the capillaries (Hoyer canals, 1877).

1834 *Vladimir A. Betz* born. A Russian anatomist and histologist from Kiev, who described the pyramidal cell in the 5th layer of the cerebral cortex (Betz cell).

1834 *Theodor Albrecht Edwin Klebs* born. A German bacteriologist who pointed out the tuberculous cavities in the lungs as a source of intestinal tuberculosis (1873), and demonstrated the peculiar property of acid fastness of the tuberculous bacilli (1896).

1834 *Otto Friedrich Karl Deiters* born. A German physician and histologist who made several contributions to neuro-auditory anatomy and the structure of the internal ear, and also described the lateral vestibular nucleus (Deiters nucleus, 1863).

1834 *Solomon Stricker* born. A German physician who studied the treatment of pain relief, and discovered that sodium salicylic acid arrests rheumatic fever.

1834 *Marie Ernst Gellé* born. A French surgeon and otologist who developed the Gellé test to demonstrate that deafness due to a bone conduction defect is not affected by pressure over the external auditory nerve.

1834 H.M.D. de Blainville of Paris demonstrated massive intravascular clotting in experimental animals, following an intravenous injection of brain tissue.

1834 *John Hughlings Jackson* born. A British neurologist who established the use of the ophthalmoscope in brain disease, proposed that areas which caused specific isolated movements existed in the cortex, and described a unilateral localized form of epilepsy.

1834 *P. Guttmann* born. A German physician who described a bruit heard over the thyroid in hyperthyroidism (Guttmann sign).

1834 A vacuum pump for compression and rarefaction of a limb was devised by French physician, Victor Theodore Junod.

1835 — Use of defibrinated blood to prevent clotting during blood transfusion was introduced by Theodor Ludwig Wilhelm Bischoff.

1835 — Diagnostic aspiration of pleural fluid was introduced by London physician, Thomas Davies. He introduced needle aspiration for empyema.

1835 — Dimness of vision due to tobacco smoking (tobacco amblyopia) was described by William Mackenzie of Scotland.

1835 — The ileopectineal fascia (Thompson fascia) was described by Alexander Thompson, professor of medical jurisprudence at London University.

1835 — *Max J. Oertel* born. A Munich physician who proposed the use of natural methods such as massage, diet, mountain climbing and exercise for the treatment of heart diseases (Oertel treatment).

1835 — *Thomas George Morton* born. A Philadelphia surgeon who carried out the successful removal of an inflamed appendix (1887), and gave a complete description of metatarsalgia (Morton disease, 1876).

1835 — *John Green* born. A St Louis ophthalmologist who described a method for the surgical correction of entropion.

1835 — *Sarcoptes scabei*, the causative agent in scabies, was discovered and described in detail by French physician, Simon François Renucci.

1835 —

Sir William Henry Broadbent

Sir William Henry Broadbent born. An eminent cardiologist and neurologist from England who described adherent pericardium (Broadbent sign), and proposed the Broadbent hypothesis for the recovery of motor power of the muscles in paralysis.

1835 — *Isaac Burney Yeo* born. A London physician who formulated Yeo treatment for obesity by giving large amounts of hot drinks and withholding carbohydrates.

1835 — *Louis Anthoine Ranvier* born. A French physician who made a special study of the peripheral nerves, and described the regular interruptions of the myelin sheath (nodes of Ranvier) in 1878.

1835 — *Valentin J.J. Magnan* born. A French psychiatrist and one of the French leaders in the school of organic psychiatry, who described the crawling sensation under the skin seen in cocaine addiction (Magnan sign).

1835   *Adam Politzer* born. A Hungarian-born professor of otology at Vienna who gave the first account of otosclerosis (1895), described the Politzer cone of light on the tympanic membrane (1889), and designed the Politzer bag to inflate the middle ear.

1835   *Frantisek Chvostek* born. An Austrian surgeon from Moravia who investigated pathology and the treatment of neurological illnesses, including the use of electrotherapy, and described the Chvostek sign of facial spasm in tetany (1876).

1835   *Christian Andreas Viktor Hensen* born. A German physiologist and pioneer in the study of hearing, who studied the morphology of the cochlea, described the Hensen duct, Hensen supporting cells, and wrote two studies on hearing, in 1880 and 1902.

1835   *Moritz Benedikt* born. A Hungarian-born Austrian physician who modernized the use of electricity for the treatment of diseases, and gave his name to Benedikt syndrome of paralysis of the oculomotor nerve (1889).

1835   The idea that weak stimuli cause strong physiological responses and strong stimuli diminish physiological activity (Arndt–Schultz law) was proposed by German psychiatrist, Rudolf Arndt.

1835   Protoplasm was discovered by French zoologist, Felix Dujardin from Tours, who named it 'sarcode'.

1835   Pierre Charles Alexandre Louis published his *Researches* which introduced statistical methods into medicine, and was fundamental to establishing modern medicine as an exact and numerate science.

1835   Irish surgeon, Abraham Colles, wrote a treatise on syphilis, *Practical Observation on the Venereal Disease*, in which he referred to immunity acquired to syphilis by a healthy mother in bearing a syphilitic child (Colles law).

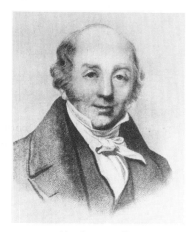

Abraham Colles

1835   *Robert von Olshausen* born. A Berlin obstetrician who devised the Olshausen operation, whereby the uterus is sutured to the anterior abdominal wall as treatment for retroverted uterus.

1835   A process of attraction of a lighter medium to a denser medium through a membrane (osmosis) was described by René Joachim Henri Dutrochet.

1835   The fungal cause of muscardine disease of the silkworm (silkworm disease) was discovered by an Italian lawyer, Agostino Bassi, considered to be the first proof for pathogenesis of germs.

1835 *Claes Gabriel Wilhelm Nylander* born. A Swedish chemist who devised a test to detect dextrose in urine (Nylander test).

1836 *Sir Thomas Clifford Allbutt* born. An English physician and medical historian who wrote an early description of joint symptoms in locomotor ataxia (1858), studied the effects of strain in producing heart diseases and aneurysms, and wrote a two-volume treatise on diseases of the arteries.

1836 Nucleosis of the ovum (Wagner spot) was described by Rudolf Wagner, professor of comparative anatomy at Göttingen.

1836 *William Tilbury Fox* born. An English dermatologist who gave the first description of dermatitis herpetiformis, or hydroa, gave the original description of epidermolysis bullosa, now named Koebner disease, and published the first important book on fungal disease.

1836 *Julius Wolff* born. A German orthopedic surgeon who proposed the Wolff law (1892) which states that all changes in the functions of the bones are accompanied by definite alteration in their internal structure.

1836 *Isodor Rosenthal* born. A professor of physiology in Germany who first described the spiral canal of the cochlea (Rosenthal canal).

1836 Myelineated nerve fibers were differentiated from the unsheathed fibers by Christian Gottfried Ehrenberg of Germany.

1836 Hermann Nasse of Germany gave a clear and detailed account of anemia in pregnancy.

1836 *Walter Butler Cheadle* born. A London pediatrician who gave his name to infantile scurvy (Cheadle disease), and differentiated between scurvy and rickets (1877).

1836 Thrity-nine cases of lead encephalopaphy were studied by Augustin Grisolle of Paris who divided them into convulsive, comatosed and delirious states.

1836 *Sir Michael Foster* born. Considered a founder of modern physiology in England, he was instrumental in establishing the *Journal of Physiology* (1878).

1836 The nucleolus was discovered by Gabriel Gustav Valentin, a German pathologist and botanist.

1836 *Claude Andre Paquelin* born. A physician from Paris who introduced a cautery made of platinum heated by the passage of a volatile hydrocarbon.

1836 Subcutaneous tenotomy was applied as treatment for most deformities arising out of muscular defects by German orthopedic and military surgeon, George Ludwig Stromeyer.

1836 *William Silver Oliver* born. A British army physician who described the sign of tracheal tug seen in thoracic aortic aneurysm, and published *A Practical Essay on the Use and Abuse of Warm Bathing in Gouty Cases.*

1836   *Eugéne Paul Gillette* born. A pathologist from Paris who described the longitudinal fibers of the esophagus around the posterior pharynx (suspensory ligament of the esophagus) in 1872.

1836   *Elizabeth Garrett Anderson* born. The first woman to qualify in medicine in England who started the New Hospital for Women at her dispensary on Euston Road in London in 1866.

1836   *Austin Flint Junior* born. A New York physiologist after whom the vascular arches at the base of the pyramid of the kidney (Flint arcade) are named.

1836   The Reichert cartilage, the second bronchial arch, was described by German professor of comparative anatomy at Dorpat, Karl Bogislaus Reichert.

1836   *Heinrich Wilhelm Gottfried Waldeyer* born. A German histologist who carried out a histological classification of cancers showing that carcinomas come from epithelial cells and sarcomas from mesodermal tissue. He suggested the terms 'chromosome' and 'neuron', and discovered the germinal epithelium in 1870.

1836   The first practical moving coil galvanometer was constructed by William Sturgeon of Lancashire, England.

1836   *Wilhelm Ebstein* born. A professor of medicine at Göttingen who described the congenital displacement of the tricuspid valve into the right ventricle (Ebstein anomaly, 1866), and the hyaline degeneration of epithelial cells in the renal tubules in diabetes mellitus (1880).

1836   The Birth and Deaths Registration Act was passed in England which made it a legal requirement to register all births and deaths with the Registrar General.

1836   *Albert von Bezold* born. A German physiologist who discovered the accelerator nerve fibers of the heart and their origin in the spinal cord (1862), described the Bezold ganglia in the interauricular system (1863), and Bezold disease of a fatal form of otitis media (1881).

1836   The New York Hospital for the Diseases of the Skin, one of the first three specialist hospitals in the United States, was founded.

1836   Cellulitis of the submandibular space usually caused by anerobic bacteria (Ludwig angina) was first observed by the German surgeon, Wilhelm Friedrich von Ludwig.

1837   *Edward Hallaran Bennett* born. A professor of surgery in Dublin who described a fracture involving the first metacarpal bone and the carpometacarpal joint, complicated by subluxation (1882).

1837   Henoch–Schönlein purpura in children was first described by Johann Schönlein and Edouard Heinrich Henoch, his pupil and a pioneer in German pediatrics, gave a classic description in 1863.

1837 The American Physiological Society was founded.

1837 *Victor André Cornil* born. A French histopathologist who wrote on the pathology of the kidneys, studied juvenile rheumatoid arthritis, and described malignant transformation of the acinar epithelium of the breast (1865).

Victor André Cornil

1837 *Bernhard Fränkel* born. A Berlin otorhinologist who designed a nasal spectrum, described mycosis of the pharynx, and performed a successful removal of an intra-laryngeal malignant growth.

1837 Gastrostomy was first performed in a case of stricture of the esophagus by Egebert, a Norwegian surgeon

1837 *Louis Felix Terrier* born. A Paris professor of surgery who described the gallbladder valve found between the gallbladder and the cystic duct (Terrier valve, 1891).

1837 *Julius August Christian Uffelmann* born. A German physician who devised the Uffelmann test which detects lactic acid in gastric juice, using ferric chloride and phenol as reagents.

1837 The first description of ciliated epithelial cells (in the bladder) was provided by Friedrich G.J. Henle.

1837 The term 'myocarditis' was introduced by German physician, Joseph Friedrich Soberheim of Berlin.

1837 Boston surgeon, John Collins Warren, published one of the first American books on tumors.

1837 Both the upper and lower jaws of a patient were excised for repair of hare lip by Alabama gynecologist, James Marion Sims.

1837 *Friedrich Wilhelm Robert Otto* born. A chemist and toxicologist at Brunswick in Germany who described a method of identifying organic poisons in biological material.

1837 *Charles Jacques Bouchard* born. A French physician who described acute gastric dilation (1884), autointoxication (1887), and Bouchard nodes in the second interphalangeal joints.

1837 *Henry Charlton Bastian* born. A founder of British neurology who worked on aphasia, publishing *A Treatment of Aphasia and Other Speech Defects* (1898), and described the abolition of the tendon reflexes in the lower extremities associated with lesions above the lumbar segment of the spinal cord (Bastian law).

1837   *Hermann Hugo Schwartze* born. A German otologist who described the mastoid cells in disease of the middle ear, which he opened with a hammer and chisel (Schwartze operation, 1873).

1837   *Moritz Kaposi* born. A Hungarian dermatologist in Vienna who gave original descriptions of pigmented sarcoma of the skin (Kaposi sarcoma, 1872), diabetic dermatitis, xeroderma pigmentosum, and lymphoderma perniciosa.

1837   The first use of an esophagoscope was reported at the Edinburgh Royal Infirmary, to extract a padlock that had been swallowed.

1837   *Berthold Stiller* born. A Hungarian physician who described general asthenia (Stiller disease) in 1907.

1837   *William Keen* born. Regarded as America's first brain surgeon, he successfully removed a meningioma (1888), tapped the ventricles (1889), and published a *System of Surgery* in eight volumes from 1906 to 1921.

1837   *Edward Greely Loring* born. A New York ophthalmologist who designed the Loring ophthalmoscope which incorporated a disc of graduated lenses and a series of introducible quadrant lenses.

1837   American pioneer in orthopedics, William Ludwig Detmold, performed the first subcutaneous tenotomy in America, and 3 years

later had reported on 167 cases, including operations on tendons other than the heel.

1837   *Wilhelm Kühne* born. A German biochemist and physiologist who coined the term 'enzyme' (1878), discovered the visual purple in the retina (rhodopsin), and described the neuromuscular spindle (Kühne, 1862).

1837   The form of lung disease caused by the inhalation of soot, anthracosis, was described by Thomas Stratton of North Shields.

1837   *Enrico Bottini* born. An Italian surgeon who described the use of galvanocautery to make a channel through an enlarged prostate.

1837   *Samuel Weissel Gross* born. An American surgeon who wrote the first comprehensive treatise on bone sarcoma in 1879.

1837   *Sir Morell MacKenzie* born. A British laryngologist who published the famous *Growths in the Larynx*, an opus entitled *Diseases of the Throat and Nose* and presented one of the earliest and largest series on congenital esophageal atresia.

1838   The occurrence of albuminuria in fevers (febrile albuminuria) was described by Martin Solon of Paris.

1838   The function of the cilia within the oviduct in moving the ovum was described by German physiologist, Gabriel Gustav Valentin.

1838   The Rathke pouch, a small diverticulum of the early embryonic pharynx giving rise to the anterior lobe of the pituitary gland, was described by German professor, Martin Heinrich Rathke.

1838 *Charles Hilton Fagge* born. A physician at Guy's Hospital, London who described sporadic cretinism, gave an exhaustive account of presystolic murmurs in 1871, and described ankylosing spondylitis as 'poker back' in 1877.

1838 The name *Bacterium tricolulare* was used by Christian Gottfried Ehrenberg of Germany in his classification of microbes.

1838 *Carl Ludwig Schroder* born. A German gynecologist who designed a method of colporrhaphy (Schroder operation), and wrote a textbook on obstetrics in 1874.

1838 *Theodor Fritsch* born. A military surgeon during the Prussian–Danish war who carried out experiments on the stimulation of the brain, proving the existence of motor control areas in the cerebral cortex (published in 1870).

1838 The Metropolitan Ear and Throat Hospital was founded by London otorhinologist James Yearsley, who described the artificial tymphanum, and identified affections of the nose and throat that cause deafness.

1838 *Richard Davy* born. A London surgeon who gave his name to a wooden sound for insertion into the rectum to stop bleeding in the iliac artery (Davy lever).

1838 *Johannes Goldscheider* born. A German neurologist who gave a complete description of epidermolysis bullosa (Goldscheider disease).

1838 The reduced excretion of urea and solids in the urine, anazoturia, was described by Robert Willis.

1838 *Hermann Schmidt-Rimpler* born. A German physician and pioneer in the routine screening of children for eye defects, who devised one of the earliest forms of optometer.

1838 *Julius Eduard Hitzig* born. A German neurologist who worked with Theodor Fritsch and experimented on the stimulation of the brain using dogs, and showed that stimulation of the motor cortex produced movements on the opposite side of the body.

1838 The pathological significance of cranial bruit, cephalic bellows sound, was explained by J.D. Fisher.

1838 Jean Etienne Dominique studied states of dementia in senile individuals and was the first lecturer in psychiatry in Paris.

1838 *Heinrich Koebner* born. A German dermatologist who described the occurrence of psoriasis following trauma of the skin, which later included lichen, warts and vitiligo (Koebner response).

1838 German botanist, Matthias Jakob Schleiden, studied the role of the nucleus in cell division and the formation of tissues.

1838 Curare was first used in medical practice to relax the muscles in rabies.

1839 *Bernard Naunyn* born. A professor of clinical medicine in Bern, Switzerland who devoted his career to the study of metabolism in diabetes (1898) and diseases of the liver and pancreas, described acidosis (1906), and founded the *Archiv für Experimentale Pathologique und Pharmakologie.*

1839 The flexible tube stethoscope was invented by American, Caspar Wistar Pennock.

1839 *William Morrant Baker* born. A surgeon at St Bartholomew's who gave a description of erythema serpens, described the formation of the synovial cyst (1877), and published a successful *Handbook of Physiology.*

1839 A classic description of spondylolithic pelvis was given by Viennese surgeon, Karl Freiherr von Rokitansky.

1839 Samuel Armstrong Lane, a surgeon at St George's Hospital, gave the first account of a successful blood transfusion to an 11-year-old boy who had a bleeding diathesis, probably hemophilia.

1839 *Georg Dieulafoy* born. A French professor of medicine who described gastric ulceration occurring as a complication of pneumonia (Dieulafoy disease), and worked on Bright disease, typhoid and appendicitis.

1839 *Charles H. Hughes* born. A neurologist from St Louis who founded the *Journal of Neurology and* Psychiatry, and gave his name to the Hughes reflex, the downward movement of the penis when the glans or prepuce are pulled upwards.

1839 The Amussat operation, a lumbar colotomy for obstruction of the colon, was performed by Jean Zulléma Amussat in Paris.

1839 Candidosis was described by Bernhard Rudolph Conrad von Langenbeck, a surgeon from Berlin.

1839 *Julius Bernstein* born. A German professor of physiology who proposed the cell membrane theory in order to explain the electrical properties of the muscles (1912).

1839 The Royal National Orthopaedic Hospital was founded by William John Little, a British orthopedic surgeon, and was originally known as the Orthopaedic Institution.

1839 *Moritz Roth* born. A professor of pathological anatomy at Basel who described the tubercle of epididymis connected with rete testis (Roth vas aberans) in 1877.

1839 Primary cuticle of dental enamel (Nasmyth membrane) was described by Alexander Nasmyth, a Scottish dental surgeon at Hanover Square, London.

1839 *Julius Friedrich Cohnheim* born. A German pathologist who pioneered histology and pathology in

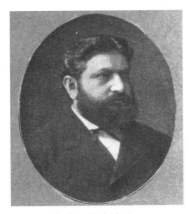

Julius Cohnheim

his dissertation on inflammation of the serous membranes (1861), introduced silver staining for the study of nerve endings in muscles (1863), and described diapedisis (1867).

1839   *Alfred von Biesiadecki* born. A Polish physician who described a recess of the peritoneum over the psoas muscle, (Biesiadecki fossa).

1839   In odontology, Sir Richard Owen, an English comparative anatomist, discovered the connection between the vascular and soft parts of the tooth tissue and the hard substance.

1839   *William Rutherford* born. A Scottish professor of physiology who pioneered the study of the mechanism of hearing, and proposed the theory that the tympanic membrane receiving the sound vibrated like a microphone, and imparted electrical impulses to the brain.

1839   The first dental school in the world was established as the Baltimore College of Dental Surgery.

1839   *Josiah Willard Gibbs* born. An American physical chemist who described the Gibbs–Donnan equilibrium which related to the movement of ions across a membrane (studied later by Frederick George Donnan).

1839   *Wilhelm Kiesselbach* born. A German otorhinologist from Erlangen who described the site of common hemorrhage in the nasal septum Kiesselbach area) in 1884.

1839   *Karl Hugo Kronecker* born. A German physiologist who described the swallowing reflex involved in the act of deglutination (1880), and a cardio-inhibitory center (Kronecker center).

1839   *H. Theodore McGraw* born. A surgeon at Detroit, Michigan who introduced a new method of ligature for performing intestinal anastomosis.

1839   A classic English description of club foot was given by William John Little, a London surgeon who suffered from it himself.

1839   Horner syndrome was first described by Edward Selleck Hare in the *London Medical Gazette*.

1840   *Giuseppe Profeta* born. A Sicilian physician in Genoa who proposed the law (Profeta law) that an apparent healthy infant will not be affected by its syphilitic mother.

1840   The procedure for enterotomy, opening an obstructed bowel above the site of the obstruction and allowing its contents to escape, was first performed in Paris by Auguste Nélaton.

1840 A clear differentiation between typhus and typhoid fever was made by Alexander Patrick Stewart.

1840 *Arnold Ludwig Heller* born. An anatomist at Kiel who described the arterial plexus in the intestinal wall (1872) and syphilitic aortitis (1899), a cause of aortic aneurysm.

1840 A bluish discoloration of the gums seen in lead toxicity (Burton line) was described by London physician, Henry Burton of St Thomas' Hospital.

1840 *John Dixon Mann* born. A Manchester physician and forensic toxicologist who described a change in electrical resistance of the skin thought to be associated with certain neuroses.

1840 *Ludwig Mauthner* born. A professor of ophthalmology in Vienna who described the membrane surrounding the axis of the nerve within the sheath of Schwann (Mauthner membrane) in 1860.

1840 *Wilhelm Heinrich Erb* born. A German neurologist who described brachial palsy (1874), syphilitic spinal paralysis (1875), discovered the absence of knee jerk in spinal syphilis, and developed electrotherapy as treatment for nervous diseases (1882).

1840 *Henry Pickering Bowditch* born. An Boston physiologist who carried out important studies on the physiology of the heart muscles

Wilhelm Erb

and nerves, including the increase in heart rate having a positive inotropic effect (Bowditch effect), developed nerve block local anesthesia, and founded the American Physiological Society (1887).

1840 *Désiré Magloire Bourneville* born. A French neurologist who described adenoma sebaceum associated with mental deficiency and epilepsy (1880), and made observations on cretinism, mongolism and myxedema.

1840 *Benjamin Douglas Howard* born. A New York physician who described a method of artificial respiration where the patient is kept in a supine position, with a roll of cloth beneath the thorax and the head below the level of thorax.

1840 The paralyzing effect of curare on the myoneural junction in frogs was demonstrated by French physiologist, Claude Bernard.

1840 The first mention of Madura foot as a specific disease was found in Brett's *Surgery of India*.

1840   *Sir Thomas Clouston* born. A British psychiatrist who lectured on mental diseases, focused on the mental aspect of adolescence, and published *The Hygiene of the Mind and Clinical Lectures on Mental Diseases*.

1840   The first scientific account of hemorrhage from dilated esophageal veins was given by Karl Freiherr von Rokitansky of Vienna.

1840   A test for detection of blood in gastric juice with guaiac and other agents (van Deen test) was devised by Dutch physiologist, Izaak Abrahamzoon van Deen.

1840   *Joseph Casimir Grynfeltt* born. A French gynecologist from Montpellier who described the superior lumbar triangle through which lumbar hernia occur (Grynfeltt triangle).

1840   *Edward Wilhelm Welander* born. A physician from Stockholm, Sweden who described chancroid or chancre found in the vulva but of nonvenereal etiology (Welander ulcer).

1840   Charles Wheatstone invented the chronoscope, an instrument to measure small intervals of time.

1840   *James N. Hyde* born. An American dermatologist who made numerous contributions to the subject, and described prurigo nodularis (Hyde disease).

1840   *Sir Dyce Duckworth* born. A London physician who first described the occurrence of respiratory arrest before cardiac arrest in certain cases of brain infection (Duckworth phenomenon).

1840   *Carlo Giacomo* born. A professor of anatomy and neurologist in Turin who gave original descriptions of several neuroanatomical structures.

1840   French psychiatrist, Joseph Gabriel François Baillarger, noticed that the line of Gennari in the cerebral cortex consisted of two bands separated by a thin dark line (the internal and external bands of Baillarger).

1840   An early successful operation for vesicovaginal fistula was performed by John Peter Mettauer.

1840   Intoxication due to poor kidney functioning (uremia) was described by French physician, Adolphe Pierre Piorry.

1840   *Ernst Abbé* born. An ophthalmologist and partner at the optical company of Carl Zeiss who worked on the improvement of microscopes, added the apochromatic objective, and developed the oil immersion method (1878).

1840   *Luigi Luciani* born. An Italian physician and professor of physiology at Siena, Florence and Rome who described hypotonia, ataxia and weakness seen in cerebellar disease (Luciani triad).

1840   The first convalescence institution in England was established at Walton-on-Thames.

1840   *Vladimir Mikhailovich Kernig* born. A Russian neurologist who first described how flexion of the thigh at the hip and extension of the leg causes pain and spasm in the hamstrings in cases of meningitis or encephalitis (Kernig sign, 1909).

1841   The Royal College of Psychiatrists, originally the Association of Medical Officers of Asylums and Hospitals for the Insane, was founded in Gloucester, England.

1841   The ciliospinal and genitospinal centers of the spinal cord were first described by Julius Ludwig Budge, a professor of physiology from Bonn, Germany.

1841   *George Oliver* born. An English pioneer in endocrinology who demonstrated the effect of injecting extracts of the suprarenal gland, producing contraction of the arteries and accelerated heart rate, thereby increasing blood pressure.

1841   Inclusion bodies in molluscum contagiosum were independently described by Scottish physician, William Henderson, and Robert Paterson (Henderson–Paterson bodies).

1841   The first case of a rupture of an aneurysm into the lung (pulmonary aneurysm) was published by Fearn in *The Lancet*.

1841   *Gustav Hugenin* born. A professor of psychiatry at Zurich who described a system of levels for motor and sensory neurons in 1879.

1841   *Albert Freeman Africanus King* born. A Washington physician who was one of the first to associate transmission of malaria with the mosquito (1883), and who published his *Manual of Obstetrics* in 1882, which ran to 11 editions.

1841   Pyelonephritis in pregnant women was described and named by French dermatologist, Pierre François Olive Rayer.

1841   *Eduard Albert* born. A surgeon from Innsbruck, Austria who developed a method of surgical fixation of a joint by fusion of joint surfaces in cases of destructive joint disease, and performed the procedure in a shoulder and in the ankle of a paralytic foot in 1893.

1841   *Observations on the Structure and Diseases of the Testis* which described the natural history of testicular cancer, and is regarded as the best presentation of testicular tumors before histology, was published by London surgeon, Sir Astley Paston Cooper.

1841   The Trommer test which detects dextrose in urine using sodium hydroxide and copper sulfate as reagents, was devised by German chemist, Karl August Trommer.

1841   *Louis Hubert Farabeuf* born. A professor of anatomy at the Faculty of Medicine in Paris who described the triangle in the upper part of the neck, bounded by the internal jugular vein, the facial vein and the hypoglossal nerve, later named after him.

1841 *Olof Hammarsten* born. A Scandinavian physician who discovered the precursor of fibrin in blood coagulation (fibrinogen).

1841 *Max Jaffe* born. A biochemist from Königsberg who introduced several biochemical techniques including those for detection of urobilin in urine(1868), and in the intestines (1871), detection of creatinine (1886), and the isolation of indican in urine (1877).

1841 The Corrigan button, an instrument used to apply counter-irritation to the skin, was first described by Dublin physician, Sir Dominic Corrigan.

1841 *Emil Theodor Kocher* born. A professor of surgery from Switzerland who demonstrated the function of the thyroid, pioneered methods of brain and spinal cord surgery, devised an operation for the reduction of subluxation of the shoulder joint, and won the Nobel prize in 1909.

1841 *Christian Friedrich Schatz* born. A German gynecologist who devised a shell-shaped pessary with perforations (Schatz pessary).

1841 St Mary's Hospital in London was founded.

1841 *Georges Hayem* born. A professor of clinical medicine from Paris who described chronic interstitial hepatitis (1874), gave the first accurate account of blood platelets (1878), identified the early stage of red cells during regeneration (1877), and Hayem–Widal disease of acquired hemolytic anemia (1898).

1841 Feeding of a patient through a gastrostomy was first proposed by C.A. Egeberg of Norway.

1841 Drainage of the pericardium in scurvy, using a trocar and canula, was performed by Karawagen at Kronstadt in Russia.

1842 The earliest description of hereditary chorea was given by American physician, Robley Dunglison.

1842 The term ovariotomy was introduced by Charles Clay of Manchester.

1842 The theory of alternation of generations was proposed by a Swedish physician, Jonannes Japetus Steenstrup. He demonstrated that certain animals produced offspring which did not resemble them, but the similarity reappeared in the next generation.

1842 Occlusion of the hepatic veins leading to portal hypertension and cirrhosis (Budd–Chiari syndrome) was observed by Czech professor, Karl Freiherr von Rokitansky.

1842 The autonomic nervous system was investigated by German anatomist at Dorpat, Friedrich Heinrich Wilhelm Bidder.

1842 *Carl Gussenbauer* born. A German surgeon who devised an internal metal splint (Gussenbauer clamp) for approximating the bones in an ununited fracture, and gave a description of the first removal of a tumor in the bladder (1875).

1842 *Richard Caton* born. An English physician who detected and identified electrical activity in the brain of living animals.

1842 *Jacques Louis Reverdin* born. A Swiss surgeon in Paris who introduced the transplantation of free skin instead of punctuated flaps (1869), and who performed early operations on the thyroid gland.

1842 *Julius Friedrich Rosenbach* born. A German surgeon who introduced the name *Streptococcus* for the cocci found in chains in 1884, and differentiated between staphylococci and streptococci.

1842 *Ludwig Bandl* born. A professor of obstetrics and gynecology at the University of Vienna who recognized that rupture of the uterus in obstructed labor was almost always confined to the lower segment of

The Bandl ring

the uterus. In 1875 he described the Bandl ring, a line of demarcation between the contracted upper segment and the thinner lower segment of the uterus in obstructed labor.

1842 The contagious nature of enteric fever was pointed out by American physician, Nathan Smith, in his work *A Practical Essay on Typhus Fever.*

1842 Oliver Wendell Holmes proposed the contagious nature of puerperal fever in his paper *On the Contagiousness of Puerperal fever* presented to the Boston Medical Society.

1842 *John Neville Davies-Colley* born. A London surgeon who described the Davies-Colley operation, in which a bone wedge is removed to correct talipes.

1842 *Vincenz Czerny* born. A professor of surgery at Heidelberg who successfully resected the esophagus in a human (1877), removed a cancer of the large bowel, and introduced the vaginal operation for carcinoma of the uterus (1878).

1842 *Charles Abadie* born. A French ophthalmologist at L'Hôtel Dieu who made contributions to the treatment of trachoma and glaucoma, introduced alcohol injection of the Gasserian ganglion to treat trigeminal neuralgia, and described the Abadie sign of spasm of the levator palpebrae muscles in exophthalmic goiter (1877).

1842 *Berthold Ernst Hadra* born. A German-born orthopedic surgeon who emigrated to Texas and performed the first spinal fusion using a silver wire to fix the 6th and 7th cervical vertebrae in 1891.

1842 *Heinrich Iranaeus Quincke* born. A German professor of medicine at Bern in Switzerland who gave an account of angioneurotic edema (1882), and distinguished between

Entamoeba histolytica and *Entamoeba coli*.

1842 *François Henri Hallipeau* born. A French dermatologist who described a variant of Neumann pemphigus vegetans (Hallipeau disease, 1889), and wrote important theses on diseases of the spinal cord, diffuse myelitis, and bulbar palsy.

1842 Karl Vierordt, a German physician, devised a method of estimating blood volume by calculating the circulation time.

1842 The first recorded use of ether as an anesthetic was by a student, William E. Clark of Berkshire Medical College, who administered it to a patient for a tooth extraction.

1842 *Charles Henry Ralfe* born. A physician at the London Hospital who devised the Ralfe test for detection of acetone in urine by adding hydroxide and iodide of potassium, and wrote *Urine* (1880) and *Diseases of the Kidney*.

1842 Constrictive pericarditis, or adherent pericarditis, was described by English physician Norman Chevers.

1842 The idea that urine formation consisted of glomerular filtration and tubular secretion, was proposed by the English physician, William Bowman.

1842 *Robert William Taylor* born. An American dermatologist who described a form of idiopathic localized atrophy of the skin (acrodermatitis chronica atrophicans).

1842 Sir James Erasmus Wilson, a dermatologist from London, described ichthyosis as fish skin or porcupine disease in his work *Diseases of the Skin*.

1842 *Robert Ultzmann* born. A German urologist who devised the Ultzmann test which detects bile pigments in urine, using potassium hydroxide as reagent.

1842 *William Anderson* born. A British urologist who described Anderson–Fabry disease (1898), relating to a burning sensation in the hands and feet, dark nodular skin lesions, and renal failure.

1842 *George Trumbell Ladd* born. An American psychologist and professor of philosophy at Yale who studied the relationship between the nervous system and mental phenomena, and published *Elements of Physiological Psychology* in 1887.

1843 *Charles Meymott Tidy* born. An English physician who devised the Tidy test to detect albumin in the urine, using phenol and glacial acetic acid as reagents.

1843 *Ludwig Georg Courvoisier* born. A professor of surgery in Switzerland who was one of the first to remove stones from the common bile duct, and formulated the Courvoisier sign relating to localized tenderness in the right hypochrondrium over an inflamed gallbladder in cholecystitis.

1843 *John Chiene* born. An Edinburgh surgeon who established several surface markings of the head and neck in surgery (Chiene lines).

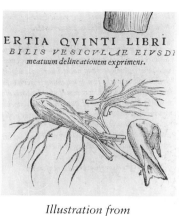

*Illustration from
Courvoisier's book*

1843 A cylindrical structure of microscopic size (urinary cast), was observed in urine by Simon of Vienna and Hermann Nasse of Germany.

1843 *Sir David Ferrier* born. A Scottish neurologist and a pioneer in study of the localization of cerebral function who wrote *Functions of the Brain* (1876) and *Localization of Cerebral Disease* (1878).

1843 British neurosurgeon, Walter Hayle Walshe of London, recognized fragments of malignant tissue in the sputum.

1843 *Warren Tay* born. A British ophthalmologist who described amaurotic familial idiocy with ocular manifestations (Tay–Sachs disease).

1843 The union of spermatozoon and ovum in a rabbit were observed by embryologist and surgeon, Martin Barry, who published his findings in *Researches in Embryology*.

1843 *Johann Otto Leonhard Heubner* born. A German professor of pediatrics who studied infant nutrition and warned against oversterilization of milk, isolated meningococci from cerebrospinal fluid (1896), described syphilitic endarteritis of cerebral vessels, and the infantile form of idiopathic steatorrhea.

1843 The role of leukocytes in inflammation and their passage through the walls of capillaries (diapedesis) were first studied by William Addison, a physician from Malvern in England, and published in seven sections in the *Transactions of the Provincial Medical and Surgical Association*.

1843 The presence of albumin in the urine (albuminuria) of mothers with puerperal convulsions was observed by John Charles Lever, lecturer in midwifery at Guy's Hospital in London.

1843 *Edmund Drechsel* born. A Swiss chemist who devised the Drechsel test for bile, using phosphoric acid and cane sugar as reagents.

1843 Peribronchitic abscesses (Fauvel granules) were described by French physician, Suplice Antoine Fauvel, who gave a classic description of mitral stenosis in the same year.

1843 *Gustavus Ludwig Thornwaldt* born. A German physician who described inflammation of the Luschka tonsil with formation of a cyst containing pus, leading to pharyngeal stenosis (Thornwaldt disease).

1843 *Friedrich Rudolf Georg Wegner* born. A German pathologist who described osteochondritic separation of the epiphyses due to secondary syphilis (Wegner disease).

1843 *Reginald Heber Fitz* born. A Harvard pathologist who described the symptoms and signs experienced during inflammation of the vermiform appendix, and named the condition appendicitis. In 1886 he published *Perforating Inflammation of the Vermiform Appendix.*

1843 The concept that urine formation in the kidneys was a simple process of filtration brought about by the hydrostatic pressure of the blood was proposed by Karl Friedrich Wilhelm Ludwig, a professor at Zurich, Switzerland.

1843 *Heinrich Hermann Robert Koch* born. A German pioneer in bacteriology and Nobel laureate (1905) who devised a staining and fixing method for bacteria (1877), developed methods of producing pure cultures (1881), discovered the tubercle bacillus (1882), and proposed the Koch postulates for determining the organism responsible for a disease.

1843 *Francke Huntington Bosworth* born. An American pioneering rhinologist who described purulent rhinitis, dislocation of the columnar cartilage of the nasal septum, and diseases involving the ethmoid cells,

1843 *William Warwick Wagstaffe* born. An English surgeon who described the Wagstaffe fracture causing separation of the internal malleolus.

1843 *Justin M.M. Lucas-Championniere* born. A Paris surgeon who introduced the Listerian system of antiseptic surgery into France (1876), and described chronic pseudomembranous bronchitis (Lucas-Championniere disease).

1843 Cirrhosis of the liver due to the parasite *Fasciolopsis buski* (Budd disease) was described by English physician, George Budd.

1843 An instrument for the exploration, dilatation and measurement of the cavity of the uterus (uterine sound) was invented by James Marion Sims, a gynecologist from South Carolina.

1843 *Julius Hirschberg* born. A Berlin ophthalmologist who introduced the use of an electromagnet for removing foreign bodies from the eye (1885), and designed a test (Hirschberg test) for measuring the angle of squint.

1843 *Clarence John Blake* born. A Boston otologist who devised a paper prosthesis for repairing a hole in the eardrum.

1843 A carcinomatous growth of the sigmoid flexure was removed, together with three inches of normal gut, during an intestinal resection by Jean François Reybard.

1843 First drainage of purulent pericarditis was performed by Hillsman at Kiel.

1843   Establishment of the diploma of the Royal College of Surgeons in England.

1843   The term relapsing fever was introduced by Scottish physician, David Craigie, during his description of an epidemic in Edinburgh.

1844   Nine cases of needle aspiration for empyema were described by Hamilton Roe, the first physician to the Brompton Hospital.

1844   The earliest recorded incision and drainage of a lung abscess was achieved by English physician, Charles Hastings.

1844   *Victor Charles Hanot* born. A French physician who described cholangiolytic biliary cirrhosis (Hanot disease, 1875), concentrated on diseases of the liver, and published on several clinical pathological aspects.

1844   *Alfred Bing* born. An Austrian otologist who devised the Bing tuning fork test to differentiate between inner and middle ear lesions.

1844   The scraping away of all dead tissue in bone necrosis, permitting a blood clot to fill the cavity, and covering it with aseptic gauze and rubber (Schede method), was first practiced by Max Schede, a surgeon in Bonn.

1844   German professor of neurology, Robert Remak, discovered the cardiac ganglia (Remak ganglia) which exert nervous control on the muscular activity of the heart.

1844   *Leopold Salkowski* born. A Berlin chemist who described pentosuria (1895), and devised tests for purine bases (1894), cholesterol (1872), creatinine (1880), bile pigments (1880), carbon monoxide in blood (1888), glucose in urine (1899), and hematoporphyrin (1891).

1844   *Paul Bunge* born. A German ophthalmologist who devised an instrument for eviscerating the eyeball (Bunge spoon).

1844   *François Alexis Albert Gombault* born. A neuropathologist from Paris who gave original descriptions of several tracts in the spinal cord in his *Etude sur la Sclerose Laterale Amyotrophique* (1877).

1844   *David Todd Gilliam* born. An American gynecologist from Ohio who designed an operation for the retrodisplacement of the uterus by fixing it to the sheath of the rectus abdominis muscle with the help of the round ligament.

1844   *Gustav Albert Schwalbe* born. A German neuroanatomist who described the vestibular nucleus and several other structures of the brain which are named after him.

1844   The Pettenkofer test for bile detection was devised by German chemist Max Joseph von Pettenkofer, and was later developed by German bacteriologist, Paul Ehrlich.

1844   *Alexander MacAlister* born. A Dublin surgeon and professor of anatomy at Cambridge who described the crico-trachealis muscle (1871).

1844 The interventricular foramen of the heart normally found in lower vertebrates (Panizza foramen), was studied in mammals by Bartolomeo Panizza, an Italian comparative anatomist at Pavia.

1844 An excellent description of pemphigus foliaceus, a form of pemphigus marked by flaccid, scabby bullae, was given by French dermatologist, Pierre Cazenove.

1844 *Ludwig Bremer* born. An American physician who used methylene and eosin as reagents in his test for detecting sugar in the blood (Bremer test).

1844 *Nicholas Senn* born. An American surgeon and pioneer in the use of X-rays in surgery who designed the Senn bone plate made of decalcified bone and used to approximate and suture the divided intestine.

1844 *Heinrich Fritsch* born. A German gynecologist who designed a double-channeled uterine catheter (Fritsch catheter).

1844 The removal of a laryngeal polyp was first carried out by Charles Henry Ehrmann of Paris.

1844 *Friedrich Trendelenburg* born. A German surgeon who described the Trendelenburg position used in surgery and anesthesia (1880), Trendelenburg sign for congenital dislocation of the hip (1895), and the Trendelenburg test for varicose veins.

1844 *Sir Patrick Manson* born. The father of tropical medicine in England who founded the London School of Tropical Medicine, published his *Tropical Diseases* (1898), proposed the extracorporeal life cycle of the malaria parasite in the mosquito (1894), and described the skin disease tinea nigra (caused by *Cladosporium mansoni*).

1844 *Adolph d'Espine* born. A Swiss pediatrician who described mediastinal lymph node enlargement causing whispering pectoriloquy over the spinous processes of 4th, 5th and 6th thoracic spines (d'Espine sign).

1844 *Henri Huchard* born. A French physician and pioneer in the study of cardiovascular disease, particularly circulation and arteriosclerosis, who described continued hypertension as a cause of athersclerosis (Huchard disease, 1887).

1844 French surgeon, Jules Aristide Gely, described a method of intestinal suture.

1844 *Heinrich Leopold Scholer* born. A German ophthalmologist who described an operative treatment for detachment of the retina (1889).

1844 *Alexander Ogston* born. A Scottish surgeon and professor who discovered *Staphylococcus* bacteria (1881), and described the imaginary line used in surgery (Ogston line, 1876)) that extends from the tubercle of the femur to the intercondylar notch.

1844 The induction of anesthesia by inhalation of nitrous oxide during

156

dental extraction was demonstrated by Boston dentist, Horace Wells, at Massachusetts General Hospital.

1844 Friedrich Gustave Jacob Henle, the celebrated German anatomist, was the first to demonstrate that urinary casts originated in the kidney.

1844 *Charles Emile Troisier* born. A French physician who described the enlargement of the lymph gland above the clavicle in cases of intra-abdominal malignancy (Troisier sign).

1844 *Emmanuel Aufrecht* born. A German physician who first observed infectious jaundice and changes in the parenchyma of the liver and kidney (Aurfrecht disease or hepatorenal syndrome).

1844 *Camillo Golgi* born. An Italian histologist and Nobel Prize winner who described nerve axons and dendrites, the tactile end-organs (Golgi corpuscules, 1878), and developed staining techniques that led to the discovery of the subcellular Golgi bodies (1898).

Illustration of nerve axions

1844 The first clear description of pneumopericardium was given by French physician, Isidore Bricheteau.

1844 *Edoardo Bassini* born. An Italian surgeon who described an operation for inguinal (1887) and femoral (1893) hernia.

1845 *Caesar Peter Moeller Boeck* born. The first dermatologist in Norway to be appointed professor of medicine at the University of Oslo, who is remembered for his description of acne varioliformis, and Boeck sarcoidosis (1899).

1845 *Karl Weigert* born. A German pathologist who devised some of the earliest and best staining methods for bacteria and tissues (myelin sheath in 1884 and elastic fibers in 1898), gave an account of myocardial infarction (1880), and described the pathological anatomy in Bright disease (1879).

1845 The term 'leukemia' was first used for the cellular disorder of blood by German anatomist, Rudolf Virchow, and the first description was provided in the same year by John Hughes Bennett of Edinburgh.

1845 *Edward Nettleship* born. An English dermatologist who studied the incidence of eye disease and ophthalmia, and described urticaria pigmentosa (Nettleship disease or syndrome, 1869).

1845 *Moritz Litten* born. A German physician who described visible depression of the lower part of the sides of the thoracic wall in respiratory effort or distress (Litten sign).

1845   Emil Heinrich Du Bois Reymond, a German professor of physiology from Berlin, demonstrated the existence of resting current in nerves.

1845   *Samuel Doty Risley* born. An ophthalmologist from Philadelphia who devised a rotating prism in a metal frame with scales (Risley prism) to measure imbalance of the ocular muscles.

1845   *Charles Louis Alphonse Laveran* born. A French parasitologist, professor of military medicine and epidemic diseases, and Nobel laureate (1907), who studied malaria in Algiers (1880), and discovered the causative organism, a protozoan parasite, *Plasmodium*.

1845   *Eduard Joseph Louis Marie Beneden* born. A Belgian cytologist and embryologist who discovered that the number of chromosomes was constant for each cell in a given body, and was characteristic of each species.

1845   *Angelo Maffucci* born. An Italian pathologist and pioneer in the study of tuberculosis who isolated the avian tubercle bacillus (*B. gallinaceous*) in 1890, and described Maffucci syndrome, endochondromatosis with cutaneous hemangioma.

1845   *Elie Metchnikoff* born. An immunologist and embryologist from the Ukraine who, while director of the Pasteur Institute in Paris, discovered the phagocytic function of white blood cells and demonstrated their role in combating bacterial invasion, successfully transmitted syphilis from man to a higher animal, and was awarded the Nobel Prize in 1908.

1845   *George Alexander Turner* born. A Scottish physician who described tinea imbricata, a severe form of ringworm occurring in tropical countries.

1845   *Paul Berger* born. A surgeon who wrote an extensive monograph on interscapulothoracic amputation, the Berger operation (1887).

1845   *John Elliot Woodbridge* born. An American physician who used an intestinal antiseptic containing calomel (Woodbridge treatment) in the treatment of typhoid.

1845   *Lawson Robert Tait* born. A surgeon from Edinburgh who performed a successful operation for ruptured tubal pregnancy (1883), introduced a method of dilating the cervix (1880), pioneered the flap-splitting operation for plastic repair of the perineum (1879), and performed the first hepatomy (1880).

1845   The first medical directory, a guide to recognized medical practitioners, was produced by James Yearsley, an otorhinologist from London.

1845   Nitroprusside was discovered by a Scottish chemist, Lord Lyon Playfair.

1845   *Urban Pritchard* born. A London otorhinologist who first described the intercellular membrane in the ampulla of the semicircular canals (1876).

1845   *Gabriel Jonas Lippmann* born. A French physicist and Nobel laureate (1908) who invented a mercury capillary electrometer, an astatic galvanometer, a seismograph, and pioneered color photography.

1845   *Wilhelm Konrad Röntgen* born. A German physicist and Nobel laureate (1901) who discovered X-rays (1895) now used for visualization of bones and soft tissues, therefore making a fundamental leap in diagnostic aids.

1845   A pewter spoon was used as a vaginal speculum by American gynecologist, James Marion Sims, which was later developed into Sims duck-billed speculum.

1845   *Friedrich Wilhelm Zahn* born. A German pathologist who described the corrugations on the free surface of a thrombus formed by the projecting edges of the lamellae of blood platelets (Zahn lines).

1845   *Friedrich Sigmund Merkel* born. A German anatomist who described sensory tactile nerve endings in the skin (Merkel corpuscles, 1880), and the meniscus tactus.

1845   The component of blood that facilitates coagulation, fibrin, was extracted by Andrew Buchanan of London.

1845   The skin condition with blebs or bullae (pemphigus) was studied in detail in thousands of patients by Viennese dermatologist, Ferdinand von Hebra, who published his *Atlas of Skin Diseases* in the same year.

1845   *David Daniel Palmer* born. The founder of chiropractic medicine from Toronto, Canada who established his School of Chiropractic Medicine at Davenport, Iowa in 1899.

1845   Lewis Durlacher, a surgeon chiropodist to Queen Victoria, published *A Treatise on Corns, Bunions, the Diseases of the Nails and the General Management of the Feet.*

1845   *Charles Karsner Mills* born. An early professor of neurology at the University of Pennsylvania who described unilateral progressive ascending paralysis (Mill disease, 1900).

1845   *Carl Anton Ewald* born. A Berlin gastroenterologist who worked on secretions of the stomach by intubation, and designed the Ewald test meal which was commonly used for gastric analysis.

1845   The germ layers were classified into ectoderm, endoderm and mesoderm by Polish-born German physician, Robert Remak.

1845   *William Richard Gowers* born. The eminent London neurologist who gave the name 'knee jerk' to the tendon reflex of the knee, introduced colorimetric estimation of hemoglobin, pioneered the ophthalmoscope in neurology, and wrote *Pseudo-hypertrophic Muscu-*

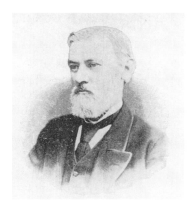

William Gowers

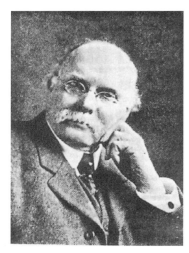

De Forest Willard

lar Paralysis (1879) and *Epilepsy and other Chronic Conditions* (1881).

1845 *Anton Weichelsbaum* born. An Austrian pathologist who isolated meningococcus or *Diplococcus intercellularis meningitides* from the cerebrospinal fluid of patients with meningitis (1887).

1846 *De Forest Willard* born. An American surgeon and a pioneer in skin and nerve grafting and suture techniques, who was a great advocate of Listerism, and did a costotransversectomy for abscesses in Pott disease.

1846 William Stokes, an eminent Irish physician, gave an account of heart block with syncopal attacks, later named Stokes–Adams syndrome.

1846 *Richard Clement Lucas* born. A surgeon at Guy's Hospital, London who was the first to describe the groove made by the chorda tymphani nerve on the spine of sphenoid (Lucas groove, 1894).

1846 The amino acid, tyrosine, was observed as a product of pancreatic digestion by Justus von Liebig of Germany.

1846 Danish pathologist, Adolph Hanover, published *On the Anatomy, Physiology and Pathology of the Eye.*

1846 *The Australian Medical Journal* was first published in Sydney.

1846 *Angelo Mosso* born. An Italian physiologist who carried out one of the first studies on the mechanism of apnoea (1903), and whose laboratory worked on effects of high altitude on health.

1846 The term 'typhoid' for enteric fever was coined by Charles Ritchie of England.

1846 The first physician to devote time to study mentally deficient children was Edouard Séguin of the Bîcetre Hospital in Paris, who published *Traitément Moral, Hygiene et Education des Idiots et des Autres Enfants Arriers.*

1846   *Henry Ashby* born. A physician at the Manchester Children's Hospital who made great contributions to the improvement of children's living conditions in the city.

1846   The first textbook on histology in English, *The Microscopical Anatomy of the Human Body in Health and Disease*, was published by English physician, Arthur Hill Hassall.

1846   Henry Jacob Bigelow and John Collins Warren, surgeons at the Massachusetts General Hospital, demonstrated ether as a surgical anesthetic.

1846   *Hans Curschmann* born. A German physician who described the spiral threads of mucus expectorated by an asthmatic (Curschmann spirals), and a rare hereditary syndrome with myotonia of lingual and thenar muscles (1912).

1846   *Otto Wilhelm Madelung* born. A German surgeon and professor at Strasburg who first described congenital dislocation of the wrist.

1846   The fungus *Malassezia furfur* (*Cladosporium mansonii*), the causative agent of tinea versicolor, was discovered by German dermatologist, Carl Ferdinand Eichstedt.

1846   *Bernhard Moritz Carl Ludwig Riedel* born. A German surgeon who described chronic thyroiditis with localized areas of stony, hard fibromas (Riedel thyroiditis, 1896), and the Riedel lobe in the liver (1893).

1846   Apparatus to measure the vital capacity of the lung, the spirometer, was invented by English physician, John Hutchison.

1846   The protoplasm of living cells was shown to be the same in plants and animals by the German botanist, Hugo von Mohl.

1846   A microscopic examination of bone tissue in a blood disorder (bone marrow biopsy) was done by English ophthalmologist, John Dalrymple.

1846   *George Henry Fox* born. A New York dermatologist who published a photographic atlas of skin diseases (1880), and described a form of itchy papular eruption at the sites of the apocrine glands, especially in the axilla, (Fox–Fordyce disease, 1902).

1846   Classic research on cerebral circulation was conducted by London physician, George Burrowes, in his work *On the Disorders of the Cerebral Circulation and the Connections between the Affections of the Brain and Diseases of the Heart.*

1846   *Felix Jacob Marchand* born. A German pathologist who used a crude differential rheotome connected to a galvanometer to measure the electrical variation of the frog's heart (1872), described parotid tumors (1891), and introduced the term 'atherosclerosis'.

1846   *Edmond Landolt* born. A French ophthalmologist of Swiss origin who devised an incomplete circle used to test for visual acuity (Landolt ring).

1846 *James Jackson Putnam* born. A Harvard neurologist who studied circumscribed analgesia, neuritis from lead poisoning, polio, myxedema and spinal cord tumors. He was a founder of the American Neurological Association.

1846 *Carl Johann August Langenbuch* born. A German surgeon who was the first to successfully remove a gallbladder (1882), and to perform a duodenostomy (1879).

1846 The anesthetic properties of ether were observed by Boston chemist, Charles T. Jackson.

1846 *John Brown Buist* born. A pathologist from the Edinburgh Medical School who described the elementary body in skin lesions seen in smallpox and vaccinia (Buist–Paschen).

1846 *Arthur Ferguson McGill* born. An English surgeon who performed the first suprapubic prostatectomy (1887).

1846 *Giulio Cesare Bizzozero* born. An Italian physician who described the platelets as the third elementary constituent of blood (1882), and discovered their role in blood coagulation (1887).

1846 The term 'bronchiectasis' was introduced by Hasse.

1847 Different stages of anesthesia were described by F. Plomley in *The Lancet*.

1847 The first description of the pharmacological and clinical properties of ether were given by John Snow in *On the Inhalation of Ether Vapor*.

1847 T. Sluyter described human pulmonary aspergillosis.

1847 *August Martin* born. A Berlin gynecologist who performed an incision of the cervix in a case of difficult delivery due to an unyielding cervix (1883), and designed a caliper for pelvimetry.

1847 *William Bevan-Lewis* born. A professor of mental diseases at Leeds who described the large cells of the motor cortex (Bevan-Lewis cells, 1879).

1847 *Paul Reclus* born. A French gynecologist who described the painless swelling of the mammary glands due to multiple dilation of the acini and ducts (Reclus disease).

1847 *Marcellus von Nencki* born. A Polish physician who devised a test using nitric and nitrous acid to detect indole (Nencki test).

1847 The American Medical Association was founded.

1847 *Paul Frederick Emmanuel Vogt* born. A German surgeon who defined the Vogt point in the skull where trephination can be performed for traumatic meningeal hemorrhage.

1847 *John Howard Mummery* born. A physician and dentist from London and president of the British

Dental Association and the Odontological Society who described the fibrillar structures of developing dentine (fibers of Mummery, 1891).

1847   *Aurel von Szily* born. A German ophthalmologist who performed chemical cauterization of the choroid.

1847   The term scleroderma was coined by E. Gintrac, after an early attempt to differentiate scleroderma from leprosy and other skin diseases was made by Italian physician, Carlo Curzio.

1847   *William Rose* born. An English surgeon who performed excision of the Gasserian ganglion as treatment for trigeminal neuralgia.

1847   *Karl Friedländer* born. A German pathologist and bacteriologist who discovered the Friedländer bacillus (*Klebsiella pneumoniae*) in 1882, a pneumonia caused by this bacillus, and the cells of the uterine decidua (Friedländer cells, 1870).

1847   The American Association for the Advancement of Science was founded.

1847   *Edmund Delorme* born. A French surgeon who advocated the decortication of the lung in empyema to allow the lung to expand fully (Delorme method).

1847   *Paul Emil Flechsig* born. A German neurologist who mapped the brain, was the first to describe the auditory radiation, and described the dorsal spinocerebellar tract (Flechsig tract).

1847   *Ettore Marchiafava* born. An Italian pathologist who described malarial parasites in red blood cells as 'hemocytozoa' (1885), gave the first description of *Plasmodium* (1880), and the neurological disorder, Marchiafava–Bignami syndrome in 1903, and the Marchiafava–Micheli syndrome.

1847   *Isaac Ott* born. An American neurologist who worked on nervous regulation of body temperature for over 30 years, leading to the discovery of the thermoregulatory center in the hypothalamus.

1847   *Carl Nicoladoni* born. An orthopedic surgeon from Austria who transplanted the achilles tendon in a case of calf paralysis.

1847   English physician, Henry Bence Jones, noted the presence of albuminoid protein in the urine of a patient with two fractured ribs, calling it myelopathic albuminuria and later named Bence Jones proteinuria.

1847   The symptoms and signs of tabes dorsalis (locomotor ataxia) were given by British physician, Robert Bentley Todd of King's College, London.

1847   *Sir Byrom Bramwell* born. A British physician who suggested that obesity, polyuria and glycosuria in pituitary tumors may be caused by disturbance of the hypothalamus.

1847   Russian pediatrician, *Nils Feodorovitch Filatov* born. He described the characteristic features of lymphadenopathy and fever seen in infectious mononucleosis (1887), and Koplik spots in measles.

1847 In searching for a better agent than ether for anesthesia, James Young Simpson, a Scottish obstetrician, began successfully using chloroform.

1847 *Richard Thoma* born. A German histologist who described small terminal expansions of the splenic pulp of the interlobar artery of the spleen (Thoma ampulla).

1847 *Carlo Forlanini* born. An Italian surgeon who established induction of pneumothorax as a regular treatment for pulmonary tuberculosis (1888).

1847 *Walter Holbrook Gaskell* born. An English physiologist who introduced the term 'block' in cardiology, described the accelerator nerves of the heart (1881), and laid the foundation for an understanding of the autonomic nervous system.

1847 *Johannes Orth* born. A German pathologist who first described kernicterus (1875), and introduced lithium and carmine into histology (Orth stain).

1847 *Nikolai Vladimirovich Eck* born. A Russian physiologist who performed pioneering surgery to study the metabolism of the body in relation to the liver, and described anastomosis of the portal vein to the inferior vena cava (Eck fistula, 1877).

1847 *Virgil Pendleton Gibney* born. A New York surgeon who described

painful fibrositis of the spinal muscles (Gibney perispondylitis).

1847 Nitroglycerin was prepared by Italian chemist, Ascanio Sobrero of Turin.

1847 *Paul Langerhans* born. A German pathologist from Berlin who discovered the islets in the pancreas which produce insulin (islet of Langerhans, 1869), cells in the epidermis involved in contact dermatitis (Langerhans cells, 1869), and insulinoma (Langerhans adenoma).

Paul Langerhans

1847 *Hans Christian Saxtroph Helvig* born. A psychiatrist and director of the Institute for the Insane in Odense who described the tractus-olivospinalis of the nervous system in 1887.

1847 Erasmus Wilson, founder of the chair of dermatology at the Royal College of Surgeons, described acrodynia, mercury poisoning, which manifests itself as painful dermatitis affecting the extremities.

1847   An acute inflammatory condition of the finer bronchioles causing asthma (bronchiolitis) was described by Berlin professor of medicine, Ludwig Traube.

1848   German chemist, Hermann Christian von Fehling, devised a test for sugar in the urine (Fehling test).

1848   *Leonardo Bianchi* born. An Italian neuropsychiatrist who described Bianchi syndrome, relating to sensory aphasia accompanied by alexia and apraxia, and seen in lesions of the left parietal lobe.

1848   *Edward Livingston Trudeau* born. A New York physician and a pioneer in the study of tuberculosis in America.

1848   *Alfonso Poggi* born. An Italian orthopedic surgeon who was the first to achieve acetabular reconstruction.

1848   *Alexander Hughes Bennet* born. An English neurologist who performed the diagnosis and operative removal of a brain tumor in 1884.

1848   The ultramicroscope, devised by Siedentopf and Austrian chemist, Richard Zsigmondy, projected light onto suspended particles in solution which were then viewed on a dark background through the microscope.

1848   *Cornelius Adrianus Peckelharing* born. A physiologist from Utrecht who suggested the existence of accessory food factors (vitamins, 1905), and proposed a blood coagulation theory.

1848   *Edouard Kirmisson* born. An orthopedic surgeon from Paris who wrote on congenital deformities, disorders of the locomotor system, acquired deformities, and devised the Kirmisson operation.

1848   *Karl Wernicke* born. A German neurologist who described Wernicke encephalopathy, ophthalmoplegia, nystagmus, ataxia with tremors from thiamine deficiency, and described aphasias.

Karl Wernicke

1848   *W. Gill Wylie* born. A New York gynecologist who shortened the round ligaments by folding them on themselves and suturing (Wylie operation) as treatment for uterine retroflexion.

1848   Despite the antiquity of leprosy, the first medical treatise was written by Norwegian physician, Cornelius Daniel Danielsson and Carl Wilhelm Boeck.

1848   Vincent Alexander Bochdalek described a congenital hernia through the remnant of the pleuroperitoneal canal in the left posterolateral part of the diaphragm (Bochdalek hernia).

1848   *Jean Albert Pitres* born. A Bordeaux physician who defined several specific areas in the prefrontal cortex (Pitres areas).

1848   *Vladimir Karlovitch Roth* born. A Russian neurologist who described septic retinitis (Roth disease).

1848   *Viktor Meyer* born. A German chemist who coined the term 'stereochemistry' for the study of molecular shapes, and devised a method of determining vapor density.

1848   *Max Nitze* born. A Berlin pioneer in urology who invented the modern electrically-lit cystoscope in 1879.

1848   *Sir William MacEwen* born. A professor of surgery from Scotland who was one of the first to successfully operate on brain tumors (1879), abscesses and trauma, removed a tumor involving the meninges of the brain and carried out some of the first bone grafts.

1848   The term 'embolism' was first used by German pathological anatomist, Rudolph Virchow.

1848   *Edward Hickling Bradford* born. A Boston orthopedic surgeon who designed a bed frame for patients with tuberculosis of the spine and leg fractures, and wrote *Treatise on Orthopedic Surgery* which contained detailed analyses of hip diseases.

1848   The eminent French chemist Louis Pasteur discovered anerobic bacteria, a group of bacteria that exist without oxygen and were harmed by its presence.

1848   *George Ryerson Fowler* born. A New York surgeon who described a head-up position to allow drainage of fluid into the pelvis in cases of peritonitis (Fowler position).

1848   *Thomas Morgan Rotch* born. A Boston physician who described dullness due to percussion over the right 5th intercostal space in pericardial effusion (Rotch sign).

1848   *Truman William Brophy* born. An American oral surgeon who designed an operation for cleft palate (Brophy operation).

1848   *Auguste-Henri Forel* born. A professor of psychiatry at Zurich who pioneered the study of subthalamic areas of the central nervous system, described the decussation between the red nuclei of the brain (Forel decussation), and wrote *The Sexual Problem* in 1905.

1848   *Hugo de Vries* born. A Dutch physiologist and geneticist who confirmed Mendel's theories, and devised a theory of mutation which proposed that new species arise by single mutation (1890).

1848   *Paul Yvon* born. A French physician who devised the Yvon test for detection of acetanilide in urine, with chloroform and mercurous nitrate as reagents.

1848   *Carl Furstner* born. A German psychiatrist who described pseudo-

166

spastic paralysis with tremors (Furstner disease).

1848 The transverse curved ridge joining the internal openings of the urethra within the bladder (Mercier bar) was described by Louis Auguste Mercier, a urinary surgeon from Paris.

1848 *William Ewart* born. An English physician who described pulmonary collapse at the left base in pericardial effusion (Ewart sign, 1896).

1848 *Observations on Certain Pathological Conditions of the Blood and Urine, in Gout, Rheumatism, and Bright's Disease* was published by the distinguished British rheumatologist, Sir Alfred Baring Garrod.

1848 *Henry Newell Martin* born. An American physiologist who studied the intercostal muscles in respiration, and described the effects of varying arterial pressure on the heart rate after devising perfusion for an isolated heart.

1848 The term 'notochord' was coined by English anatomist, Richard Owen.

1848 The first recorded death following chloroform anesthesia was that of Hannah Greener, aged 15, at Durham.

1848 The first use of ethyl chloride as a local anesthetic was by Heyfelder of Erlangen, Germany.

1848 Use of hypnosis for surgical operations in India was introduced by Scotsman, James Esdaile.

William Ewart

1848 An early description of the diverticula of the colon was given by French physician, Jean Cruveilheir.

1849 *Emil Zuckerkandl* born. A Hungarian-born anatomist in Vienna who wrote an important monograph on the pathology and anatomy of the accessory sinuses, and described the fascia of Zuckerkandl (retrorenal fascia, 1883).

1849 *Frederick Akbar Mahomed* born. A physician from Guy's Hospital, London who pioneered the study of blood pressure in clinical medicine, and developed his own modified sphygmograph.

Mahomed's sphygmograph

1849 *Sir Felix Semon* born. A German-born laryngologist working in London who described the retraction or fixation of the umbilicus in upper airway disease (Semon sign).

1849 *Louis Adolphus Duhring* born. An American dermatologist who wrote the first textbook on dermatology in America, and described dermatitis herpetiformis (Duhring disease, 1884).

1849 *Joseph Jules Dejerine* born. A French neurologist and one of the pioneers of localization of function in the brain, who described a form of hypertrophic interstitial neuritis in infants (Dejerine disease, 1893), a form of arthritis (Dejerine–Sottas disease, 1890), and a thalamic syndrome (Dejerine–Roussy syndrome, 1906).

1849 *Friedrich Schauta* born. An Viennese gynecologist who devised a radical hysterectomy for carcinoma of the cervix (Schauta operation) in 1908.

1849 *Joseph Grasset* born. A French neurologist who described drawing of the head to the side in cases of unilateral cerebral lesions, producing flaccid hemiplegia (Grasset law).

1849 *M. Oberst* born. A German surgeon who devised the Oberst operation for ascites, whereby a flap of skin is projected into the abdomen to provide drainage of ascitic fluid.

1849 Struthers ligament, attached to the medial condyle of the humerus, was described by Sir John Struthers, a professor of anatomy at Aberdeen.

1849 *Henry Duret* born. A French neurosurgeon who described the arteries supplying the nuclei of the cranial nerves, and the subarachnoid canals.

1849 The earliest neurological study on spinal muscular atrophy (Aran–Duchenne disease) was written by Guillaume Duchenne of Paris.

1849 Neurofibromatosis, characterized by developmental changes in the nervous system, skin and bones with soft tumors and areas of pigmentation (von Recklinghausen disease), was originally described by Robert Smith from Dublin.

1849 *Hermann Eichorst* born. A physician from Zurich who gave a comprehensive account of pernicious anemia (1878), and described a type of progressive muscular atrophy (Eichorst type) affecting the femoral and tibial muscles.

1849 *Charles Émile François Franck* born. A French physiologist and neurologist who studied the excitability of the cerebral cortex, and localization of its activity.

1849 *Oskar Lassar* born. A German dermatologist who formulated acetylsalicylic acid and zinc oxide (Lassar paste).

1849 *Ivan Petrovitch Pavlov* born. An experimental physiologist from central Russia who discovered the secretory nerves of the pancreas (1888), worked on the circulatory system, digestive glands and conditioned reflexes, and was awarded the Nobel Prize in 1904.

1849   *Franz Christian Boll* born. A Swiss anatomist who discovered the basal cells of the lachrymal glands (1869), and the photosensitive pigment in the retina (rhodopsin, 1877).

1849   *Otto Kahler* born. A German physician who described the course of the posterior nerve roots that enter the posterior columns so that fibers at higher levels medially displace those from lower levels, and multiple myeloma (Kahler disease).

1849   *Arthur Hartmann* born. A German otorhinologist who devised the Hartmann curette in adenoidectomy, and the first audiometer.

1849

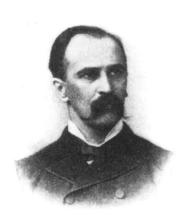

Sir William Osler

Sir William Osler born. A regius professor of medicine at Oxford, originally from Canada, who described one of the first cases of actinomycosis (1886), effective treatment of Addison disease (1896), hereditary angioneurotic edema (1888), familial hemorrhagic telengiectasis (1907), wrote *Principles and Practice of Medicine*,

and reformed American medical education.

1849   *Thomas Lewis Gilmer* born. A dentist in Chicago who devised a splint (Gilmer splint) for treating fracture of the mandible.

1849   London dermatologist, Erasmus Wilson, described trichorrhexis nodosa (trichodasis).

1849   *Oscar Wilhelm August Hertwig* born. An anatomy professor from Jena who described the cells at the roots of teeth responsible for the formation of enamel, and demonstrated that fusion of the nuclei of ovum and spermatozoa was essential for fertilization.

1849   *August Froriep* born. A physiologist from Tübingen who described a dorsal root ganglion (Froriep ganglion) found inconsistently at a position posterior to the hypoglossal nerve.

1850   *George Edward Fell* born. An American physician who devised apparatus for performing artificial respiration during surgery without collapsing the lung.

1850   *George Gaffky* born. A German bacteriologist who obtained a pure culture of *Salmonella typhi* and demonstrated it to be the cause of typhoid (1884).

1850   *Carl Richard Greef* born. An ophthalmologist in Berlin who described a type of intracellular body (Prowazek–Greef body), found in trachomotous secretions.

1850   Amyotrophic lateral sclerosis was later described by François Amilcar Aran as progressive muscular atrophy.

1850   The true nature of the pathological process of fatty degeneration of the heart was described by Richard Quain in the *Medico-Chirugical Transactions*.

1850   The modern uterine curette was developed by French gynecologist, Joseph C.A. Recamier, who obtained endometrium for analysis.

1850   *Woldemar von Schroeder* born. A German physician who devised the Schroeder test (1882) for urea, with a solution of bromine in chloroform as reagent.

1850   *Johann von Mikulicz-Radecki* born. A Polish professor of surgery and an early advocate of antiseptic surgery who was one of the first to use gloves and a mask, described large vacuolated phagocytes with small pyknotic nuclei in rhinoscleroma (Mikulicz cell), and Mikulicz syndrome associated with hypertrophy of the salivary glands (1892).

1850   The visible S-shaped line on the chest, demarcating the upper border of a pleural effusion (Damoiseau sign), was noted by French physician, Louis Hyacinthe Celeste Damoiseau.

1850   *Paul Albert Grawitz* born. A German surgeon and pathologist who carried out early work on the origin of hypernephroma, or renal cell carcinoma (Grawitz tumor, 1884).

1850   *George Huntington* born. A Baltimore neurologist who was the first to recognize adult hereditary chorea (Huntington chorea or disease, 1872), and to describe its symptoms.

1850   *Theodor Schott* born. A physician from Nauheim in Germany who advocated a treatment for heart disease using warm saline baths with exercise (Schott treatment).

1850   The absence of a thymus, or multiple abscesses in it, in cases of congenital syphilis (Dubois disease), was described by Paul Dubois of Paris.

1850   *Moritz Nussbaum* born. A professor of biology and histologist at Bonn, Germany who described the Nussbaum cells in the pyloric gastric glands (1877).

1850   *Anton Wölfler* born. A physician from Prague who devised the Wölfler operation, whereby an opening between the stomach and the distal part of the duodenum is created in cases of pyloric obstruction.

1850   *Robert Marcus Gunn* born. A London ophthalmologist who described unilateral ptosis of the eyelid and exaggerated opening of the eye, related to jaw movement (jaw-winking phenomenon, or Gunn syndrome, 1883).

1850   *Arthur Edward James Barker* born. A London surgeon who devised a method of excision of the hip by an anterior approach (Barker operation).

1850 Dentinal fibrils (Tomes fibers) were described by London dental surgeon, Sir John Tomes.

1850 *Adolf Jarisch* born. An Austrian dermatologist famous for his *Textbook of Skin Diseases*, who published on many areas of skin disease and syphilis, and is remembered for his description of the Jarisch–Herxheimer reaction (1895).

1850 *Sir Edward Sharpey-Schäfer* born. A pioneer in endocrinology who demonstrated the effects of suprarenal gland extract (1895), and showed that it produced artery contraction and accelerated heart rate, thus increasing blood pressure (epinephrine).

1850 An instrument for determining the velocity of the nerve current (myographion) was invented by German surgeon and professor of physiology, Hermann von Helmholtz.

1850 *Ivan Michailovitch Setchenov* born. Considered the father of Russian physiology and neurology, who described the reflex inhibitory center in the medulla oblongata (Setchenov center), and several other structures of the nervous system.

1850 *Charles Robert Richet* born. A French physiologist and Nobel laureate (1913) who did pioneering work on serum therapy, having noted that the blood of animals which are resistant to a harmful bacterium may contain an element that could confer immunity, and also worked on hypnosis, digestion, pain and muscle contraction.

1850 Retinal changes in hypertension were observed by Viennese neurologist, Ludwig Türck.

1850 *Daniel Elmer Salmon* born. An American veterinary pathologist who famously described gram negative rod-shaped bacteria, a genus which includes the bacteria causing typhoid fever, and named *Salmonella* in his honor.

1850 Bulldog forceps or spring clips were introduced to occlude veins.

1850 *Hans Büchner* born. A German bacteriologist who did pioneering work on proteins in the blood (gammaglobulins), that combine with invading organisms and protect against infections.

1850 *Alfred Eddowes* born. A dermatologist from St Johns Hospital for Diseases of the Skin in London who described osteogenesis imperfecta (Eddowes disease or syndrome, 1873).

1850 *William Harrison Cripps* born. An English surgeon who described a method of colotomy in the iliac region (Cripps operation) in 1880.

1850 *Paul Gerson Unna* born. A dermatologist from Hamburg who described Unna dermatosis (seborrheic eczema, 1887), and introduced the use of icthyol, resorcin and zinc oxide paste in dermatology.

1850 *Otto Haab* born. A Swiss ophthalmologist who described a method of extracting foreign metal particles from the eye using a magnet.

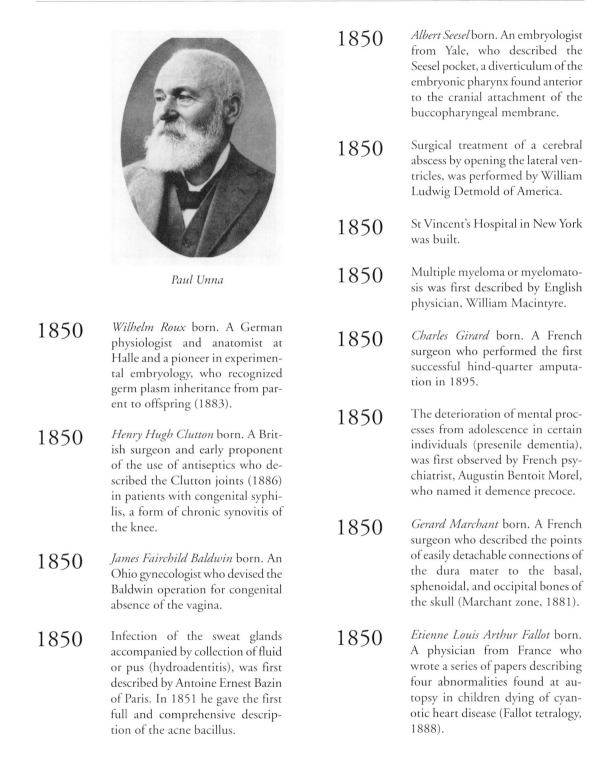

Paul Unna

1850   *Wilhelm Roux* born. A German physiologist and anatomist at Halle and a pioneer in experimental embryology, who recognized germ plasm inheritance from parent to offspring (1883).

1850   *Henry Hugh Clutton* born. A British surgeon and early proponent of the use of antiseptics who described the Clutton joints (1886) in patients with congenital syphilis, a form of chronic synovitis of the knee.

1850   *James Fairchild Baldwin* born. An Ohio gynecologist who devised the Baldwin operation for congenital absence of the vagina.

1850   Infection of the sweat glands accompanied by collection of fluid or pus (hydroadentitis), was first described by Antoine Ernest Bazin of Paris. In 1851 he gave the first full and comprehensive description of the acne bacillus.

1850   *Albert Seesel* born. An embryologist from Yale, who described the Seesel pocket, a diverticulum of the embryonic pharynx found anterior to the cranial attachment of the buccopharyngeal membrane.

1850   Surgical treatment of a cerebral abscess by opening the lateral ventricles, was performed by William Ludwig Detmold of America.

1850   St Vincent's Hospital in New York was built.

1850   Multiple myeloma or myelomatosis was first described by English physician, William Macintyre.

1850   *Charles Girard* born. A French surgeon who performed the first successful hind-quarter amputation in 1895.

1850   The deterioration of mental processes from adolescence in certain individuals (presenile dementia), was first observed by French psychiatrist, Augustin Bentoit Morel, who named it demence precoce.

1850   *Gerard Marchant* born. A French surgeon who described the points of easily detachable connections of the dura mater to the basal, sphenoidal, and occipital bones of the skull (Marchant zone, 1881).

1850   *Etienne Louis Arthur Fallot* born. A physician from France who wrote a series of papers describing four abnormalities found at autopsy in children dying of cyanotic heart disease (Fallot tetralogy, 1888).

1850   *George Martin Kober* born. One of the first in America to point out that flies are carriers of disease in a report on typhoid fever, and a pioneer in industrial hygiene in America.

1850   Experimental studies on electrical stimulation of the heart were carried out by M. Hoffa and Karl Friedrich Wilhelm Ludwig.

1850   Iodine deficiency as the cause of endemic goiter was proposed by French physician, Gaspard Adolphe Chatin.

1851   An ice and salt mixture for refrigeration local anesthesia was introduced by Scottish physician, Neils Arnott.

1851

Karl Ludwig

Nerves of the salivary glands were described by German physiologist, Karl Wilhelm Ludwig.

1851   The distinction between carcinoma and hypertrophy of the prostate was made by English surgeon, John Adams.

1851   The first hospital in Britain to be devoted to cancer, The Cancer Hospital, was established by William Marsden, a London surgeon. It became the Royal Cancer Hospital (Free) in 1936, and later the Royal Marsden Hospital.

1851   *Graham Steell* born. A Scottish cardiologist famous for *Physical Signs of Cardiac Diseases, Physical Signs of Pulmonary Diseases*, and *Textbook of the Diseases of the Heart*.

1851   *Charles Chamberland* born. A pioneer in methods of sterilizing medical equipment who invented the autoclave.

1851   *Arnold Pick* born. A psychiatrist from Prague who, in 1892, described aperceptive blindness with central atrophy, where the patient cannot fix reflexly on objects within his gaze (Arnold Pick syndrome).

1851   The receptor organ of sound (organ of Corti) was described by Italian anatomist, Alfonso Corti.

1851   *Ernest Fuchs* born. A Viennese ophthalmologist who described depressions on the anterior surface of the iris near the pupillary border (stomata of Fuchs, 1885), and peripheral atrophy of the optic nerve.

1851   *Frank Thomas Paul* born. A graduate of Guy's Hospital, London, who employed the Paul tube in 1892 to temporarily drain fecal matter after colostomy in cases of obstruction of the large bowel.

1851 *George Thompson Elliot* born. An American dermatologist who described the Elliot sign of induration at the periphery of certain syphilitic skin lesions.

1851 The mechanism of production of the first and second heart sounds were explained by Arthur Leared of the University of Dublin, who also devised a binaural stethoscope.

1851 The membrana vestibularis of the cochlea separating scala vestibuli and scala media (Reissner membrane) was described by Ernst Reissner, professor of anatomy at Breslau.

1851 *Moritz Loewit* born. A professor of pathology at Innsbruck, Austria who described erythroblasts (Loewit cells) and other cellular elements of blood.

1851 *Albert Florence* born. A surgeon from France who devised the Florence test for detecting spermatic fluid using iodine.

1851 Felix Adolph Richard, a surgeon from Paris, described ovarian fimbria of the ostium of the fallopian tube.

1851 *Charles Bent Ball* born. A surgeon from Dublin, Ireland who described the rectal valves (Ball valves) in *The Rectum and Anus, their Diseases and Treatment* (1887), and devised an operation for the relief of pruritis.

1851 *Robert Abbe* born. A New York surgeon who devised a method of dilating esophageal stricture, and introduced catgut for suturing the intestines (1889).

1851 *Samuel James Meltzer* born. An American physiologist who pioneered endotracheal insufflation using ether as anesthetic for thoracic surgery, and described the mechanisms of bronchial asthma.

1851 Emile Pierre Marie van Ermengen isolated the etiological agent for botulism, *Clostridium botulinum*.

1851 *Ferdinand C. Valentine* born. A New York surgeon who described the patient supine at the edge of the operating table with legs hanging down, used for irrigating the urethra (Valentine position).

1851 *Theodor Weyle* born. A chemist from France who devised the Weyle test to detect creatinine, using sodium nitroprusside as reagent.

1851 *André Chantemmesse* born. A French bacteriologist who worked on typhoid toxin, antityphoid serum, and isolated the dysentery bacillus (1888).

1851 An account of the presystolic component of mitral murmur in mitral stenosis and hypertrophy of the heart, including clinical signs, was given by Walter Hayle Walshe of the University College of London.

1851 *J.P. Bjerrum* born. An ophthalmologist from Denmark who devised the Bjerrum chart for testing vision.

1851 Plaster of Paris was introduced as a bandage by Danish military surgeon, Anthonius Mathijsen.

1851 *Paul Kraske* born. A surgeon from Freiburg who described the Kraske operation for carcinoma of the rectum, where the surgical approach is gained by excision of the sacrum and coccyx.

1852 *Charles Euchariste de Medici Sajous* born. An American physician who wrote the first monograph in the United States on internal secretions, and proposed the role of the adrenals in the body's defense mechanism.

1852 *Sir David Drummond* born. An English surgeon who devised an operation for ascites in which the surface of the parietal peritoneum was roughened to facilitate adhesions.

1851 *Richard Julius Petri* born. German bacteriologist who designed the shallow glass dish for culturing bacteria (Petri dish).

1852 *Joseph Disse* born. A German anatomist who described the perisinusoidal space in the liver (Disse space).

1852 *Samuel Vulfovich Goldflam* born. A neurologist in Warsaw who described myasthenia gravis (1893) or Erb–Goldflam disease.

1852 The first description of periarteritis nodosa (or polyarteritis nodosa) was given by Czech physician, Karl Freiherr von Rokitansky.

1852 Synthesis of salicylic acid was reported by H. Gerland. This was one of several important publications on previously isolated active medicinals.

1852 *Edward Charles Spitzka* born. A New York neurologist who described the fibers of the posterior longitudinal bundle connecting the 3rd and 6th nerve cranial nuclei (bundle of Spitzka, 1876).

1852 *Theodor Kaes* born. A German neurologist who described a new layer in the cerebral cortex (Kaes–Bekhterev layer, 1907), later described by Russian neurologist, Vladimir Mikhailovitch Bekhterev.

1852 The maximum velocity of nerve conduction in experimental animals was found to be 30 meters per second by Hermann von Helmholtz of the University of Bonn, Germany.

1852 *Baron Shibasaburo Kitasato* born. A Japanese bacteriologist who isolated the causative organism of bubonic plague, *Pasteurella pestis*, in 1894, independently of Alexandre Yersin.

1852 An instrument for determining the number of blood cells in a given volume (hemacytometer) was first devised by Karl Vierordt.

Karl Vierordt

1852 Utero-sacral and utero-recto-sacral ligaments of the broad ligament (Jarjavay ligaments) were described by French physician, Jean François Jarjavay.

1852 *Charles Sedgwick Minot* born. A professor of comparative anatomy at Harvard who designed a rotary microtome, studied the placenta, and published a theory on aging, The problem of age, growth and death (1908).

1852 *Charles Loomes Dana* born. A New York neurologist who designed an operation for resection the posterior roots of the spinal nerves as treatment for intractable pain, athetosis, or spastic paralysis (Dana operation).

1852

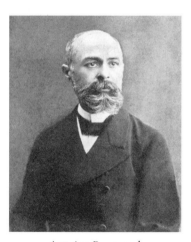

Antoine Becquerel

Antoine Henri Becquerel born. A French physicist who discovered that certain substances emit radiation and who shared the Nobel Prize in 1903 with Pierre and Marie Curie.

1852 *Max Schäffer* born. German physician who described the extension of the great toe on pinching the achilles tendon (Schäffer reflex).

1852 *Ivar Victor Sandström* born. A Swedish physician who discovered and described the parathyroid, and demonstrated its necessity for sustaining life.

1852 *John Newport Langley* born. A neurophysiologist from Newbury, England who coined the terms preganglionic, postganglionic and autonomic during work on the nervous system, and was the founder-owner of the *Journal of Physiology*.

1852 *Emil Hermann Fischer* born. A Prussian chemist and Nobel laureate, who discovered hydraxane

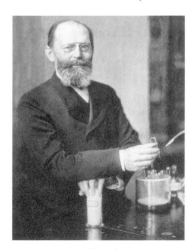

Emil Fischer

(1875), showed that albumin was composed of amino acids (1889), studied purine metabolism, and developed barbital depressants (1902).

1852   *Moritz Holl* born. A physician from Vienna who described the intercrural ligament found in front of the urinary meatus of the female (1896).

1852   A congenital condition considered to be incurable (epispadias) was successfully treated using reversed flap surgery by Auguste Nélaton of Paris.

1852   Leon Bassereau of Paris studied sexually transmitted infection, characterized by ulceration of the male and female external genitalia (chancroid).

1852   *Sir James Kingston Fowler* born. A London physician who noted the association between throat infections and acute rheumatism, and proposed that pulmonary tuberculosis spread from the apex of the dorsal lobe along the greater fissure to the periphery.

1852   *Edouard Brissaud* born. A French neurologist who described infantile myxedema (1907), and a condition of uncontrolled tic spasms in children (1896).

1852   *Arthur Tracy Cabot* born. A Boston surgeon who designed a posterior wire splint for immobilizing the lower limb.

1852   *William Stewart Halstead* born. An American surgeon who performed the first successful ligation of the subclavian artery in America, pioneered circular sutures for intestines (1887), introduced cocaine for local anesthesia (1885), and introduced rubber gloves into surgery (1894).

1852   *Guillaume Vignal* born. A French histologist who described the embryonic connective tissue on the axis cylinders of the fetal nerve fibers (Vignal cells, 1889).

1852   *Achille Etienne Malecot* born. A French surgeon who designed a large-bore suprapubic urinary catheter (Malecot catheter).

1852   The term 'epithelioma' was coined by Adolph Hanover, to denote the skin lesions.

1852   *Edouard Victor Alfred Quenu* born. A professor of surgical pathology in Paris, who devised an operation to divide the ribs in order to promote retraction of the chest wall in empyema (Quenu thoracoplasty), and described a series of lymphatic plexuses in the mucous membrane of the anus (1893).

1852   *Arthur Henry Benson* born. An Irish ophthalmologist who described the small degenerative white spherical bodies in the vitreous eye in advanced age.

1852   *Santiago Ramon y Cajal* born. A Spanish physician and a professor of anatomy who studied the microstructure of the nervous system (including nerve degeneration and regeneration), developed many histological stains, and shared the Nobel Prize in 1906.

1852   The Great Ormond Street Hospital for Sick Children was founded by a London physician, Charles West.

1852   Tactile sensory nerve endings (Meissner corpuscles) were de-

Illustration of nerve fibers

scribed by Georg Meissner and Rudolf Wagner, professors of physiology at Göttingen, Germany.

1852   *Viktor von Hacker* born. A Viennese surgeon who devised an operation for hypospasias and described a method for gastrostomy (1886).

1852   *Henry Eales* born. An English physician who wrote a review of the appearance of the retina in patients with renal disease, and on recurrent retinal and vitreous hemorrhage (Eales disease).

1852   *Francis Henry Williams* born. An American physician who estimated the heart size using a fluoroscope (1896), the first application of X-rays to cardiology.

1852   An operative treatment for vesicovaginal fistula was popularized by American gynecologist, James Marion Sims.

1852   The ganglionic cells (Bidder ganglia) were discovered at the junc-

tion of the auricles and ventricles by German anatomist, Friedrich Heinrich Wilhelm Bidder.

1852   William Senhouse Kirkes gave a classical description of dislodged arterial emboli from the heart.

1852   Histology was defined as 'the science of the minute structure of the organs of the animals and plants' by John Thomas Queckett.

1852   The first hypodermic needle was developed by Scottish physician, Alexander Wood.

1852   *Alexander Stanislavovic Dogiel* born. A Russian neurologist who described nerve endings of the bulb type in the cardiovascular system (1903), and created a classification of spinal and other ganglia.

1852   Successful resection of a gangrenous lung following trauma in an American sailor in Hong Kong, was done by W.A. Harland.

1852   The occurrence of slow pulse in jaundice was observed by French physician, Jules Edouard A. Monneret.

1852   The first recorded excision of the head of the femur in America was undertaken by Henry Jacob Bigelow.

1853   *Robert Marston* born. A dentist from Leicester, England who patented the first modern anesthetic injector for regulating the strength of anesthetic vapor (1898).

1853   *Sir Frederick Treves* born. A notable English surgeon who wrote *Manual*

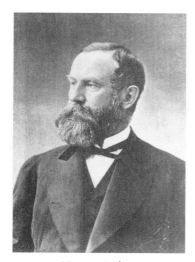

Henry Bigelow

of *Surgical Anatomy* (1881) and *The Elephant Man and other Reminiscences*, the true story of Joseph Merrick, a man suffering from neurofibromatosis.

1853   *Jules Comby* born. A French pediatrician who described the whitish yellow patches seen in the inflamed buccal mucosa before the onset of Koplik spots in measles (Comby sign).

1853   The fungus responsible for candidosis was named *Oidium albicans* by Charles P. Robin.

1853   *William Murrell* born. An English physician whose special interest was therapeutics, he introduced nitroglycerin as treatment for angina (1879), published *Manual of Pharmacology and Therapeutics* (1896) and several other books.

1853   *Ambrosius Arnold Willem Hubrecht* born. A comparative anatomist at Leiden who described a thickening

at the site of first formation of the primitive streak (1905).

1853   *Albrecht Kossel* born. A Swiss-born German physiological chemist and Nobel laureate (1910) who separated protein and nucleic acid and showed that the latter was composed of four bases, adenine, thiamine, cytosine and guanine.

1853   *Robert Tigerstedt* born. A physiologist from Finland who discovered a pressor substance formed in the kidneys (renin), and carried out studies on nerve response to mechanical stimulation.

1853   *Themistokles Gluck* born. A professor of surgery in Bucharest who

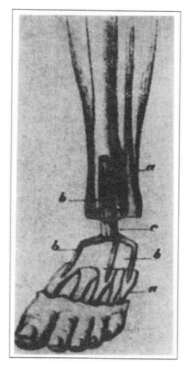

Illustration of joint replacement procedure

pioneered joint replacement, and prostheses for joints, using intramedullary nails and an ivory intramedullary peg.

1853   Claude Bernard, the French physiologist, discovered and explained glycogen and its metabolism.

1853   *Hans Christian Joachim Gram* born. A physician from Denmark who developed the Gram stain for bacteria, and was one of the first to recognize macrocytes in pernicious anemia and jaundice.

1853   *Sir James Mackenzie* born. One of the greatest British cardiologists who noted the loss of effective atrial contraction (atrial paralysis), described the functional pathology of cardiac tissue (1907), and published the famous *Diseases of the Heart* (1908).

1853   *Alexander Hugh Ferguson* born. A Chicago surgeon who specialized in the treatment of hernia and described a radical cure for femoral hernia (1895).

1853   *George Stevenson Middleton* born. A Scottish physician who gave a description of erythema elevatum diutinum, a skin disease marked by persistent, painless nodules, first noted on the hands of a rheumatic patient.

1853   The Y-shaped iliofemoral ligament of the hip joint (Gunn ligament) was described by American surgeon, Moses Gunn.

1853   *John Elmer Weeks* born. A New York ophthalmologist who discov-

ered the bacillus (Koch–Weeks bacillus, *Haemophilus aegyptius*) of epidemic mucopurulent bilateral conjunctivitis (pink disease) in 1886.

1853

Pierre Marie

Pierre Marie born. A French surgeon who was the first to observe a pituitary disorder associated with gigantism (1886), and described the condition now known as ankylosing spondylitis (1898) in *La Spondylose rhizomelique*.

1853   The first successful abdominal hysterectomy was performed by American surgeon, Walter Burnham.

1853   *Joseph Thomayer* born. A German surgeon who described inflammatory conditions of the pelvis, where percussion showed tympany on the right side and dullness on the left side, with the patient lying on their back.

1853   Protoporphyrin or hematin was used as an indicator for detection of blood in forensic medicine by

German histologist, Ludwig Teichmann.

1853 *James Rutherford Morison* born. A surgeon in Newcastle, England who pioneered pelvic surgery for women, published *Abdominal and Pelvic Surgery* (1925), and pioneered surgical treatment for gallstones and gastric cancer.

1853 *George Michael Edebohls* born. A New York surgeon who introduced decortication to treat chronic nephritis (1901), and performed nephropexy in a movable kidney with chronic nephritis (1899).

1853 *Paul Julius Poirier* born. A French surgeon who described the lymphatic gland situated on the uterine artery where it crosses the urethra (Poirier gland).

1853 Identification of malignant cells in body fluids was made by F. Donaldson, who described his findings in *The Practical Application of the Microscope to Cancer*.

1853 *Karel Maydl* born. A surgeon at Prague and Vienna who performed the first successful colostomy (1888), and uretero-intestinal anastomosis with insertion of the extroverted bladder into the rectum for ectopic vesicae (1894).

1853 *Oskar Langendorf* born. A professor of physiology at Rostock in Germany who described the principal cells of the thyroid (Langendorf cells) in 1889.

1853 *Wilhelm Uhthoff* born. A German physician and ophthalmologist who described the occurrence of nystagmus in multiple sclerosis (Uhthoff sign).

1853 The Women's Hospital in New York was founded by American gynecologist, James Marion Sims.

1853 *Gilbert Ballet* born. A Paris physician who described Ballet disease, paralysis of the extraocular muscles in thyrotoxic exophthalmos.

1853 *Ernest Gustav Adolf von Strümpell* born. A German physician and psychologist who distinguished psychogenic from organic symptoms of disease, and described rheumatoid spondylitis or spondylitis deformans (Marie–Strümpell disease) in *Textbook for Medical Students* (1891).

1854 Neuroglia, the supporting structures of the nerve tissue, were described by German pathological anatomist, Rudolph Virchow.

1854 The quadrate ligament of the superior ulnar articulation was described by Jean Louis Paul Denuce, professor of clinical surgery at the University of Bordeaux, France.

1854 *Adolf Lorenz* born. A leading orthopedic surgeon from Austria who designed an osteotomy operation and manipulative reduction for congenital dislocation of the hip.

1854 *Richard Frommel* born. A German gynecologist who devised a treatment for retroversion of the uterus by shortening the uterosacral ligaments (Frommel operation, 1890).

1854   *Charles Edward Beevor* born. An English neurologist who described upward displacement of the umbilicus from paralysis of the lower rectus abdominal muscle (Beevor sign).

1854   The discovery of a practical method of frequently measuring blood pressure by applying counter pressure to the artery was developed by Karl Vierordt, a German clinician.

1854   A granular form of trachoma (Arlt trachoma) was described by Austrian ophthalmologist, Carl Ferdinand von Arlt.

1854   The peritoneal folds of the uterus (Duncan folds) were described by Scottish obstetrician, James Matthews Duncan.

1854   *Friedrich Karl Adolf Neelsen* born. A German pathologist from Dresden who developed the acid-fast method of staining mycobacteria.

1854   *Paul Julius Möbius* born. A physician from Leipzig in Germany who described the incomplete convergence of the eyes in toxic goiter (Möbius sign).

1854   *Hayward Warren Cushing* born. A Boston surgeon who introduced a mattress-type of continuous invaginating intestinal suture (Cushing suture).

1854   The center of the brain, acting as the 'master switchboard' for controlling and regulating the circulatory system, was located by German physiologist, Karl Friedrich Wilhelm Ludwig.

1854   *Paul Ehrlich* born. A German bacteriologist, Nobel laureate (1908) and pioneer in hematology and chemotherapy who developed staining techniques for blood cells, the side-chain theory of immunity, enzyme action and drug action, and the drug salvarsan for treating syphilis.

1854   A form of rapid fatal congenital osteogenesis imperfecta (Vrolik syndrome) was described by Dutch anatomist, Willem Vrolik.

1854   *Henry Ambrose Grundy Brooke* born. An English dermatologist who described basal cell tumors, most commonly around the eyelids and on the face and scalp, and inherited as an autosomal dominant (Brooke epithelioma, 1892).

1854   *George Lincoln Walton* born. An American surgeon who described a method of reducing dislocation of the cervical vertebra (1895).

1854   Acute or chronic fungal infection generally seen in males and affecting the groin, perineum and perineal area (tinea cruris) was described by Friedrich von Bärensprung.

1854   *Emil von Behring* born. An army surgeon from western Prussia who demonstrated the first successful clinical use of diphtheria antitoxin (1890), and used serum therapy against tetanus and diphtheria (1891). He was awarded the first Nobel Prize in 1901.

1854   *James Carroll* born. An English-born physician in America who pioneered the study of yellow fever and typhoid bacteria.

1854 *Max Rubner* born. A German physiologist who measured metabolic changes in the body using the animal body as a calorimeter (1891), and described the specific dynamic action of food.

1854 *James Mescheter Anders* born. An American physician who described adiposa tuberosa simplex (Anders disease), consisting of small subcutaneous fatty nodules which are tender to the touch and usually found in the extremities or the abdomen.

1854 *Victor Babes* born. A Rumanian bacteriologist who devised the mallein test for diagnosis of glanders (1891).

1854 *Arnaldo Angelucci* born. An Italian ophthalmologist who described vernal conjunctivitis, hyperexcitability, tachycardia and vasomotor liability (Angelucci syndrome), and maintained a life-long interest in trachoma.

1854 *Philippe Charles Ernest Gaucher* born. A French physician who described a familial disorder of cerebroside metabolism with large pale cells in the spleen, as epithelioma primitif de la rate (1882).

1854 One of the greatest eye surgeons, Albrecht von Graefe of Berlin, founded the *Archiv für Ophthalmologie*, introduced iridectomy as treatment for glaucoma and iritis, and the cataract operation a year later.

1854 The differentiation between pulmonary collapse and post-operative pneumonia was given by William Gairdner, regius professor of medicine at Glasgow University.

1854 The causative organism of cholera, *Vibrio cholerae*, was discovered by Italian professor of anatomy at Pisa, Filippo Pacini.

1854 The difference between serous and purulent effusions in the chest were clarified by J.A. Marotte of Paris.

1854 Caisson disease was described by French surgeon, Brian Pol.

1854 Use of galvanocautery in major surgery was developed by Albrecht Theodor von Middeldorpf of Breslau.

1854 A modern laryngoscope was designed by Manuel Garcia, a Spanish music teacher working in London.

1854 Combined cephalic version in obstetrics was introduced by American obstetrician, Marmaduke Burr Wright.

1855 Lateral illumination in examination of the eye was introduced by German ophthalmologist, Richard Liebreich.

1855 The concept of an equilibrium within the body despite changes in external environment (homeostasis) was developed by the eminent French physiologist, Claude Bernard.

1855 *Warren Plimpton Lombard* born. An American physiologist who pioneered studies in the physiology

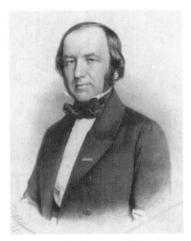

Claude Bernard

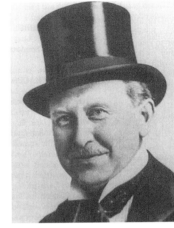

John Pringle

of the capillaries, vessels in the arterioles, and small veins of the human skin.

1855   *William Henry Battle* born. An English surgeon who described the blue discoloration of the skin over the mastoid process in cases of fracture of the base of the skull.

1855   *Gustav Riehl* born. An Austrian dermatologist, and an early protagonist of blood transfusion in the treatment of shock after burns, who described idiopathic hyperpigmentation of the skin (Riehl melanosis).

1855   *Rudolf von Jaksch* born. An Austrian physician in Prague who described acute hemolytic anemia in children (von Jaksch anemia), and was one of the first to investigate the presence of acetone bodies in urine.

1855   *John James Pringle* born. An English dermatologist who described

sebaceous adenoma (type Pringle), granularis rubra nasi, and edited a color atlas of dermatology, *Dermachromes*.

1855   *Ludwig Edinger* born. A German anatomist, regarded as the founder of comparative neuroanatomy, who described the nucleus of the third cranial nerve, the Edinger–Westphal nucleus.

1855   *Emil Berger* born. An Austrian ophthalmologist who described irregular pupils (Berger sign) seen in cases of early neurosyphilis.

1855   *Caesar A. von Ramdohr* born. An American surgeon who devised the Ramdhor suture, relating to the upper part of the divided intestine being invaginated into the lower part during intestinal anastomosis.

1855   The theory of hearing that proposed that the transverse fibers of the basilar membrane in the cochlea of the inner ear acted as a tuned resonator (resonance theory) was developed by Hermann von Helmholtz of Berlin, Germany.

1855 The symptomology of tabes dorsalis (locomotor ataxia) was described by Sir John Russell Reynolds, professor of medicine in London, in *Diagnosis of the Diseases of the Spinal Cord and Nerves*.

1855 *Henry Luc* born. An otorhinologist from Paris who designed several operations for diseases of the maxillary and frontal sinuses.

1855 *Anatole Marie Emile Chauffard* born. A French physician who named the point of tenderness below the right clavicle (Chauffard point) in cholecystitis, described a form of rheumatoid arthritis in children between first and second dentition (Still–Chauffard syndrome), psuedoxanthoma elasticum (1889), and acholuric familial jaundice (1907).

1855 *Christian Bohr* born. A Danish physician who described the effect of carbon dioxide on the dissociation of oxygen from hemoglobin (1904).

1855 *Georges Edouard Albert Brutus* born. A French neurologist who described the syndrome of echolalia, coprolalia, and chorea in children.

1855 *Albert Ludwig Siegmund Neisser* born. A German bacteriologist who discovered the gonorrhea bacterium (*Neisseria gonorrhoeae*), and wrote a complete review of hydatid disease in *Die Echinococcenkrankheit* (1877).

1855 *Sir John Bland-Sutton* born. An English pathologist, gynecologist and pioneer in the study of cancer who showed rickets could be cured by adding crushed bone to the diet, and wrote *Cancer Clinically Considered and Tumors, Innocent and Malignant* (1922).

1855 The Luschka foramen found at the lateral recesses of the fourth ventricle of the brain, was first described by Hubert von Luschka, a professor of anatomy at Tübingen.

1855 *Friedrich Dimmer* born. A Viennese ophthalmologist who described a special operation for treating ectropion, and a form of unilateral keratitis.

1855 *John Blair Deaver* born. An American surgeon who described the fat-free portions of the gut and their relation to the vascular arcade (1902), and devised the Deaver incision for appendectomy through the sheath of the right rectus muscle.

1855 The Rinnie test, using a tuning fork to differentiate between sensorimotor deafness and conduction deafness, was devised by German otologist, Heinrich Adolf Rinnie.

1855 *George Edouard Albert Gilles de La Tourette* born. A French neurologist who described the syndrome of violent muscle jerks of the face, shoulders, and extremities (Tourette syndrome, 1885), and worked on hysteria and hypnotism.

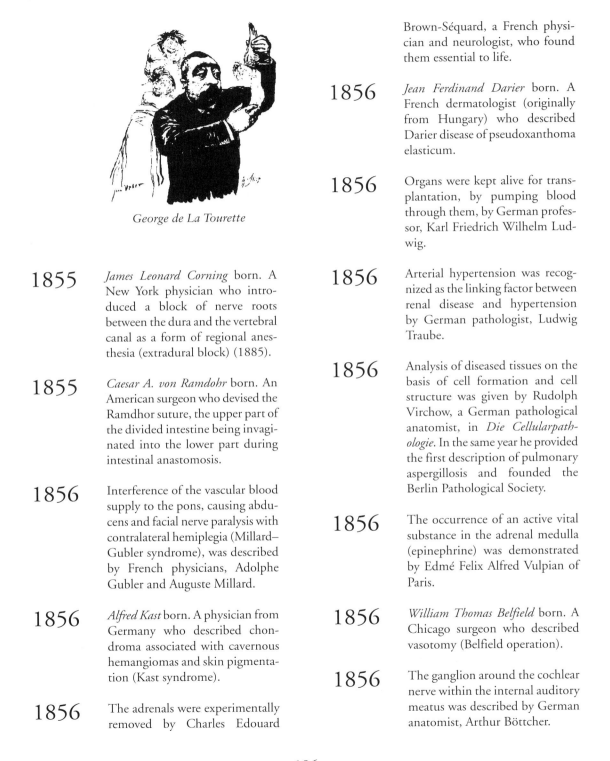

George de La Tourette

1855   *James Leonard Corning* born. A New York physician who introduced a block of nerve roots between the dura and the vertebral canal as a form of regional anesthesia (extradural block) (1885).

1855   *Caesar A. von Ramdohr* born. An American surgeon who devised the Ramdhor suture, the upper part of the divided intestine being invaginated into the lower part during intestinal anastomosis.

1856   Interference of the vascular blood supply to the pons, causing abducens and facial nerve paralysis with contralateral hemiplegia (Millard–Gubler syndrome), was described by French physicians, Adolphe Gubler and Auguste Millard.

1856   *Alfred Kast* born. A physician from Germany who described chondroma associated with cavernous hemangiomas and skin pigmentation (Kast syndrome).

1856   The adrenals were experimentally removed by Charles Edouard Brown-Séquard, a French physician and neurologist, who found them essential to life.

1856   *Jean Ferdinand Darier* born. A French dermatologist (originally from Hungary) who described Darier disease of pseudoxanthoma elasticum.

1856   Organs were kept alive for transplantation, by pumping blood through them, by German professor, Karl Friedrich Wilhelm Ludwig.

1856   Arterial hypertension was recognized as the linking factor between renal disease and hypertension by German pathologist, Ludwig Traube.

1856   Analysis of diseased tissues on the basis of cell formation and cell structure was given by Rudolph Virchow, a German pathological anatomist, in *Die Cellularpathologie*. In the same year he provided the first description of pulmonary aspergillosis and founded the Berlin Pathological Society.

1856   The occurrence of an active vital substance in the adrenal medulla (epinephrine) was demonstrated by Edmé Felix Alfred Vulpian of Paris.

1856   *William Thomas Belfield* born. A Chicago surgeon who described vasotomy (Belfield operation).

1856   The ganglion around the cochlear nerve within the internal auditory meatus was described by German anatomist, Arthur Böttcher.

1856   *Sir William Arbuthnot Lane* born. A surgeon at Guy's Hospital, London who treated empyema in a child by resecting a rib (1883), devised an operation for cleft palate (1897), and introduced internal fixation for fractured long bones (1893).

1856   The minute nodules at the margins of the tricuspid and mitral valves of the heart were described by Guiseppe Albini, professor of physiology at Naples.

1856   *Albert Einhorn* born. A German chemist who discovered the local anesthetic, novocaine, in 1899.

1856   *Nicolai Kulchitsky* born. A Russian anatomist and histologist who described the argentaffin cells (Kulchitsky cells, 1897) between the crypts of Lieberkühn in the intestinal mucosa and the neural crest cells, believed to be the origin of small cell cancer of the lung.

1856   *Charles Barrett Lockwood* born. A surgeon at St Bartholomew's Hospital and founder of the Anatomical Society of Great Britain and Ireland (1887), who described the suspensory ligament of the globe of the eye (Lockwood suspensory ligament, 1886).

1856   *Russel Henry Chittenden* born. An American physiologist who is considered to be the founder of physiological chemistry and nutrition in the US, his important works include *Nutrition of Man* (1907) and *Physiological Economy in Nutrition* (1905).

1856   *Jacob Franck* born. A Chicago physician who described the prolongation of clotting time in some cases of cirrhosis of the liver.

1856   *Friedrich Oskar Witzel* born. A German surgeon who described a method of gastrotomy through a thoracic incision (Witzel operation).

1856   The circular fibers of the ciliary muscles (Rouget muscle) were described by French professor of physiology at Montpellier, Charles Marie Benjamin Rouget.

1856   *Karl August Schuchardt* born. A German surgeon who practiced extended mediolateral paravaginal incision (Schuchardt incision, 1893).

1856   *Howard Henry Tooth* born. An English physician who described the peroneal form of progressive muscular dystrophy (Charcot–Marie–Tooth–Hoffmann syndrome, 1886).

1856   Epileptic hemiplegia affecting the epileptic side (Todd paralysis) was described by Robert Bentley Todd, an English physician and professor of physiology at King's College.

1856   The first accurate measurement of blood pressure in man was made by French physician, J. Faivre, using a mercury manometer attached to an artery.

1856   The first pharyngotomy in England was done by Edward Cock, for removal of a foreign body.

1856   Respiratory obstruction due to swallowing the tongue was described by British neurophysiologist, Marshall Hall. He described the body-rolling method for external chest compression during resuscitation.

1856 First drainage of a lung abscess in the United States was carried out by A.M. Leonard at Buffalo.

1857 Acetone in urine in cases of diabetes was shown by Prague physician, Wilhelm Petters.

1857 *Sir Victor Alexander Haden Horsley* born. The founder of neurosurgery in Britain who proved that myxedema and cretinism are due to thyroid deficiency (1886), performed the first successful removal of a spinal tumor (1887), and produced a stereotactic apparatus for accurate location of electrodes in the brain (1908).

1857 *Eugéne Gley* born. A French physician and endocrinologist who used oral thyroid extract, showed iodine in thyroid and blood, rediscovered the parathyroids, and was the first to understand their significance.

1857 *Frederick Byron Robinson* born. An American anatomist who described the Robinson circle, formed by anastomosis of the abdominal aorta, common iliac, hypogastric, uterine and ovarian arteries.

1857 *John Benjamin Murphy* born. An American pioneer in vascular surgery who demonstrated that severed arteries and veins could be reunited by end to end anastomosis (1896), performed artificial pneumothorax,

Murphy's button

designed the Murphy button for intestinal anastomosis, and introduced the Murphy saline drip.

1857 The superficial fascia of the neck, through which the external jugular vein penetrates behind the sternomastoid muscle, was described by Leopold Ritter Dittel, professor of surgery in Vienna.

1857 *Oscar Harrison Rogers* born. A physician from New York who designed an early aneroid manometer (Rogers sphygmomanometer).

1857 The ciliary glands (Moll glands) were described by an ophthalmologist from the Hague in Holland, Jacob Antonius Moll.

1857 *Sigard Adolphus Knopf* born. A New York physician and pioneer in the treatment of tuberculosis who promoted the Knopf method of breathing using diaphragmatic muscles rather than intercostal muscles in apical lobe tuberculosis.

1857 Peptic ulcer was described in detail by William Brinton of St Thomas' Hospital, London, with over 7000 postmortem findings.

1857

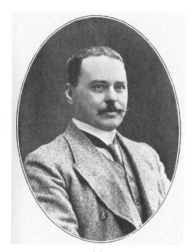

Ronald Ross

Ronald Ross born. A British physiologist who carried out much of his research in India where he elucidated the life cycle of the malaria parasite in 1897 (identifying the mosquito as carrier), the transmission of malaria to birds by bites of infected insects (1898), and was awarded the Nobel Prize in 1904.

1857   *Louis Bard* born. A physician from Switzerland who described pulmonary metastasis in cancer of the stomach (Bard syndrome, 1888).

1857   The Higginson syringe, consisting of a nozzle, rubber reservoir and pump used for giving enemas, was devised by English surgeon, Alfred Higginson.

1857   *Sir Charles Scott Sherrington* born. An English physiologist and neurologist who demonstrated decerebrate rigidity by transection of the spinal cord through the upper part of the midbrain (1897), established the knee jerk reflex as an

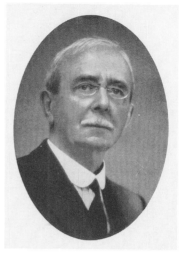

Sir Charles Scott Sherrington

inherited phenomenon (1893), and first used the term motor unit (1925).

1857   Louis Pasteur proved that microorganisms were the cause of fermentation, undermining the theory of spontaneous generation.

1857   *Robert Tuttle Morris* born. A surgeon in New York who described the point of maximum tenderness (Morris point) in acute appendicitis.

1857   *Pierre Félix Lagrange* born. A French ophthalmologist who devised a drainage procedure (cyclodialysis) for glaucoma in 1907.

1857   *John MacIntyre* born. A laryngologist in Scotland and a pioneer in clinical radiology, who established a department of radiology, and constructed the first portable X-ray unit.

1857 *Jules François Babinski* born. A Paris physician from Poland who is recognized for his work on hysteria, described dystrophia adiposa genitalis (1900), the Babinski reflex, and Babinski syndrome.

1857 Uremic pericarditis in cases of renal failure was studied by Heinrich von Bamberger of Germany.

1857 *Hendrick Zwaardemaker* born. A German physiologist who made careful and detailed studies on the functional aspects of the sense of smell.

1857 *Sir Archibald Edward Garrod* born. A London physician who was a pioneer in the study of inborn errors of metabolism, including alkaptonuria, cystinuria and pentosuria (1909).

1857 *John Templeton Bowen* born. An American dermatologist who described a variant of basal cell epithelioma which occurred as a precancerous lesion of the skin (intra-epidermal epithelioma, or Bowen disease, 1912).

1857 *John Jacob Abel* born. An American biochemist who constructed the first membrane for artificial kidneys, and did the first extraction of epinephrine, found posterior pituitary hormones, specific amino acids from the blood, determined the molecular weight of cholesterol, and crystallized insulin.

1857 *Otto Tiger Freer* born. A surgeon from Chicago who described the surgical correction of deflected nasal septum (Freer operation) in 1903.

1857 *Royal Whitman* born. An orthopedic surgeon from New York who described an operation for ununited fracture of the neck of the femur (1921).

1857 *Wilhelm Ludwig Johannsen* born. A Danish botanist and geneticist who coined the term gene to denote the unit of heredity, introduced the concepts genotype and phenotype (1902), and wrote the influential work, *Elements of Heredity* (1909).

1857 The stratum lucidum of the epidermis (Oehl layer) was described by Eusebio Oehl, professor of histology at Pavia in Italy.

1857 *Julius Wagner-Jauregg* born. An Austrian neurologist and Nobel laureate (1927) who investigated the relationship between cretinism and goiter, and treated late stage paralysis in syphilis by inducing malarial fever.

1857 *Sir Frederick William Hewitt* born. A London physician and pioneer in anesthetics who designed the first portable apparatus for administering nitrous oxide and oxygen for dental and other short operations (1888).

1857 Swedish physician, Pehr Henrick Malmsten, described *Balantidium coli*, a protozoan parasite in the large intestine.

1857 *Vladimir M. Bekhterev* born. A Russian neurologist who studied brain morphology, discovered the superior vestibular nucleus, described numbness of the spine and a new form of spondylitis.

1857   *John Alexander MacWilliam* born. A professor of physiology at Aberdeen, Scotland who gave the first account of death due to ventricular fibrillation, and devised the MacWilliam test for albuminuria.

1857   *Eugene Bleuler* born. An Austrian psychiatrist from Vienna who used the term 'schizophrenia' to include dementia praecox (1911), and developed the concepts autism and ambivalence.

1857   *James Percivall Tuttle* born. A New York surgeon who designed a rectal speculum with an electric light attached to its extremity, and capable of inflating the rectal ampulla (Tuttle proctoscope).

1857   *Fedor Victor Krause* born. A Berlin surgeon who described the Krause operation for trigeminal neuralgia, involving extra-dural excision of the gasserian ganglion.

1857   *Carl Garré* born. A surgeon from Switzerland who described a form of chronic non-suppurative sclerosing osteomyelitis (Garré disease).

1857   An early description of pityriasis rubra (Hebra pityriasis or tinea cruris) was given by Austrian dermatologist, Ferdinand Ritter von Hebra.

1857   *Sir Robert William Philip* born. A Scottish pioneer in the study and control of tuberculosis, who established the first tuberculosis dispensary in the world in Edinburgh in 1888.

1857   The central fossa between the two cavities of the larynx (Merkel fossa) was described by Carl Ludwig Merkel, a professor of laryngology at Leipzig, Germany.

1858   Professor of pathology at Dresden, Friedrich August von Ammon, described the cilia on the inner surface of the ciliary body of the eye (Ammon filaments).

1858   *Willard Myson Allen* born. A Berlin physician who devised the cornet forceps for holding litmus paper while testing urine.

1858   *Edmond Weill* born. A French pediatrician who described the absence of expansion in the subclavicular region of the affected side in infantile pneumonia (Weill sign).

1858   Interstitial keratitis, deafness, and pegged incisor teeth in congenital syphilis (Hutchinson triad) were described by Jonathan Hutchinson.

1858   *Bernard Parney Sachs* born. An American neurologist who worked on mental and nervous diseases, wrote on amaurotic familial idiocy, and published *Nervous Diseases of Children*.

1858   *Ludwig Bruns* born. A German neurologist from Hannover who described vertigo as a result of sudden movements of the head, caused by cysticercosis of the 4th ventricle in the brain (Bruns syndrome).

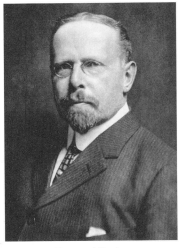

Bernard Sachs

1858   The first official publication of the *British Phamacopeia*.

1858   *Richard Friedrich Johannes Pfeiffer* born. A Polish bacteriologist who discovered *Haemophilus influenzae*, and demonstrated bacteriolysis which provided the first scientific evidence for the presence of antibodies.

1858   *Christian Eijkman* born. A Dutch physician and Nobel laureate (1929) who proposed the cause (and cure) of beriberi while serving in the Dutch East Indies, and described the concept of essential food factors (vitamins).

1858   French physiologist, Claude Bernard discovered the vasodilator fibers in the chorda tympani, and by stimulating this nerve demonstrated an increase in blood flow to the area.

1858   *Sir Robert Jones* born. An English orthopedic surgeon who advocated active surgical intervention, and pioneered bone grafting and other reconstructive procedures.

1858   *Carl Harko von Noorden* born. A Viennese co-worker with Bernard Naunyn who studied diabetes and laid down the principles of the antidiabetic diet before the insulin era.

1858   *Gabriel Anton* born. An Austrian neurologist who linked brain pathology with psychology in pioneering work on the lack of self-perception of deficits in patients with cortical blindness and deafness, Anton syndrome (1899).

1858   *Alexander Duane* born. A New York oculist who used a candle flame and prism to measure the degree of ocular heterophoria (Duane test), and described congenital fibrosis of the external rectus (Duane syndrome).

1858   *Max Friedmann* born. A German physician who described a form of relapsing infantile spinal paralysis (Friedmann disease).

1858   Experiments were conducted on chloroform by John Snow of London, who specialized in anesthesia, and wrote *On Chloroform and other Anaesthetics* in the same year.

1858   *Paul Taenzer* born. A German dermatologist who described ulerythema ophryogenes (keratosis pilaris), a skin disease characterized by the formation of a hard nodule around each hair follicle (Taenzer disease).

1858   The occurrence of pulmonary atresia together with dextroposition of the aorta was described in a treatise by Thomas Bevill Peacock of London.

1858   Tabes dorsalis was described as locomotor ataxia by Guillaume Duchenne, an eminent neurologist from Paris.

1858   Ernst Leberecht Wagner, a German surgeon, published a treatise on uterine cancer based on autopsy material, and described the path of metastases of cancer of the cervix.

1858   *Xavier Oswald Werder* born. An American surgeon who described a radical method of hysterectomy for cancer of the cervix (1898) which involved the total removal of vagina and uterus by suprapubic approach.

1858   *Pyotr V. Nikolsky* born. A Russian dermatologist who wrote extensively on syphilis, venereal disease and skin diseases, and described a clinical sign of easy dislodgment of normal epidermis under shearing stress (Nikolsky sign).

1858   *Antoine Edouard Jeanselme* born. A Paris dermatologist who described pityriasis versicolor and published a history of syphilis (1931).

1858   *John Addison Fordyce* born. A New York dermatologist who described the white or yellow spots (sebaceous cysts) on the mucosal surface of the lips, tongue or cheeks (Fordyce disease, 1896).

1858   *Harold Gifford* born. A Milwaukee ophthalmologist who described constriction of the pupils occurring when the orbicularis occuli muscle is contracted with open eyelids (Gifford reflex).

1858

Ismar Boas

Ismar Isidor Boas born. A German gastroenterologist who described hyperaesthesia below the right scapula posteriorly, and the 9th and 11th ribs, in acute cholecystitis (Boas sign).

1858   *Oskar Minkowski* born. A Lithuanian professor of medicine who established the role of the pancreas in diabetes, and showed pituitary enlargement in acromegaly.

1858   Curare was first used in medical practice to relax the muscles in tetanus.

1858   The forerunner of the General Medical Council (GMC) of the United Kingdom, the General Council of Medical Education and Registration of the United Kingdom, was established.

1858   *Nicolas Augustine Gilbert* born. A Paris hematologist who described a form of congenital hemolytic anemia (1901), Gilbert disease.

1858   Swiss physiologist Kölliker and German anatomist, Müller noted that contraction of heart muscle was accompanied by electrical activity (electrocardiography).

1858   *Ernst Tavel* born. A Swiss surgeon who prepared one of the first antistreptococcal sera (Tavel serum), and devised a method of gastrotomy (1906).

1858   The term 'rheumatoid arthritis' was coined by a consulting physician from London, Alfred Baring Garrod, to denote a form of arthritis which differed from gout. In 1859 he published a treatise on his findings, *Treatise on Gout and Rheumatism*.

1858   *Erasme Bonnaire* born. A Paris obstetrician who described dilatation of the cervix using the fingers of one hand while pressing above the pubic symphysis with the other hand.

1858   Gastrostomy was introduced into England by John Cooper Forster of Guy's Hospital.

1858   *Daniel Hale Williams* born. An American physician and founder of Provident Hospital in Chicago (1891) to provide training for black interns and the first school for black nurses in the US. He is credited with the first successful American heart surgery.

1858   Complete recovery of a patient given 6 minutes of external cardiac massage was reported by Janos Balassa of Hungary.

1858   Treatment of aneurysm by ligation of the iliac and femoral arteries was carried out by Gurdon Buck, a surgeon from New York.

1858   A method of artificial respiration in first aid (Silvester method) was devised by English physician, Henry Robert Silvester.

1859   The first operation for relief of a gastric fistula was performed by Albrecht Theodor von Middeldorpf of Breslau.

1859   *Svante August Arrhenius* born. A Swedish chemist who established the dissociation constant (1883), advanced the theory of electrolyte dissociation, formulated the effect of temperature on the rate of chemical reaction, and received the Nobel Prize for Chemistry in 1903.

1859   The National Hospital for the Relief of Paralysis, Epilepsy and Allied Disorders, the first neurological center in the world, was started in London by Louisa Chandler and her sister.

1859   *Ernst Francke* born. A German physician who described red streaks near the border of the gums in influenza (Francke sign).

1859   *Sir St Clair Thompson* born. A laryngologist from London who designed bayonet-shaped forceps (St Clair Thompson quinsy opener) to drain peritonsillar abscesses, and wrote *Cancer of the Larynx* (1930).

1859 Acute febrile polyneuritis (Landry paralysis) was described in two cases of acute ascending paralysis by German professor, Adolf Kussmaul, and later in the same year was described by Jean Baptiste Octave Landry.

Adolf Kussmaul

1859 A depression in the internal surface of the lachrymal sac (Maier sinus) was described by Rudolf Maier, professor of pathological anatomy at Freiburg, Germany.

1859 The active principle of cocaine was obtained by Albert Niemann of Germany.

1859 A detailed description of sunstroke was given by Sir Thomas Longmire, a British army surgeon in India.

1859 The Sappey vein in the venous plexus of the falciform ligament of the liver was described by Marie Philibert Constant Sappey, chair of anatomy in Paris.

1859 *William Guy* born. A pioneer of modern dentistry in Britain and a founder of the dental school at Edinburgh.

1859 The theory of vision which ascribed separate functions to rods and cones in the retina was proposed by German zoologist, Max Johann Sigismund Schultze.

1859 Jerky movements and alcholalia, in hysteria and schizophrenia (Bamberger disease), were described by Viennese physician, Heinrich von Bamberger.

1859 *Augusta Dejerine-Klumpke* born. A French neurologist who wrote an important treatise on the neurological features of lead poisoning, and described lower brachial plexus palsy (Dejerine-Klumpke paralysis, or waiter's tip).

1859 *Theobald Smith* born. An eminent American bacteriologist who distinguished human and bovine tuberculosis, demonstrated the tick was a vector of Texas cattle fever, and formulated the principle of antibody–antigen reaction.

1859 *Albert Hoffa* born. A German orthopedic surgeon who wrote a textbook of surgery, resected the prominent ribs in scoliosis, devised machines for its correction, and described solitary traumatic lipoma of the knee (Hoffa disease).

1859 *Mark Armand Ruiffer* born. A pioneer in paleopathology who studied conditions such as tuberculosis, arteriosclerosis, and gallstones.

1859 Vomiting of blood due to gastric ulcer (hematemesis) was described by William Brinton, a physician at St Thomas' Hospital, London.

1859 *Josiah Newhall Hall* born. A physician from Colorado who described diastolic shock transmitted to the trachea due to aortic aneurysm in the thorax (Hall sign).

1859 *Ludwig Stacke* born. A German otologist who devised an operation for the removal of the mastoid and the contents of the tympanum so that the antrum, tympanum and meatus forms a single cavity (Stacke operation).

1859 *William Evans Casselberry* born. A Chicago laryngologist who devised the Casselberry position to allow swallowing following intubation.

1859 *Albert Kuntz* born. A professor of histology at St Louis University, Kentucky who described the gray ramus running from the second thoracic ganglion to the first thoracic nerve (1927).

1859 *Hermann Wolfgang Freund* born. A German gynecologist who described a limitation in expansion of the apex of the lung, occurring because of shortening of the first rib and leading to narrowing of the thoracic inlet (Freund anomaly).

1859 *William Nisbet* born. An English physician who described nodular abscess in the penis following acute lymphangitis of soft chancre (Nisbet chancre).

1859 *Julius von Hochenegg* born. A surgeon from Vienna who described

an operation for the removal of a malignant rectum through the sacral route.

1860 *Streptobacillus monoliformis* was shown as the cause of rat bite fever by a physician in the Indian Medical Service, Henry Vandyke Carter, 47 years after the first report was made by Whitman Wilcox.

1860 *Sir William Withey Gull* born. A physician at Guy's Hospital, London who described the cretinoid state in the adult (Gull disease) or myxedema (in a woman), and gave a clear description of arteriosclerotic atrophy of the kidney.

1860 Catatonia was described and named by Karl L. Kahlbaum of Germany.

1860 Early right heart catheterisation was undertaken by Frederick Pavy of Guy's Hospital to obtain blood samples for study of carbohydrate metabolism.

1860 An operating chair for surgical and gynecological procedures was devised by American surgeon, Christopher Johnston.

1860 Repeated rib resection for chronic empyema was described by A. G. Walter of Pittsburgh.

1860 *Robert Cochrane Buist* born. A Scottish lecturer in midwifery and gynecology who described the method of resuscitating an asphyxiated newborn baby by alternately holding the child on the back and stomach (Buist method).

1860   *Sir James Berry* born. A Canadian-born British surgeon who described an aneurysm of the circle of Willis which may rupture and cause subarachnoid hemorrhage (Berry aneurysm), and specialized in surgery of the cleft palate and thyroid gland.

1860   *Alexander Crever Abbott* born. A bacteriologist from Philadelphia who designed a process for detecting spores in bacteria using methylene blue and fuchsin stains.

1860   *Waldemar Mordecai Wolfe Haffkine* born. A Russian-born British physician who pioneered inoculation against cholera in India, and conducted an antiplague vaccination program using live vaccine in the Indian village of Mulkowal, accidentally killing 19 people with tetanus.

1860   *Joaquin Dominguez Albarrán* born. A Cuban-born professor of medicine who emigrated to France, and whose name is associated with the Albarrán gland in the prostate, Albarrán operation for nephropexy, and Albarrán test for kidney function.

1860   *George Neil Stewart* born. A graduate of the University of Edinburgh who (with Julius Moses Rogoff) used adrenocortical extract for treatment of adrenal insufficiency (1929).

1860   Hugh Lennox Hodge of Philadelphia published *Diseases Peculiar to Women* in which he discussed displacement of the uterus, and advocated the use of pessaries for its correction

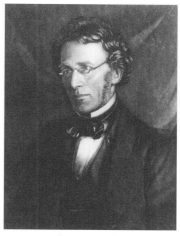

Hugh Lennox Hodge

1860   *Eduard Kaufmann* born. A German physician who undertook the first study of cartilage changes in achondroplasia.

1860   The clinical state of nervous exhaustion and asthenia was named 'nervosisme' by Paris physician, Jean Eugéne Bouchut.

1860   *Ernest Edmund Maddox* born. An English ophthalmologist who devised several visual tests and designed a number of eye instruments.

1860   *Joseph Merrick* born. A British victim of neurofibromatosis who was rescued from being a public exhibit by Frederick Treves, and was later the subject of Treves' biography, *The Elephant Man.*

1860   *William Henry Howell* born. A professor of physiology at Johns Hopkins University who discovered and isolated heparin from the liver, was the first to observe that blood pressure fell significantly during sleep, and described Howell–Jolly bodies in the blood.

1860 Enucleation of the enlarged lateral lobes of the prostate through an external incision was carried out by Austrian surgeon, Leopold Ritter von Ditte.

1860 *Augusto Ducrey* born. An Italian dermatologist who described the sexually transmitted Ducrey disease (1889), characterized by ulceration of the male and female external genitalia.

1860 *Vittorio Mibelli* born. An Italian dermatologist who described angiokeratoma (Mibelli disease), and porokeratosis.

1860 *Johannes Fabry* born. A German dermatologist who described an X-linked condition resulting in kidney failure, corneal opacities and multiple skin lesions (Fabry disease, 1898).

1860 The Delore method of forcible manual correction of genu valgum was proposed by French physician, Xavier Delore.

1860 Inflammation of the fallopian tubes (salpingitis) was described by Scottish obstetrician, Sir James Young Simpson, and was rectified by opening the abdomen and removing the ovaries and fallopian tubes by his counterpart, Lawson Tait.

1860 A classical account of eczema was given by Ferdinand von Hebra, a Viennese dermatologist.

1860 *Henri Albert Charles Antoine Hartmann* born. A professor of surgery in Paris who described the outpouch of the gallbladder near its junction with the cystic duct (Hartmann pouch, 1891), and the Hartmann operation for rectal cancer (1909).

1860 *John Scott Haldane* born. An eminent Scottish respiratory physiologist who demonstrated the physiological mechanism and toxic effects of carbon monoxide, described silicosis, the role of ferricyanide in releasing oxygen from oxyhemoglobin, examined blood gases, and produced a respiratory gas analyzer.

1860 *Mathieu Jaboulay* born. A French neurosurgeon who performed the first sympathetectomy for the relief of vascular disease (1900), interpelviabdominal amputation, and introduced gastroduodectomy (1892).

1860 *Gustav Killian* born. An otolaryngologist from Berlin, Germany who described radical treatment for diseased frontal air sinuses through an incision in the eyebrow (Killian operation, 1903).

1860 *Julian Mannaberg* born. A Viennese physician who described the accentuation of the second heart sound (Mannaberg sign) in appendicitis and abdominal disease.

1860 Prague physician, Vitem Dusan Lambl, discovered the protozoan parasite, *Giardia lamblia*, of the small intestine.

1860   *Charles Émile Achard* born. A Paris physician who introduced one of the first tests for renal function, coined the term paratyphoid fever, wrote on encephalitis lethargica, and edema in Bright disease.

1860   *S. Heinrich Frenkel* born. A medical superintendent from Switzerland who advocated the use of extensive physiotherapy for neurological disease with his introduction of exercises for tabetic ataxia (1890).

1860   *Curt Schimmelbusch* born. A German pathologist and surgeon who wrote on thrombosis, aseptic treatment of wounds, bacteria contaminating wounds, and gave a description of cystic dysplasia of the breast (Schimmelbusch disease).

1860   *Otto Lubarsch* born. A German pathologist who (with Ludwig Pick) described scleroderma macroglossia and skeletal muscle involvement with amyloid and scleroderma (Lubarsch–Pick syndrome), and introduced the term hypernephroma to describe Grawitz tumors.

1860   *Louis F. Wickham* born. A French dermatologist who described striation on the top of pruritic papular rash of lichen planus (Wickham striae), appearing as lines or small white dots among the classically itchy and shiny polygonal papules.

1860   *K.W. Hurthle* born. A German histologist who described thyroid adenoma, composed of large epithelial cells with acidophilic cytoplasm (Hurthle cell adenoma).

1860   *Diseases of the Ear* was published by Joseph Toynbee, a British pioneer in otology, who also devised a speculum for examination of the ear.

1860   *Willem Einthoven* born. A Dutch physiologist and Nobel laureate (1924) who simplified measuring time-related electrical changes in tissues with his string galvanometer (1903).

1860   *Arthur Dean Bevan* born. A Chicago surgeon who devised the Bevan operation for undescended testis (1899).

1860   *Sir William Maddock Bayliss* born. A physiologist from England who developed the concept of the hormone and the feedback mechanism, during pioneering studies on secretin and other hormones.

1860   The modern otoscope was invented by Anton Friedrich von Tröltsch of Germany.

1860   Eugéne Joseph Woillez of France devised an instrument made of jointed whale bone (cyrtometer), for tracing the outline of the chest wall on paper during respiration.

1860   Curare was first used in medical practice to relax the muscles in epilepsy.

1860   A familial liver disease accompanied by cirrhosis and involuntary movements, caused by a disorder in copper metabolism (hepatolenticular degeneration), was described by Friedrich Theodor von Frerichs.

1860 *Robert H. Russell* born. An Australian orthopedic surgeon who was the first to resect an osteostoma of the lower ulnar, and substitute a cadaveric graft.

1860 *William Dobinson Halliburton* born. A professor of physiology from King's College, London who wrote *The Essentials of Chemical Physiology* (1892), and was the first to study the chemical composition of cerebrospinal fluid.

1860 *Thoma Jonnesco* born. A professor of surgery at Bucharest who described the retro-duodenal fossa (Jonnesco fossa or fold, 1889), and carried out an operation for removal of the cervical ganglia of the sympathetic trunk (Jonnesco operation).

1860 The first complete life history and morphology of *Echinococcus* was provided by German zoologist, Karl Georg Friedrich Rudolph Leuckart.

1860 *Eduard Spiegler* born. A dermatologist from Vienna who (with German dermatologist, Heinrich Fendt) described lymphocytoma cutis (Spiegler–Fendt sarcoid).

1860 Malignant cells in sputum were identified by Lionel Smith Beale of King's College, England, his findings formed the basis for analysis for malignant cells in the diagnosis of lung carcinoma

1861 *Clinical Notes on Pericarditis* was published by Sir William Tennant Gairdner, professor of medicine in Glasgow, Scotland.

1861 *Jean Danysz* born. A Polish bacteriologist who studied plague, used radium to treat malignant tumors, described a decrease in antitoxin neutralizing capacity when toxin is added incrementally rather than all at once (Danysz phenomenon), and discovered a group of paratyphoid bacilli named after him.

1861 *Archiv für Klinische Chirurgie* was founded by German surgeon, Bernard Conrad von Langenbeck.

1861 Simultaneous right heart and left arterial catheterisation in horses was performed by Etienne Marey and Auguste Chauveau of France.

1861 Defibrinated blood to prevent clotting during experimental blood transfusions on animals was used by Jean Louis Prevost, a physiologist from Switzerland.

1861 Cerebral palsy with mental deficiency and muscle weakness in the newborn (Little disease) due to a variety of causes such as asphyxia, birth injury, and prematurity was described by William John Little of London.

1861 *Sir Almroth Edward Wright* born. An English bacteriologist who

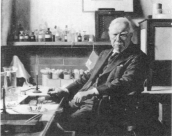

Sir Almroth Wright

developed a typhoid vaccine, worked on parasitic diseases, and contributed to the discovery of a thermolabile substance in the serum acting on bacteria during phagocytosis (opsonin, 1903).

1861   *Eugen Steinach* born. A Viennese surgeon who proposed the role of hormonal factors in the female reproductive cycle (1911), and attempted experimental ligation of the vas deferens for impotence (1920).

1861   *Dimitri Leonidovitch Romanovsky* born. A Russian physician who devised Romanovsky stain (eosin and methylene blue stain for studying blood films) to demonstrate that malarial parasites were damaged during treatment with quinine, a landmark in chemotherapy.

1861   American neurologist, Charles Gilbert Chaddock, described an extensor plantar response obtained by stroking the skin in the area of the external malleolus in cases of pyramidal tract lesions (Chaddock sign).

1861   The association between gallstones and cancer was suggested by Friedrich Theodor von Frerichs in *Clinical Treatise on Diseases of the Liver.*

1861   *Gilford Hastings* born. An English surgeon who described mixed premature and immature development, progeria.

1861   American surgeon from Benton, New York, Erastus Bradley Wolcot,

was the first to perform nephrectomy.

1861   *Arthur van Gehuchten* born. A Belgian anatomist who devised a fixing method for tissue in a mixture of glacial acetic acid and chloroform (van Gehuchten method).

1861   *On Scrofulous Diseases of the External Lymphatic Glands* was written by P.C. Price, a surgeon to the Great Northern Hospital and the Metropolitan Infirmary at Margate, England.

1861   *Carl Fraenkel* born. A German bacteriologist who described the characteristic pathology in smaller arteries and arterioles found in lesions resulting from typhus, and demonstrated artificial immunity to diphtheria in guinea pigs injected with an attenuated strain of the bacillus (1890).

1861   *Fred Neufeld* born. A German bacteriologist who described bacteriotrophins (1904), and demonstrated lysis of pneumococci by bile salts.

1861   *Karl Herxheimer* born. A German dermatologist who described chronic atrophic acrodermatitis and acute exacerbation of syphilitic lesions (Herxheimer reaction).

1861   Erythema induratum scrophulosorum accompanied by a positive tuberculin test (Bazin disease) was described by French dermatologist, Antoine Bazin.

1861   Louis Pasteur prepared a modern medium for bacterial culture.

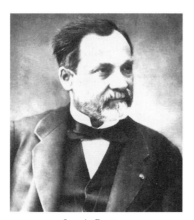

Louis Pasteur

1861   *Alessandro Codivilla* born. An Italian orthopedic surgeon who wrote on tendon transplantation and the redistribution of muscles power around the joints, using this in treatment of spastic paralysis.

1861   *John William Ballantyne* born. A Scottish gynecologist, regarded as the father of antenatal care in Britain, who wrote *Deformities of Foetus* (1895), and campaigned for improved antenatal care.

1861   *James Bryan Herrick* born. A physician and cardiologist from Illinois who described the clinical features of sudden coronary artery occlusion (1912), and gave the first description of sickle-cell anemia (1910).

1861   Two separate murmurs heard over the femoral or brachial artery during diastolic and systolic phases of the heart in cases of aortic insufficiency were described by French physician, Louis Paul Duroziez (Duroziez sign).

1861   *Sir Henry Head* born. A London neurologist who mapped the cutaneous areas of the sensory nerve roots related to visceral organs (1893), and published an important work on speech defects, *Aphasia and Kindred Disorders of Speech (1926)*.

1861   *Samuel Louis Ziegler* born. A Philadelphia ophthalmologist who designed a V-shaped iridectomy for creating artificial pupils (Ziegler operation).

1861   *Christian Georg Schmorl* born. A German professor of pathology who found small cartilaginous intervertebral disc protrusions, believed to be degenerative in nature (Schmorl nodes, 1926), during postmortem examination.

1861   *Friedrich Obermayer* born. An Austrian physiological chemist who devised the Obermayer test to detect indican in urine, using lead acetate as reagent.

1861   British surgeon and gynecologist, Sir Spencer Wells, performed the first hysterectomy for myoma.

1861   J.H. Salisbury of Ohio attempted to establish a diagnosis of Farmer's lung by skin testing.

1861   A classic account of pyemia or septicemia was given by Sir Samuel Wilks of Guy's Hospital, London.

1861   The first experiments on dialysis were carried out by Thomas Graham, a chemist from Glasgow, who used a simple dialyzer made of parchment tied to the end of a large-mouthed funnel.

1861   A condition of painful spasm of the vaginal muscles during sexual intercourse (vaginismus) was described by American gynecologist, James Marion Sims.

1861   The lines of normal tension in the skin indicating the direction along which the skin stretches least were noted and mapped by Austrian anatomist, Carl von Langer.

1861   *Achille Sclavo* born. An Italian bacteriologist in Rome who developed an antiserum for anthrax.

1861   *G.E. Brewer* born. A New York surgeon who described Brewer kidney, related to hematogenous abscesses following septicemia.

1861   *William James Mayo* born. One of the great reformers of American medicine and co-founder of the Mayo clinic who devised a new procedure of partial gastrectomy for carcinoma of the pyloric end of the stomach (1900).

1861   *Hugo von Feleki* born. A Hungarian urologist who devised an instrument for massaging the prostate gland (Feleki instrument).

1861   Ménière syndrome, characterized by episodic vertigo, tinnitus and progressive deafness, was described by French otorhinologist, Prosper Ménière.

1861   *Pierre Luis Ernest Delbet* born. A Paris surgeon who described an operation for fractured neck of the femur in which a bone graft was applied to the femoral neck.

1861   A systematic account of various operative methods for induction of labor in the recent past, was given by English obstetrician, Robert Barnes.

1861   *Alfred Theodore MacConkey* born. An English bacteriologist who developed MacConkey agar for culture of bacteria, consisting of a mixture of malachite green, bile, dextrose, and meat.

1861   *Wilhelm Hendrix Cox* born. A Dutch bacteriologist who introduced a process of impregnating nerve cells and neuroglia with potassium salts, mercuric chloride and ammonia for histological studies.

1861   *Sir Frederick Gowland Hopkins* born. Nobel laureate (1929) and regarded as the father of British biochemistry, he discovered the amino acid, tryptophane (1901), first noted additional dietary

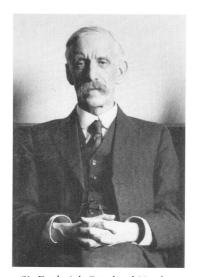

Sir Frederick Gowland Hopkins

factors (vitamins) were required to maintain good health (1906), and studied lactic acid accumulation in muscle fatigue.

1861 *Charles Henry May* born. Chief of the eye clinic of Colombia University who designed a simple self-illuminating ophthalmoscope and published *Manual of Diseases of the Eye* (1906).

1861 *August Karl Gustav Bier* born. A German surgeon from Kiel who studied tissue response to local asphyxia produced by the deprivation of blood (1887), and used cocaine as a spinal anesthetic (1889).

1861 The deep and superficial lymphatic plexus on the wall of the stomach (Teichmann plexus) was described by Ludwig Carl Teichmann-Stawiarski, professor of anatomy at Cracow, Poland.

1861 The role of the eustachian tube in swallowing was described by Joseph Toynbee, the first aural surgeon at St Mary's Hospital in London.

1862 *Maurice Nicholas Arthus* born. A French physiologist who discovered the antigen-antibody (IgE) reaction which results in local reaction and tissue damage (1903).

1862 A test for visual acuity (Snellen chart) was devised by Hermann Snellen, a Dutch ophthalmologist from Utrecht.

1862 The muscle spindle or the stretch afferent, a neuromuscular end organ of the muscle (Ruffini corpuscle), was studied by Willy Kühne, and later in detail by Italian professor, Angelo Ruffini.

1862 *Adolf Wallenberg* born. A German neurologist who described Wallenberg syndrome of ipsilateral loss of pain sensations in the face, with contralateral hypoesthesia for pain and temperature of the trunk due to occlusion of the posterior cerebellar artery (1895).

1862 *Rudolf Frank* born. An Austrian surgeon who described a method of gastrotomy in which a part of the stomach was drawn through the chest wall and a tube inserted into it to maintain a passage.

1862 *James Haig Fergusson* born. A Scottish obstetrician who designed the Haig Fergusson forceps, with a pelvic and cephalic curve and axis traction handle fitting on to the handles of the blades.

1862 A domette-covered, wire-framed mask for administration of volatile anesthetics was introduced by English obstetrician, Thomas Skinner.

1862 *Franklin Burr Mallory* born. An American pathologist who pioneered the study of stains in histology and devised the Mallory stain for collagen fibers (1900).

1862 *László Udránsky* born. A physiologist from Hungary who devised the Udránsky test for detecting bile, using furfurol as reagent. (1890)

1862 *Edwin Ellen Goldmann* born. A surgeon from Freiburg who described a two-stage operation for the removal of a pharyngeal diverticulum (1909).

1862   *Henry Smith* born. A British surgeon in the Indian Medical Service who devised the clamp and cautery treatment of hemorrhoids, and described a method of extracting cataracts in the capsule (1905).

1862   *Ernest Dupré* born. A French physician who described a form of psychoneurosis in which the patient makes a conscious effort to control his symptoms (Dupré disease).

1862

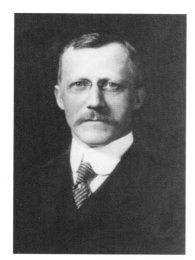

Thomas Gilchrist

Thomas Casper Gilchrist born. A Baltimore dermatologist at the Johns Hopkins University who described a chronic granulomatous lesion of the skin associated with bony lesions, caused by a fungus (1897).

1862   The alimentary enzyme trypsin was discovered by German biochemist, Willy Friedrich Kühne.

1862   *Hans Kehr* born. A German surgeon who described pain in the left shoulder in cases of splenic rupture due to diaphragmatic irritations from free blood in the peritoneum.

1862   The Austin Flint murmur, an apical mid-diastolic or presystolic functional murmur originating from the mitral valve in patients with aortic stenosis, was described by Austin Flint of New York.

1862   A network of autonomic nerve fibers in the intestinal wall (Auerbach plexus) was described by German neuropathologist, Leopold Auerbach.

1862   An operative treatment of the condition, phimosis, by rupturing the mucous membrane of the prepuce, was described by American surgeon, Joseph Pancoast.

1862   *George Ferdinand Isidore Widal* born. A French microbiologist who devised the Widal test for typhoid fever based on the agglutination reaction observed previously by von Gruber and Durham,

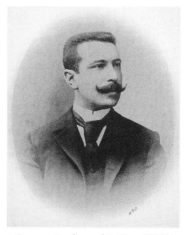

George Ferdinand Isidore Widal

which showed that the reaction was to infection rather than to immunity.

1862 *Alfred Dührssen* born. A German gynecologist who introduced a vaginal operation for myomectomy and other gynecological conditions.

1862 *Knud Heldge Faber* born. A Danish physician who described microcytic hypochromic red blood cells, acholorhydria and glossitis associated with chronic iron deficiency anemia (Faber syndrome, 1909).

1862 Raynaud disease was described by French physician, Maurice Raynaud of Paris, who presented several cases of intermittent cyanosis on exposure to cold, as local asphyxia of extremities.

1862 One of the first books on orthopedics, *Lectures on Orthopedic Surgery*, was published in America by Louis Bauer.

1862 *Malcolm La Salle Harris* born. A Chicago surgeon who described the hepatoduodenal band consisting of a fold of peritoneum from the gallbladder to the cystic duct across the transverse colon (Harris band).

1862 A systematic study of hemoglobins or metalloporphyrins was carried out by German physiological chemist, Felix Immanuel Hoppe-Seyler.

1862 Thomas Joseph Clover, a leading English anesthetist, invented a quantitative chloroform inhaler.

1862 *Lothar von Frankel-Hochwart* born. An Austrian neurologist who described cochlear, vestibular and trigeminal lesions (Frankel-Hochwart disease) seen in early syphilis.

1862 *Alvar Gullstrand* born. A Swedish professor of ophthalmology and Nobel laureate (1911) who analyzed the mechanism of visual accommodation and invented the slit lamp (1903) which made microscopic study of the living eye possible.

1862 *Franklin Paine Mall* born. A professor of anatomy at the Johns Hopkins University who described the small areas of splenic pulps (Mall lobules) within the spleen (1898).

1862 *American Journal of Obstetrics*, the first specialized journal published in America, was founded by Abraham Jacobi and Emil Noeggerath.

1863 A self-registering clinical thermometer was introduced by English physician, William Aitkin, of the Royal Victoria Hospital, Netley.

1863 *Leonardo Gigli* born. An Italian gynecologist who devised the Gigli operation for sectioning the pubis in cases of difficult labor.

1863 *Alexandre Émile John Yersin* born. A Swiss-born bacteriologist who isolated bubonic plague bacillus, *Yersinia pestis*, from humans in Hong Kong, and developed an antiserum for plague.

1863 Leptospirosis (Weil disease) was described by Jeffrey Allen Marston after Adolf Weil had published four cases of infectious jaundice with hemorrhage.

1863 Silver stain, used to study nerve endings in muscles, was introduced by Julius Friedrich Cohnheim, a German pathologist from Poland.

1863 *Charles Lyman Greene* born. A Minnesota physician who described the physical sign of cardiac borders being displaced during respiration in cases of pleural effusion.

1863 Paralysis of the vocal cords due to a recurrent laryngeal nerve lesion was noted by Berlin physician, Carl Adolf Christian Jacob Gerhardt.

1863 A syndrome of hemiplegia with contralateral paralysis of the oculomotor nerve secondary to a lesion in the cerebral peduncle (Weber syndrome) was described by London physician of German origin, Sir Herman Weber.

1863 Leading London dermatologist, William Tilbury Fox, published the first book on fungi of medical importance, *Skin Diseases of Parasitic Origin*, and the following year published *A Treatise on Skin Diseases*.

1863 *Thomas James Watkins* born. A Chicago gynecologist who designed the Watkins operation for prolapse of the uterus where the bladder is separated from the wall of the uterus, so that the uterus is left in position to support the entire bladder.

1863

Simon Flexner

Simon Flexner born. A Louisville bacteriologist and the first director of the Rockefeller Institute (1903) who discussed *Shigella flexneri* (the causative agent of dysentery), and prepared antiserum to treat cerebrospinal meningitis (1908).

1863 Franz Ernst Christian Neuman, professor of pathological anatomy at Königsberg, Germany, described the semicalcified layer of the matrix (Neuman layer) surrounding dentine.

1863 The lateral nucleus of the eighth nerve was described by German physician, Otto Friedrich Carl Deiters, who also discovered astrocytes in nervous tissue in the same year.

1863 *Georges Marinesco* born. A neurologist from Bucharest, Rumania who described trophic changes in the skin of the hand in cases of syringomyelia, and showed that the pituitary was essential for life.

1863 *Edvard Ehlers* born. A German dermatologist who gave a description of a hereditary connective tissue disorder characterized by hyperelasticity and skin fragility, the formation of pseudotumors and overextensibility of joints, Ehlers-Danlos syndrome.

1863   *Wilhelm His Jr* born. A German physician who described trench fever (Volhynia fever), and the atrioventricular bundle which conducts impulses to the heart and which bears his name (1893).

1863   The mechanism of hearing based on resonance, previously mentioned by Albrecht von Haller, was analyzed and explained by German professor of physiology, Hermann von Helmholtz.

1863   *Theodore Fisher* born. A London physician who described a systolic murmur heard in cases of adherent pericardium which was later found to be associated with mitral stenosis.

1863   *Alfred Kirstein* born. A laryngologist in Berlin who developed the first direct laryngoscope (1895).

1863   *Adalbert Czerny* born. A Berlin pediatrician who described deficiency anemia (Czerny anemia) in infants with a deficient diet.

1863   The five branches of nerves arising from the spheno-palatine ganglion (Randacio nerves) were described by an anatomist at the University of Palermo, Francesco Randacio.

1863   The spaces in the anterior section of the retina near the ora serrata were described by Robert Blassig, director of the Ophthalmic Hospital at St Petersburg.

1863   *Albert Abrams* born. A German physician in San Francisco who invented spondylotherapy (1910) in which he applied pressure to various points in the spine as treatment for a variety of illnesses.

1863   *Donald Ross Paterson* born. A British otorhinologist who designed the bronchoscopic forceps for the removal of foreign bodies or biopsy, and described Kelly–Paterson syndrome (1919).

1863   The complete resection of the hip joint with creation of an artificial joint was first performed by Lewes Albert Sayre, an orthopedic surgeon from New Jersey.

1863   *Cecil Price Jones* born. A pioneer in hematology from Guy's Hospital whose first set of papers on the diameters of red blood cells led to the establishment of normal values of red cell size and hemoglobin concentration.

1863   A rise in blood pressure due to carbon dioxide in asphyxia was noted by Ludwig Traube, professor of medicine from Berlin.

1863   German physiologist, Eduard Pflüger, showed linear arrangement of sex cells during the development of the ovary.

1863   German physiologist, Albert von Bezold, described the nerve ganglia in the interauricular septum, the Bezold ganglia.

1863   *Albert Frank Stanley Kent* born. An English physiologist who carried out research on the mammalian heart, and described the specialized band of cardiac connective tissue at the atrioventricular junction (bundle of Kent, 1893)

1863   *John Clarence Webster* born. An American gynecologist from the Rush Medical College, Chicago who described an operation for retroversion of the uterus (1901).

1863   Speech impairment, lateral curvature of the spine, and swaying of the body with irregular movements (Friedrich ataxia) was described by Nikolaus Friedrich, a German physician from Heidelberg.

1863   *Leo M. Crafts* born. A Minneapolis neurologist who described dorsiflexion of the great toe occurring when the anterior surface of the ankle is stroked in cases of pyramidal tract lesions.

1863   *William Phillips Dunbar* born. An American physician who studied the role of pollen in hay fever and introduced a serum against pollen (1905).

1863   Dermatomyositis, a form of connective tissue disease involving inflammation of muscle and overlying tissue, was described by Ernest Leberecht Wagner.

1863   *William Gibson Spiller* born. An American neurologist who described arachnoiditis and chronic inflammation of the spine in a patient as meningitis circumscripta spinalis, one of the earliest descriptions.

1863   *Charles Donovan* born. A Scottish physician and microbiologist who demonstrated the characteristic staining bodies in the spleen of patients with kala azar at autopsy (1903), and was the first to identify these in the splenic blood of live patients.

1863

Leon Charles Albert Calmette

Leon Charles Albert Calmette born. A French bacteriologist and follower of Pasteur who is best remembered for his work with Camille Guérin in the development of the first vaccine against tuberculosis (BCG: Bacillus Calmette–Guérin, 1908).

1864   Use of wire thread to stimulate clot formation in an aneurysm was introduced by English surgeon, Charles Hewitt Moore.

1864   Rib resection for empyema was suggested by W. Roser of Germany.

1864   *Henri Triboulet* born. A French physician who isolated streptococci from patients with acute rheumatism (1898), and devised a fecal test for intestinal tuberculosis, which is now obsolete.

1864 A collective study of speech defects was carried out by English neurologist, John Hughlings Jackson.

1864

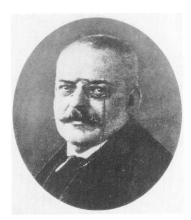

Alois Alzheimer

Alois Alzheimer born. A German psychiatrist who described the most common cause of senile dementia (Alzheimer disease) after carrying out research on the brains of demented and senile patients in Munich.

1864 *George Washington Crile* born. An Ohio surgeon and physiologist who pioneered the study of electrical shock, was one of the first to use blood transfusion and epinephrine in its treatment, and published a monograph on the subject (1899).

1864 German bacteriologist, Robert Koch, isolated *Bacillus anthracis*.

1864 *Raymond Jacques Adrien Sabouraud* born. A French dermatologist who attained a world reputation for his work on ringworm and dermatophytes, developed X-ray treatment for ringworm (1904), and devised the Sabouraud culture medium for pathogenic fungi.

1864 *Davide Giordano* born. An Italian surgeon who described the sphincter (Giordano sphincter) at the opening of the common bile duct into the duodenum.

1864 The Contagious Diseases Act, an Act of Parliament designed to combat the spread of venereal diseases, was passed in England.

1864 *William Sydney Thayer* born. An American professor at the Johns Hopkins Hospital in Baltimore who studied and described the third heart sound.

1864 An exhaustive treatise on carbolic acid was written by Parisian chemist, François Jules Lemaire.

1864 *Frederick George Novy* born. A professor of bacteriology in Michigan who identified the causative organism of American relapsing fever, the body louse (*Pediculus humanis corporis*).

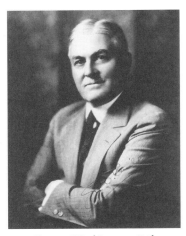

George Washington Crile

1864

Karel Wenckebach

Karel Frederick Wenckebach born. A Dutch physician who described a form of progressive atrioventricular heart block until a drop in ventricular beat occurred (Wenckebach phenomenon), and wrote on the beneficial effects of quinine in treating arrhythmias.

1864   Rarefaction of the bone due to parathyroid tumors (osteitis fibrosa cystica) was observed by Gerhard Engel of Germany.

1864   Cortical areas responsible for specific isolated movements in the body were proposed by British neurologist, John Hughlings Jackson, who described the unilateral localized form of epilepsy (Jacksonian fits).

1864   Hemoglobin was obtained in crystalline form and given its present name by Ernst Felix Emanuel Hoppe-Seyler of Germany

1864   *Antonin Poncet* born. A French surgeon who described tuberclous polyarthritis (Poncet disease).

1864   The first diagnosis of mesenteric embolism in a living subject was made by Adolf Kussmaul, an eminent professor of surgery from Germany.

1864   *Willy Sachs* born. A surgeon from Bern, Switzerland who modified Senn's bone plates for suturing intestines.

1864   The American Ophthalmological and Otological Society was founded.

1864   *Henri Fraenkel* born. A Paris ophthalmologist who described the upward rolling movement of the eye during an attempt to close the eyelids in cases of lower motor neuron paralysis of the facial nerve.

1864   An early sign of pregnancy, where softness and flexibility of the cervix could be felt on digital examination (Hegar sign), was described by Alfred Hegar, professor of obstetrics at Freiburg.

1864   *Louis Fisher* born. A New York physician who gave his name to the systolic murmur heard in the anterior fontanel of the temporal region in cases of rickets.

1864   *Ernst Wertheim* born. A German gynecologist working in Vienna who devised a radical panhysterectomy for cervical cancer (1898).

1864   German ophthalmologist, Edwin Theodor Saemisch, described cataract due to the effect of lightning.

1864   *Victor Eisenmenger* born. A German physician who described any left to right shunt which develops pulmonary hypertension with consequent reversal of the shunt and cyanosis e.g. patent ductus arteriosus, (Eisenmenger syndrome, 1897).

1865

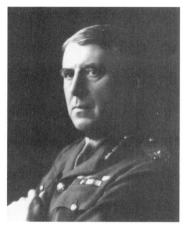

Baron Berkeley Moynihan

Baron Berkeley George Andrew Moynihan born. A British surgeon who carried out extensive work on surgical pathology of gastric and duodenal ulcers, and identified chronic gastric ulcer as a precursor of gastric carcinoma (1923).

1865   *William Edward Fothergill* born. An English gynecologist who designed a procedure involving anterior colporrhaphy combined with amputation of the cervix (Fothergill operation).

1865   *Heinrich Ernst Albers-Schönberg* born. A pioneer radiologist from Germany who described osteopoikilosis, and osteopetrosis with accompanying leukoerythroblastic anemia and hepatosplenomegaly (Albers-Schönberg disease, 1903).

1865

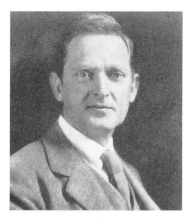

Ferdinand Zinsser

Ferdinand Zinsser born. A German dermatologist from Cologne who, with Martin F. Engman and Harold Cole, described a rare sex-linked recessive disorder, dyskeratosis congenita.

1865   *Edson Brady Fowler* born. A surgeon from Illinois who described osteotomy of metatarsal heads (Fowler procedure).

1865   The supporting cells of the testicular epithelium (Sertoli cells) were described by Enrico Sertoli, professor of experimental physiology in Milan, Italy.

1865   *Robert Heinz* born. A professor of pharmacology and toxicology in Erlangen, Germany who observed small deep purple, irregular bodies within red blood cells after staining with crystal violet (Heinz bodies, 1906).

1865   *Sir Charles Alfred Ballance* born. An English neurosurgeon who researched nerve generation and grafting, performed a mastoidectomy, and contributed towards the first removal of a spinal tumor.

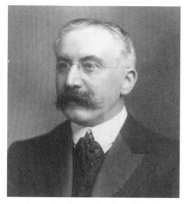

Sir Charles Alfred Ballance

1865 A locking device, introduced by French surgeons, Eugéne Koeberle and Emile Jules Pean, modified the artery forceps.

1865 *Egmont Munzer* born. A professor of medicine at Prague who described the tract from the internal geniculate body to the lateral part of the pons (Munzer tract, 1895).

1865 Malignant transformation of the acinar epithelium of the breast was described by French histopathologist, Victor André Cornil.

1865 *Ira van Gieson* born. A New York neuropathologist who devised a histological staining method for tissues, using alum–hematoxylin (van Gieson stain).

1865 *Adolf Schmidt* born. A physician from Halle, Germany who developed the Schmidt test for detection of bilirubin in feces, with mercuric chloride as reagent.

1865 Russian physiologist, Elie de Cyon, showed that stimulation of the aortic depressor nerve caused a drop in blood pressure.

1865 *Adolf Magnus-Levy* born. An American physiologist who pioneered the study of the thyroid, administered thyroid extract from animals to humans, and found that their basal metabolic rate was elevated (1895).

1865 The pathway through which food is converted to energy was shown by German physiologist, Karl von Voit, who later developed a test for basal metabolism.

1865 *Sir George Lenthal Cheatle* born. A London surgeon who devised the Cheatle forceps for removal of instruments from a steam sterilizer.

1865 *Sir William Boog Leishman* born. A Scottish parasitologist who devised Leishman stain to detect parasites in blood films of patients with kala azar (leishmaniasis), and developed an anti-typhoid vaccine.

1865 *Norbert Ortner* born. A professor of medicine in Vienna, Austria who described paralysis of the left vocal cord due to an enlarged left atrium in mitral stenosis (Ortner syndrome).

1865 Incremental lines in the substance of dentine in the teeth (Salter lines) were described by Sir Samuel James Salter of Guy's Hospital in London.

1865 The electroretinogram was devised by Alarik Frithiof Holmgren, a physiologist from Sweden.

1865 *Christian Archibald Herter* born. A pathologist in New York who described infantilism due to chronic intestinal infection (Herter disease, 1908), published studies of experimental myelitis (1889), and founded the *Journal of Biological Chemistry* (1905).

1865   Iodism, caused by chronic iodine poisoning, with an acute reaction involving the mucous membranes, was first described by Boinet in his thesis *Iodotherapie*.

1865   *Charles Franklin Hoover* born. A Cleveland physician who investigated pulmonary and hepatic disease, and the ventilatory functions of the diaphragm.

1865   *Max Askanazy* born. A German physician who was the first to relate the findings of osteitis fibrosa cystica to parathyroid tumors (1904).

1866   *Johan Albin Dalen* born. A Swedish ophthalmologist who described small white spots on the retina (Dalen spots), and nodules in the pigmented epithelium of the choroid and iris (Dalen nodules) in sympathetic ophthalmitis.

1866   Miliary aneurysms were described by Abel Henry Bouchard, who associated these with cerebral hemorrhage.

1866   *Ernest Henry Starling* born. One of the great British physiologists who devised the heart–lung preparation (1910), formulated the law of contraction for heart muscle, Starling law of the heart, and coined the term 'hormone'.

1866   Artificial insemination was used successfully in a patient with a history of 9 years of infertility by American gynecologist, James Marion Sims.

1866   *John Whitridge Williams* born. A Boston obstetrician who reported a case of chloriocarcinoma (1895), and published a textbook of obstetrics for students and practitioners (1903).

1866   Hereditary autosomal recessive disease manifesting as retinitis pigmentosa, mental retardation, polydactyly and hypogonadism was described by London ophthalmologist John Laurence and Philadelphia ophthalmologist Robert Moon.

1866   *Jesse William Lazear* born. A Baltimore doctor who deliberately and fatally allowed a mosquito to bite him during an outbreak of yellow fever in Havana in 1900, thus helping to establish the mosquito as a transmitter of the disease

1866   *Leonard Erskin Hill* born. A British physiologist who worked on respiratory physiology of caisson disease (1915) at the London Hospital.

1866   The vasomotor reflex was first discovered by Russian physiologist, Elie de Cyon and German physiologist, Carl Friedrich Wilhelm Ludwig.

1866   Carbolic acid was used as a disinfectant during the cholera epidemic in London, and was also employed for the deodorization of sewage.

1866   The recapitulation theory that the series of embryonic stages through which an animal passes during its development represents its evolutionary ancestry was advocated by the German father of modern morphology, Ernst Haeckel.

1866   *Albin Lambotte* born. A Belgian surgeon who was the first to operate for gastric ulcer, carried out an early craniotomy, and created osteosynthesis (including instruments for this).

1866   *Charles Jules Henri Nicolle* born. A French physician who became director of the Pasteur Institute in Tunis, and identified the body louse as a transmitter of typhus fever (1911), for which he was awarded the Nobel Prize in 1928.

1866   Whiplash injury was first noticed with the introduction of high speed railway travel and was described by Sir John Eric Erichson of University College, London.

1866   *Karl Albert Ludwig Aschoff* born. A German pathologist who named the endothelial system (1913), and described a characteristic histological lesion found in rheumatic carditis, the Aschoff body (1904).

1866   An attempt to view the esophagus was made by otorhinologists F. Semeleder and Karl Stoerk of Vienna.

1866   A calcified area of the lung (Ghon focus), shown on chest X-ray and due to healed primary tuberculosis, was described by Austrian pathologist, Anton Ghon.

Karl Albert Ludwig Aschoff

1866   *Jean Nageotte* born. A French physician who became professor of comparative histology at the College of France (1912), and worked on nerve grafting and the myelin sheath.

1866   The short-stemmed clinical thermometer was invented by Sir Thomas Clifford Allbutt, a British clinician.

1866   Complete excision of the larynx (laryngectomy) was performed in a case of stenosis of the larynx (due to syphilis) by Patrick Heron Watson.

1866   Tabetic gastric crisis with paroxysms of severe abdominal pain in patients with tabetic syphilis, were described by Georges Delmarre of Paris.

1866   *Paul F. Strassman* born. A German obstetrician who described engorgement of the umbilical vein following pressure on the fundus of the uterus, showing the placenta has not separated (Strassman phenomenon).

1866 The V-shaped fracture of the distal tibia (Gosselin fracture) was described by French surgeon, Leon Athanese Gosselin.

1866 *Sinding Larsen* born. A Norwegian orthopedic surgeon who gave the first description of osteochondritis of the patella, and was a director of a clinic specializing in tuberculosis.

1866 *August Paul von Wasserman* born. A German bacteriologist and director of the Institute of Experimental Therapy in Berlin who developed the complementation test for diagnosis of syphilis (Wasserman test, 1906).

1866 *Hans Held* born. A Prussian professor of anatomy at Leipzig who described the decussation of certain specific acoustic nerve fibers in the lateral fillet (a lemniscus in the trapezoid body) in 1891.

1866 *Sir Arthur Keith* born. An anatomist and anthropologist from Scotland who discovered the sino-atrial node of the heart (1907), and made many contributions to surgical pathology and anatomy, including 14 cases of esophageal atresia.

1866 French cardiologist, Pierre Carl Eduard Potain, explained the mechanism and physiology of heart sounds.

1866 *Arthur Cushny* born. A British pharmacologist at London, and Edinburgh who analyzed urinary secretion and wrote *The Secretion of Urine* (1917).

1866 *Adolf Meyer* born. A psychiatrist and neurologist from Switzerland who emigrated to America and proposed the concept of psycho-biology which integrated medicine and psychiatry, and sought to explain mental disorders on the basis of maladjustment.

1866 A classification for the mentally retarded, according to facial and body features, including one group he named Mongol, was proposed by John Langdon Haydon Down of England.

1866 *James Ewing* born. An oncologist from Cornell University Medical College in New York who described an endothelial tumor of the shaft of long bones (Ewing sarcoma, 1920), and is recognized for his work on cancer.

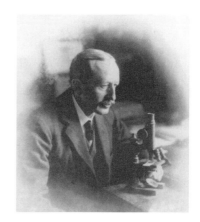

James Ewing

1866 *Claudien Phillipe* born. A director of the Pathological Anatomy Laboratory in the Salpétrérie Hospital in Paris who described the septomarginal tract in the sacral region of the cord (1901).

1866 The ophthalmic clinic at the New York College of Physicians and Surgeons was established by Rea Agnew, a professor of ophthalmology at the same clinic.

1866 *Thomas Hunt Morgan* born. A pioneer in modern genetics from Kentucky who established sex-linked inheritance while working on the *Drosophila* fly, for which he received the Nobel Prize in 1933.

1866 *Heinrich Ewald Hering Jr* born. An Austrian pathologist who studied the physiology and pathology of the heart vessels, described irregular pulse as auricular fibrillation (1903), and the branch of the glossopharyngeal nerve to the carotid sinus (1924).

1866 *Joel Ernest Goldthwait* born. A Massachusetts orthopedic surgeon who invented a procedure for recurrent patella displacement (1899), and wrote on the lumbar disc prolapse operation.

1866 The first attempt to view the interior of the chest (thoracoscopy) was made by S. Gordon of Dublin.

1867 An underwater system for closed drainage of empyema was devised by T. Hillier of London.

1867 The first use of galvanocautery in laryngeal surgery was by Swedish physician, Gustaf Samuel Crusell.

1867 A study of nitrogen metabolism in muscular work was carried out by German physician, Ludimar Hermann.

1867 Thomas Lauder Brunton, a physician from St Bartholomew's Hospital, used amyl nitrate as treatment for angina pectoris, and recognized quinism, the toxic state due to the use of quinine or cinchona and its symptoms.

1867 The Canadian Medical Association was founded.

1867 *Arthur Whitfield* born. A London dermatologist who formulated Whitfield ointment from benzoic and salicylic acid, to treat fungal infections.

1867 American surgeon, John Stough Bobbs from Indianapolis, performed cholecystostomy.

1867 *Aldred Scott Warthin* born. An Indiana pathologist who described exaggerated pulmonary sounds in cases of acute pericarditis (Warthin sign).

1867 *Michel Victor Pachon* born. A French physician from Bordeaux who designed a sensitive oscillometer (1909) to record arterial pulsation of the extremities.

1867 Magitot disease, a form of osteoperiostitis of the alveoli of the teeth, was described by French dentist, Emile Magitot.

1867 The first medical international congress was held in Paris.

1867   *Johannes Andreas Grib Fibiger* born. A Danish pathologist, Nobel laureate (1926), and pioneer of experimental carcinogenesis, who discovered a squamous cell carcinoma of the stomach caused by larvae of the nematode *Spiroptera neoplastica* (Fibiger tumor, 1913).

1867   The Gunning splint for fracture of the mandible was devised by American dentist, Thomas Brian Gunning.

1867   *Eugen von Hippel* born. An ophthalmologist in Göttingen, Germany who gave the first description of angiomatosis of the retina (Hippel disease, 1895).

1867   The Junker inhaler for chloroform or methylene anesthesia was introduced by German surgeon, Ferdinand Ethelbert Junker of the Samaritan Hospital, London.

1867   Louis Emil Javal of France invented the astigmometer for measuring the degree of astigmatism.

1867   *Dumitru Gerota* born. A professor of experimental surgery at the University of Bucharest, Rumania who demonstrated the technique of injecting the lymphatic system in order to visualize lymph glands.

1867   Theodor Fritsch, a military surgeon during the Franco-Prussian war, noted in studies of soldiers suffering from brain damage, that stimulation of one side of the brain caused the opposite side to twitch.

1867   *Karl Theodor Paul Polykarpos Axenfield* born. An ophthalmologist from Freiburg who designed an operation for ptosis, and described the causative bacteria of angular conjunctivitis (1896).

1867   Eminent English psychiatrist, Henry Maudsley, maintained that insanity was fundamentally a bodily disease in *The Physiology and Pathology of Human Mind*.

1867

Max Wilms

Max Wilms born. A German surgeon who studied a kidney tumor which bears his name (1899), and a unilateral tumor in children that gives rise to secondary tumors in the lungs and liver.

1867   *Harris Peyton Morsher* born. A professor of laryngology at Harvard and chief of the laryngological unit at Massachusetts General Hospital, who described the ethmoidal sinus beneath the bulla ethmoidalis (Morsher cells, 1902).

1867   *Franz von Hofmeister* born. A surgeon in Stuttgart who described a method of partial gastrectomy, where end-to-end anastomosis of the gastric remnant with the jejunum is made with the remnant being partly closed and used as a valve.

1867 A laryngoscope was used to remove a polyp on the vocal cord by American surgeon, Jacob da Silva Solis-Cohen.

1867 The spread of a tumor by metastasis (metastatic carcinoma) was first investigated by German anatomist, Heinrich Wilhelm Gottfried Waldeyer.

1867 *Edmund Biernacki* born. A Polish physician in Austria who described analgesia of the ulnar nerve in dementia paralytica and tabes dorsalis (Biernacki syndrome).

1867 *Hugo Schottmuller* born. A German professor of medicine at Hamburg who isolated *Streptococcus viridans* from the blood of patients with bacterial endocarditis (1910), and described paratyphoid (1900).

1867 *Berthold Gustav Carl Giemsa* born. A pharmacist from Germany who devised a method (Giemsa stain, 1890) for staining blood cells, and was a pioneer in chemotherapy.

1867 *Otto Knut Olof Folin* born. A Swedish professor of biochemistry who demonstrated the importance of amino acids in human digestion and metabolism (1906), and described procedures for the analysis of uric acid, sugar (1913), urea, nonprotein nitrogen and creatine (1913).

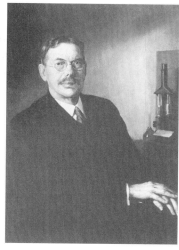

Otto Knut Olof Folin

1868 *Sir John Herbert Parsons* born. An ophthalmic surgeon and pathologist in London who published *The Pathology of the Eye*, and several other important works.

1868 Deviation of the eyes to the side of the lesion of the cerebral hemisphere was described by Swiss physician, Jean Louis Prevost.

1868 *Richard Clark Cabot* born. A Harvard professor who described the cytoplasmic ring arrangement within the red blood cells in peripheral blood of patients with megaloblastic anemia. (Cabot rings, 1897).

1868 *Eugéne Apert* born. A Paris endocrinologist and pediatrician who (with Octave Crouzon) described a condition associated with craniostenosis with oxycephaly, syndactyl, mental retardation, and visual loss (Crouzon–Apert syndrome, 1906).

1868   Friedrich Albrecht von Graefe from Berlin, the first great eye specialist, introduced linear extraction of a cataract.

1868   In *On Asthma, its Pathology and Treatment*, Henry Hyde Salter pointed out that contact with animals, foods and hayfever could all be causes of asthma, and described intrinsic asthma, and cells in sputum.

1868   *Erich Hoffmann* born. A German dermatologist and syphilologist who prepared the serum for the historic discovery of *Treponema pallidum* in 1905.

1868   *Christen Thorel* born. A German physician who described the myocardial bundle (Thorel bundle) connecting the atrial and atrioventricular nodes beside the inferior vena cava, and reported talcosis of the lung.

1868   Jean-Antoine Villemin, a French surgeon, demonstrated the infectious nature of tuberculosis by transferring it from man to rabbit.

1868   Progressive joint damage due to excessive movement range, caused by loss of pain sensation secondary to neuropathy or other neurological disease (Charcot joints) was described by French neurologist, Jean Martin Charcot.

1868   *Jabez North Jackson* born. A professor of anatomy in Kansas who described the peritoneal attachment of the cecum and the ascending colon to the right abdominal wall (Jackson membrane, 1913) producing obstruction of the bowel.

1868   *John Forssman* born. A Swedish pathologist who prepared a heterophile antigen for producing sheep red cell hemolysin (Forssman antigen) in 1929.

1868   *Felix Pinkus* born. A German dermatologist who described a rare skin disease characterized by small, flat papules, and named it lichen nitidus, or Pinkus disease.

1868   *Walter Bernard Coffey* born. A San Francisco surgeon who treated cancer by injecting an extract from the suprarenal cortex of the sheep.

1868   The first adenoidectomy was performed by Wilhelm Meyer, believing that removal of the adenoids would improve hearing.

1868   The causative spirochete of relapsing fever transmitted by the human louse (Obermeyer spirillum or *Borrelia obermeyeri*), was discovered by German physician, Otto Hugo Franz Obermeyer.

1868   A method of partial heat sterilization (pasteurization) to prevent fermentation by microorganisms or vinegar formation in wine, was demonstrated by Louis Pasteur.

1868   A treatise on the application of clinical thermometry was published by Carl Reinhold August Wunderlich, professor of medicine at Leipzig.

1868   The fasciculus gracilis or the posterior column of the spinal cord was described by a neuroanatomist from Zurich in Switzerland, Friedrich Goll.

1868

Guy Hunner

Guy L.R. Hunner born. A Baltimore surgeon and gynecologist, and one of the first students at the Johns Hopkins Hospital, who described the Hunner ulcer, a chronic vesical ulcer at the vertex of the bladder.

1868 *Korbinian Brodmann* born. A German neuropsychiatrist and pioneer in the localization of cerebral function who classified the cortical areas of the brain in numerical terms (Brodmann areas).

1868 *Ludwig Pick* born. A pediatrician and professor of pathological anatomy in Berlin who described a disorder of sphingomyelin (Niemann–Pick disease, 1926), and scleroderma macroglossia with German pathologist, Otto Lubarsch.

1868 *Alfred Simpson Taylor* born. A New York surgeon who described a method of treatment for fracture dislocation of the cervical spine in 1924.

1868 Auguste Chauveau of Paris was the first to demonstrate experimentally in animals that swallowing tubercular matter led to ulceration in the intestines (intestinal tuberculosis).

1868 *The American Journal of Obstetrics* was the first specialized journal to be published in America, later its name changed to *American Journal of Obstetrics and Gynecology*.

1868 *Thomas Stephen Cullen* born. A Canadian gynecologist who gave the first description of pathological and clinical endometrial hyperplasia, edited several gynecological textbooks, and described discoloration of the umbilicus (Cullen sign, 1916).

1868 *Leonard Wheeler Ely* born. A San Francisco orthopedic surgeon who described a sign for detecting hip lesion or psoas muscle irritation by flexing the hip (Ely sign).

1868 A detailed review of cardiac aneurysm was given by M. Pelvet of Paris, in his paper, *Des Aneurysmes du Coeur*.

1868 *Sir Frederick Still* born. A London physician at the Hospital for Sick Children at Great Ormond Street, who published *A Form of Chronic Joint Disease in Children* (1896) which contained a description of juvenile rheumatoid arthritis, known today as Still disease.

1868 *Fritz de Quervain* born. A Swiss surgeon who first used the medullary nail in a femur fracture, first described tendon sheath thickening, and described subacute thyroiditis (de Quervain thyroiditis, 1904).

1868   The gelatinous material in the external meatus in infants who are born dead (Wreden sign) was described by Robert Robertovitch Wreden, an otologist from St Petersburg Russia.

1868

Karl Landsteiner

Karl Landsteiner born. An Austrian-born American pathologist and Nobel laureate (1930) who discovered isoagglutinins in human blood (1900), and published a paper on specific blood groups, so making blood transfusion a safer option.

1868   Langerhans cells, epidermal cells involved in the immune response in contact dermatitis and which contain tubular granules whose function is unknown, were discovered by German pathologist, Paul Langerhans.

1868   *Alfred Walter Campbell* born. An Australian pathologist who defined the precentral area of the cerebral cortex (Campbell area, 1905), and carried out studies related to localization of function in the cerebral cortex.

1868   *Sir Leonard Rogers* born. A British physician who first gave emetine injections for amebic dysentery and hepatitis (1912), advocated intravenous saline in the treatment of dehydration due to cholera, and wrote *Fevers in the Tropics*.

1868   An early American classic on gynecology, *A Practical Treatise on the Diseases of Women*, was published by Theodore Thomas Gaillard of South Carolina.

1868   The concept of muscle biopsy for diagnostic studies was introduced by Guillaume Duchenne of France.

1868   An early esophagoscope consisting of two telescopic tubes was designed by Louis Waldenburg .

1869   Repair of cervical laceration was done by American gynecologist, Thomas Addis Emmet.

1869   First American university hospital was established at the University of Michigan.

1869   A more radical resection. including lower third of the pectoralis muscle for breast cancer, was described by R. Sweeting.

1869   Use of galvanopuncture to stimulate clot formation in an aneurysm was introduced by Italian surgeon, Luigi Cinicelli.

1869 The first attempt at a human electrocardiogram was made by Alexander Muirhead at St Bartholomew's Hospital.

1869 Use of a first-aid package on the battlefield was introduced by German army surgeon, Johann von Esmarch.

1869 *Henri C.J. Claude* born. A French neurologist who described ipsilateral oculomotor palsy with contralateral ataxia and hemichorea due to a lesion in the red nucleus (Claude syndrome, 1912).

1869 *Nicholas Constantin Paulesco* born. A Rumanian physician and pioneer in the study of diabetes who pointed out the causal relationship between diabetes and lesions of the pancreas.

1869 Meynert decussation on the tracts of tegmenti within the spinal canal was described by Theodor Herman Meynert, professor of neurology at Vienna, Austria.

1869 The Passavant bar, a ridge on the posterior wall of the pharynx produced by the contraction of the palatopharyngeus muscle, was described by German surgeon, Philip Gustav Passavant.

1869 The theory that the tympanic membrane of the ear, on receiving the sound, vibrated like a microphone and imparted electrical impulses to the brain, was put forward by William Rutherford of King's College, London.

1869 *John Hammond Teacher* born. A Scottish pathologist from Glasgow who reported a case of sciatica due to rupture of the intervertebral disc (1911), and wrote an early work on the human embryo.

1869 Transplantation of free skin instead of pedunculated flaps was introduced by a surgeon from Switzerland and a pioneer in skin grafting techniques, Jacques Louis Reverdin.

1869 Trichorrhexis nodosa (*Tinea nodosa*), a condition in which swellings are formed along hair shafts, was described by English physician, Francis Valentine Paxton.

1869 A form of chronic skin disease which leaves brown stains, occurring mainly in children and named urticaria pigmentosa (Nettleship disease), was described by London dermatologist, Edward Nettleship.

1869 *Georg Clemens Perthes* born. A German surgeon at Tübingen who described osteochondritis deformis juvenilis (Perthe disease), and used deep X-ray therapy in the treatment of cancer.

1869 The periodic table was proposed by Russian chemist, Dimitri Mendeleeff in his *Principles of Chemistry*, which accurately predicted the subsequent discovery of several elements.

1869 Endotracheal anesthesia through a canula after a tracheostomy was administered by German surgeon, Friedrich Trendelenburg.

1869 A form of arthritis of the hands and fingers in patients with rheumatic fever (Jaccoud disease) was described by Paris professor of pathology, Sigismond Jaccoud.

1869   *A.A. Hymans Van Den Berg* born. A Dutch physician who described the Van Den Bergh test which detects unconjugated bilirubin using diazo reagent (1900).

1869   George Miller Beard, an American physician, established the concept of asthenia and nervous exhaustion.

1869   *Artur Biedl* born. A German physician who worked on neural control of the viscera through splanchnic centers (1895), and demonstrated the importance of adrenal glands in internal secretions (1910).

1869   Sensory aphasia was described by British neurologist Henry Charlton Bastian.

1869   *Russel Aubra Hibbs* born. An orthopedic surgeon from Kentucky who described the first spinal fusion operation (1911), and designed a frame (Hibbs frame) used for the application of plaster in treatment of spinal scoliosis.

1869   *Leo Loeb* born. A German–American pathologist who, during his studies on carcinogenesis, experimentally transmitted carcinoma through several generations of animals, and showed that extirpation of the corpora lutea accelerated ovulation (1911).

1869   *Wilfred Harris* born. A neurologist from London who was the first to perform alcohol injection of the gasserian ganglion through the foramen ovale for treatment of trigeminal neuralgia.

1869   *Harvey Williams Cushing* born. An Ohio neurosurgeon who made important contributions to the study of the pituitary gland and its tumors, and classified cerebral tumors, gliomas and meningiomas, describing techniques for their removal.

Harvey Williams Cushing

1869   *Luther Crouse Peter* born. A Philadelphia ophthalmologist who designed an operation for oculomotor paralysis, which involved the transplantation of the tendon of the superior oblique muscle.

1869   *Nathaniel Bishop Harman* born. A London ophthalmologist who designed special prismatic spectacles for use by the surgeon during ophthalmic surgery, and the Bishop Harman diaphragm test for visual images.

1869   The organic base of apomorphine was obtained by English bacteriologists, Wright and Matthieson, by adding hydrochloride acid to morphine.

1869   Tumor of the meninges (meningioma), usually next to the dura mater, was first referred to as endothelioma by Camillo Golgi, a professor of histology at Pavia, Italy.

1869   Gastromesenteric ileus with distention of the duodenum proximal to the root of mesentery was classically described by Charles Hilton Fagge, of Guy's Hospital, London.

1869   *Elizabeth Hurdon* born. An associate in gynecology at Johns Hopkins University, Baltimore who was a pioneer in study of the pathology of cancer of the uterus and its treatment by radiation.

1869   *Joseph Bolivar DeLee* born. A New York professor of obstetrics who designed several obstetric instruments and was a leading figure in this field with the publication of *Principles and Practice of Obstetrics* (1913).

1869   *Ernest Amory Codman* born. A surgeon from Massachusetts General Hospital who devised the first anesthetic chart (with Harvey Cushing).

1869   The first anatomical description of the hip joint in relation to its dislocation was given by Henry Jacob Bigelow, of Massachusetts General Hospital.

1869   *Maude Elizabeth Seymour Abbott* born. A Canadian pioneer in pediatric cardiology and medical education for women who showed that congenital heart disease was associated with an 18% risk of other malformations.

1869   The first study of retinitis in glycosuria (diabetic retinopathy) was carried out by Henry Dewey Noyes of America.

1869   *Wilhelm Schlesinger* born. A Viennese physician who devised the Schlesinger test for detecting urobilin in the urine using Lugol iodine as reagent.

1869   Emanuel Frederick Hagbarth Winge of Norway demonstrated the bacterial origin of ulcerative endocarditis.

1869   *Sir James Purves Stewart* born. A British neurologist at the Royal National Orthopedic Hospital in London who wrote an important textbook of neurology, *The Diagnosis of Nervous Disease.*

1869   Light rigidity of the pupil (Argyll Robertson pupil) was described by Scottish ophthalmologist Douglas Argyll Robertson, in remarks made on the action of light on the pupil.

1869   *Martin F. Engman* born. A St Louis dermatologist at the Barnard Free Skin and Cancer Hospital who became one of the pioneers in use of radium and X-ray treatment of skin disease.

1870   Nephrectomy was first performed as a treatment for urinary tract fistula by Gustav Simon, a professor of surgery at Heidelberg, Germany.

1870 *Jay Frank Schamberg* born. A Philadelphia dermatologist who described progressive pigmentary dermatosis on the lower limbs and distinguished it from hemorrhagic manifestations (Schamberg disease, 1901).

1870 Adolf Eugen Fick became the first to calculate cardiac output by estimating the difference of oxygen content between arterial and venous blood.

1870 The first clear description of dermatitis exfoliativa, also known as Wilson disease, was originally described by English dermatologist, Erasmus Wilson.

1870 *Leopold Heine* born. An ophthalmologist at Kiel who designed an operation for glaucoma (Heine operation), where the ciliary body is separated from the sclera using a spatula.

1870 *James Stanfield Collier* born. A London neurologist who described that part of the medial longitudinal bundle within the tegmentum of the midbrain (Collier bundle).

1870 A definitive account of subacute bacterial endocarditis (SABE) was given by English physician, Sir Samuel Wilkes, as arterial pyemia.

1870 Irritation of the semicircular canals as a cause of vertigo was shown by German physiologist, Friedrich Leopold Goltz.

1870 The Langhans layer, or cytotrophoblast, which covers the chorionic villi beneath the syncytial layer was described by a German pathologist, Theodor Langhans.

1870 Plexiform neurofibroma was first described by German surgeon, Paul von Bruns.

1870 *Manfred Bial* born. A German physician who devised the Bial test for detecting pentose sugar in the urine, using hydrochloric acid as a reagent.

1870

Jules Bordet

Jules Jean Bordet born. A Belgian physiologist and Nobel laureate (1919) who described complement (1900), a thermolabile component of serum, and extracted the endotoxin from the whooping cough bacillus to make a vaccine.

1870 *Fritz August Momberg* born. A German surgeon who devised a belt for compressing the abdominal aorta in post-partum hemorrhage (1908).

226

1870   *Clarence Erwin McClung* born. An American cytologist who suggested that accessory chromosomes were determinants of sex (1902).

1870   *Ernest Marcel Labbe* born. A Paris physiologist who was the first to give a full description of chromaffin cell tumors of the adrenal medulla (1922).

1870   *Ross Granville Harrison* born. A Pennsylvania comparative anatomist who introduced the hanging drop method of tissue culture, and demonstrated the growth of nerve fiber from cells outside the organism for the first time (1907).

1870   *Sir Norman Godfrey Bennet* born. A London dental surgeon who proposed a classification for occlusion and malocclusion of the teeth (Bennet classification).

1870   *George Ludwig Zuelzer* born. A German research chemist who gave the first subcutaneous injection of pancreatic extract to a 50-year-old diabetic patient (1906), producing a temporary recovery, he then patented his preparation in 1912.

1870   *Artur Pappenheim* born. A German professor of hematology at Berlin who founded the journal *Folia Hematologica*, and devised the Pappenheim stain, a specific test for plasma cells.

1870   *George Hellhorn* born. A St Louis gynecologist who described a method of vaginal hysterectomy under local anesthesia.

1870   Corneal change in arcus senilis (a circular opacity surrounding the cornea) was associated with fatty degeneration of the heart by Jacob Mendes da Costa.

1870   Thomas Henry Huxley gave the name 'biogenesis' to his theory that living matter always arises by the agency of preexisting living matter.

1870   *Samuel Goodwin Gant* born. A New York surgeon who devised the Gant clamp, an angled clamp used in hemorrhoidectomy.

1870   *Jules Gonin* born. A Swiss ophthalmic surgeon who devised a method of operative treatment for detachment of the retina (1927).

1870   *Kiyoshi Shiga* born. A Japanese bacteriologist who graduated from Tokyo Medical School and discovered the bacillus of dysentery (*Shigella shigae*).

1870   Nodular hypertrophy of the skin and mucous membrane of the nose (rhinoscleroma) was described and named by Viennese dermatologists, Ferdinand von Hebra and Moriz Kaposi.

1870   Ingenious experiments were carried out by French physiologist, Paul Bert, in which he measured the elastic pressure of the lung while he simultaneously opened the chest wall of a dog.

1870   *Hugh Hampton Young* born. An American urologist who invented procedures for intravascular diverticulotomy, perineal prostatectomy, cystoscopes and retrourethral fistula.

1870 The production of localized motor movements and convulsions in the body due to stimulation of certain areas of the brain was demonstrated by Gustav Theodor Fritsch and Eduard Hitzig of Germany.

1870 *William Phillips Graves* born. An American gynecologist who devised an operation for uterine malposition (1923).

1870 A method of reduction of subluxation of the shoulder joint, was described by Nobel laureate, Emil Theodor Kocher, a Swiss professor of surgery at Bern.

1870 *Willibald Nagel* born. A German physiologist who devised the Nagel test for color vision, performed with a set of cards printed in concentric circles of color.

1870 An aneurysm of the hepatic artery was observed by German physician, Heinrich Irenaeus Quincke.

1870 Changes in bone marrow in myeloid leukemia were described by Franz Ernst Neuman.

1870 The stimulant effect of carbon dioxide in respiration was demonstrated by L. Herman and T. Escher.

1871 Jacob Mendes Da Costa, a physician from the Jefferson Medical College, Philadelphia, described irritable heart amongst soldiers during the American Civil War, known as cardiac neurasthenia (Da Costa syndrome).

1871 The Meyer glands beneath the tongue, in the hypoglossus muscle, were described by a professor of histology in Zurich, Georg Hermann von Meyer.

1871 Characteristics of childhood persisting into adult life (infantilism), were first used by Paul Joseph Lorain of Paris to denote idiopathic arrest of growth in connection with tuberculosis.

1871 *Edwin B. Claybrook* born. An American surgeon who described rupture of an abdominal viscus causing easy auscultation of the heart and breath sounds in the abdomen (Claybrook sign).

1871 *Christian Kjelland* born. An obstetrician from Norway who devised the Kjelland forceps (1915) used for rotation in deep transverse arrest during labor.

1871 *Alfred Fröhlich* born. An Austrian neurologist who described sexual infantilism (1900), obesity secondary to lesions of the hypothalamus, and studied the effects of the pituitary on the autonomic nervous system.

1871 A one-stage procedure for extensive cleft of the hard and soft palate (Whitehead operation) was devised by New York surgeon, William Riddick Whitehead.

1871 *Howard Taylor Ricketts* born. A microbiologist from the United States who showed that the causative agent of Rocky Mountain spotted fever was transmitted by ticks, and who researched the causative organism of Mexican typhus fever.

1871   *Maurice Marcelle* born. A French surgeon who designed a motor ambulance during World War I, and described the triangle in the ilioinguinal region (Marcille triangle).

1871   Adolf Ludwig Sigismund Gusserow, a German obstetrician, described pernicious anemia in pregnancy.

1871   Part of the mammary gland extending towards the axilla (Spence axillary tail) was described by James Spence, professor of surgery at Edinburgh.

1871   *Jan Schoemaker* born. A Dutch surgeon from the Hague who described the Schoemaker line, which connects the greater trochanter of the femur to the anterior superior iliac spine.

1871   *James Homer Wright* born. A Boston pathologist who developed Wright stain (1910), used for megakaryocytes and platelets, and who also prepared special stains for the malarial parasite (1902).

1871   *Erwin Payr* born. A professor of surgery at Leipzig in Germany who described a fold of the peritoneum over the splenic flexure of the colon (Payr membrane, 1910).

1871   *Robert Kienböch* born. An Austrian radiologist who introduced the concept of dosage in X-ray therapy, and published an 8-volume book on the diagnosis of disorders of bones and joints, and described Kienböch disease, consisting of osteochondrosis of the lunate bone (1910).

1871   *Sir Grafton Elliot Smith* born. An Australian neurologist who was an authority on brain anatomy and human evolution, and who published several important works on evolution, including *Human History*.

1871   *Gaston Millian* born. A French dermatologist who studied syphilis and other skin diseases, and described ear involvement seen in facial erysipelas (Millian ear sign).

1871   A bacterial filter made of porous clay, to separate anthrax bacteria from the medium, was developed by Tiegel.

1871   *William Zangemeister* born. A German gynecologist who described the Zangemeister maneuver, used during face presentation in delivery.

1871   *Karl Leiner* born. An Austrian pediatrician who described erythroderma desquamation (generalized dermatitis) in children with recurrent local and systemic infection, marked wasting and a deficiency of the central nervous system (Leiner disease).

1871   *Howard Davis Haskin* born. An Oregon surgeon who devised a test for urinary proteins using acetic acid and sodium chloride as reagents.

1871   *Friedrich Ernst Krukenberg* born. A German pathologist who described bilateral ovarian carcinoma (Krukenberg tumor) often used to denote ovarian secondaries from a gastric carcinoma.

1871   *Otto Naegeli* born. A hematologist and professor of medicine at Zurich, Switzerland who described myelomonocytic leukemia, and published *Lehrbuch der Blutkrankheiten und Blutdiagnostik* in 1913.

1871   *William Blair-Bell* born. A Liverpool obstetrician who used oxytocin in labor (1909), and was a founder of the Royal College of Obstetricians and Gynecologists.

1871   *Wilhelm Ellerman* born. A Danish pathologist who demonstrated that leukemia could be produced by a filterable agent (1908), and designed a skin test with tuberculin of various dilutions to gauge the severity of the disease.

1871   Sulcus intermedius primus of the cerebral cortex (Jensen sulcus) was described by Julius Jensen, director of the Allenburg Institute of Mental Diseases.

1871   Neurologist, Carl Friedrich Otto Westphal of Berlin, described agoraphobia.

1871   *Sir Robert Hutchinson* born. A physician at the Hospital for Sick Children at Great Ormond Street who was the first to isolate a globulin (1896), and described suprarenal sarcoma of children which led to secondary growths in the skull (1907).

1871   *Walter Bradford Cannon* born. An eminent Harvard physiologist who introduced the idea that involuntary reactions of the body in certain situations (fear, anger, etc.) are influenced by emotions, and coined the term 'homeostasis'.

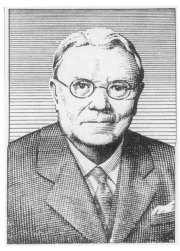

Walter Bradford Cannon

1871   An esophagoscope made of two telescopic metal tubes devised by Walderburg, was demonstrated by Stoerk at the Society of Physicians in Vienna.

1871   *Louis Dupuys-Dutemps* born. A French ophthalmologist who worked with neurologist Raymond Cestan on pupillary reflexes, and described paradoxical lid retraction present in Bell palsy (Dupuys–Dutemps phenomenon).

1871   Hammond disease, or athetosis, related to the failure to maintain a fixed posture due to abnormal involuntary movements, was described by American neurologist, William Alexander Hammond.

1871   *Alberto Barton* born. A Peruvian physician of English descent who discovered the parasite (*Bartonella*) causing Bartonellosis (1917), an acute febrile hemolytic anemia seen in South America.

1871   *Louis Ombredanne* born. An orthopedic surgeon from France who used cross-legged skin flaps, improved prostheses, and studied arthrodesis of paralyzed feet.

1871   *Charles Albert Elsberg* born. A New York pioneer in neurosurgery who published several papers on olfactory sensation and vision in 1938.

1871   *Theodore Waldemar Tallqvist* born. A physician from Finland who devised a color lithographic scale for estimating the percentage of hemoglobin in blood (Tallqvist scale).

1871

Henry Bowditch

American physiologist, Henry Pickering Bowditch, discovered all-or none phenomenon in muscle contraction and proposed a mechanism.

1871   An important monograph, *Growths in the Larynx*, was published by the father of British laryngology, Sir Morell Mackenzie.

1871   George David Pollock used skin grafts for treating contractures following burns.

1871   *Florence Rena Sabin* born. A graduate of Johns Hopkins Medical School and the first woman to be elected to the National Academy of Sciences, who studied the maturation of myeloblasts, and devised a supravital stain for leukocytes.

1871   *Fritz Richard Schaudinn* born. A German zoologist who discovered the spirochete, *Treponema pallidum*, the causative organism of syphilis (1905), and demonstrated that hookworm infection occurs through the feet.

1871   *Edville Gerhardt Abbott* born. An orthopedic surgeon from Maine who designed a treatment for scoliosis using bandages and a frame, followed by a series of plaster jackets.

1871   Henry Duret and Johann Otto Leonhardt Heubner of Germany described the distribution of blood vessels within the substance of the brain.

1871   Pulsus alterans was described and differentiated from pulsus bigeminus by Ludwig Traube, professor of pathology at Berlin, Germany.

1872   *Charles Hunter* born. A professor of medicine at the University of Manitoba who described gargoylism (1917), a hereditary disease due to a disturbance of mucopolysaccharide metabolism.

1872   Glands of the lower eyelid conjunctiva (Wolfring glands) were described by Polish ophthalmologist, Emilij Franzevic von Wolfring.

1872 *Gatian de Clérambault* born. A French psychiatrist who described a state in which the patient believes his mind is controlled by someone else or by external forces (Clérambault–Kandinsky syndrome).

1872 The first German official *Pharmacopoeia Germanica* was published.

1872 Oophorectomy for gynecological problems was used by Georgia surgeon, Robert Battey.

1872 *William Wayne Babcock* born. A surgeon in Philadelphia who described a new operative technique for thoracic aneurysm (Babcock operation, 1926), and designed a surgical method for abdominal aneurysm (1929).

1872 Intravenous chloral hydrate was tried as an anesthesia in animals by Pierre-Cyprien Orè of Bordeaux.

1872 *Wilfred Batten Lewis Trotter* born. An English neurologist who studied the pathology and symptoms of post-head injury status, defined concussion (1924), and described Trotter syndrome associated with deafness, palatal paralysis and facial neuralgia (1911).

1872 *Samuel Taylor Darling* born. An American pathologist who described histoplasmosis (Darling disease) whilst working in the Canal Zone in Panama in 1906.

1872 French surgeon, Simon Duplay, described Duplay bursitis involving the subacromial or subdeltoid bursa.

1872 The mechanism and pathology of sunstroke were explained by an American neurologist from the University of Pennsylvania, Horatio Charles Wood.

1872

Rudolph Heidenhain

Rudolph Peter Heinrich Heidenhain, a German professor of physiology and histology, demonstrated the antisalivary effects of atropine.

1872 *Fritz Steinmann* born. A Swiss surgeon who introduced the Steinmann pin (1907), which is inserted through the distal end of the fragment of a fracture, and combined with skeletal traction.

1872 A description of autumnal catarrh was given by American physician, Morrill Wyman, who also identified ragweed pollen as the cause.

1872 *Charles Laubry* born. A Paris cardiologist who pioneered the radiological method of studying the heart and blood vessels by injecting radio-opaque substances into the blood.

1872   Pericardial pseudocirrhosis of the liver was differentiated from cirrhosis by German physician, Heinrich von Bamberger.

1872   *Osvaldo Gonçalves Cruz* born. A Brazilian bacteriologist who gave his name to the causative organism of South American trypanosomiasis, *Trypanosoma cruzi*.

1872   Progressive pernicious anemia (Biermer disease) was described by Swiss professor of medicine, Anton Biermer.

1872   *Percy Theodore Herring* born. A professor of physiology from St Andrew's University in Scotland who showed the spinal origin of cervical sympathetic nerves (1903), and named the Herring bodies in the posterior lobe of the hypophysis.

1872   *Thompson Richardson Brown* born. An English physician who described the occurrence of eosinophilia and its diagnostic importance in trichinosis (1898).

1872   Impetigo herpetiformis was described by Austrian dermatologist, Ferdinand von Hebra.

1872   Julius Friedrich Cohnheim studied local or regional asphyxia (ischemia) due to blood deprivation.

1872   *Karl Ernst Wilhelm Deutschländer* born. A Hamburg surgeon who gave his name to the march fracture (Deutschländer disease) involving the metatarsal bone (usually the 2nd).

1872   *Sir Joseph Barcroft* born. A professor of physiology at Cambridge who studied changes in hemoglobin during respiration, and pioneered studies on the physiology of the developing fetus.

1872   *Hugh Cabot* born. A Minnesota urologist and specialist in the treatment of hypospadias who devised an operation for undescended testis (1936).

1872   Ablepharon, a congenital abnormality in which there are no eyebrows or palpebral fissure, and the skin is continuous from the forehead to the cheek, was described by W. Zehender.

1872   The rare familial disease accompanied by progressive involuntary movements, ataxia, and mental deterioration (Huntington chorea/disease) was observed and described by American physician, George Huntington.

1872   *Clive Rivers* born. A physician at the City of London Hospital who pioneered artificial pneumothorax in the treatment of tuberculosis, and advocated the early diagnosis and treatment of pulmonary tuberculosis.

1872   *Mervyn Henry Gordon* born. A British bacteriologist who pioneered studies on virology, described a precipitin test for differentiating between smallpox and chickenpox, and published an important study of the viruses of vaccinia and variola (1925).

1872

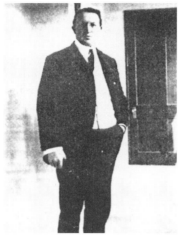

William Baer

William Stevenson Baer born. A Baltimore orthopedic surgeon who used membrane from a pig's bladder in arthroplasty, treated chronic osteomyelitis with maggots (before the advent of antibiotics), and injected oil into joints to prevent adhesions.

1872 *James Sherren* born. An English surgeon who advocated conservative management for acute appendicitis complicated by peritonitis, and studied the consequences of injury to the peripheral nerves (1905).

1872 *Ernest Hey Groves* born. An orthopedic surgeon from Britain who wrote *On the Diseases of the Joints*, detailing the use of full-thickness bone grafts.

1872 *James Ramsay Hunt* born. An American neurologist who described fresh cerebral softening in people with carotid artery lesions (1914), which led to recognition of cerebrovascular disease from extracerebral vascular involvement, and Ramsay Hunt syndrome of geniculate neuralgia.

1872 Carotid sinus syndrome, caused by an overactive carotid sinus reflex, following minimal stimulation of the carotid sinus, was described by French neurologist, Jean Marie Charcot.

1872 *Adrian Trebondeau* born. A French naval physician who proposed the theory that the sensitivity of the cells to radiation varied according to reproductive capacity and differentiation.

1872 White hemorrhagic spots seen in the retina in bacterial endocarditis (Roth spots) were described by Swiss physician, Moritz Roth.

1872 Various clinical types of lead palsy, including wrist drop, were described in detail by French neurologist, Guillaume B.A. Duchenne.

1872 *Karl Sternberg* born. An Austrian pathologist from Vienna who described Sternberg lymphoma, a mediastinal mass progressing to leukosarcoma.

1872 Pigmented sarcoma of the skin (Kaposi sarcoma) was described by Hungarian dermatologist, Moritz Kaposi.

1872 Arteriosclerotic atrophy of the kidney was described by William Withey Gull and Henry Gawen Sutton of London.

1873 The first clinical diagnosis of fat embolism was made by E. von Bergmann.

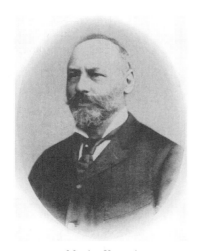

Moritz Kaposi

1873 Retinoscopy was introduced by French ophthalmologist, Ferdinand Cuignet.

1873 Local injection of carbolic acid into a lung abscess was undertaken by J. B. Saunders in America.

1873 The first removal of a foreign body (a needle) from the heart was performed by G. W. Callender in London.

1873 *Rupert Waterhouse* born. An English physician at the Royal National Hospital for Rheumatic Diseases who described suprarenal apoplexy as the cause of Waterhouse–Friderichsen syndrome.

1873 Hansen bacillus, *Mycobacterium leprae*, the causative organism of leprosy, was discovered by Norwegian bacteriologist, Gerhard Henrik Armauer Hansen.

1873 *William David Coolridge* born. A Massachusetts physicist who developed the prototype of the modern X-ray vacuum tube (Coolridge tube).

1873 A test for hearing, using a tuning fork (Gruber test) was devised by Austrian otorhinologist, Joseph Gruber at the Clinic for Ear Disease in Vienna.

1873 Tracheoesophageal fistula without esophageal atresia was recognized by D.S. Lamb of Philadelphia.

1873 Manchester physician, Charles Harrison Blackley, published his work on hay-asthma, *Experimental Researches on the Causes and Nature of Catarrhus Aestivus*.

1873 An original description of erysipeloid, a dermatitis caused by infection with *Erysipelothrix rhusiopathine*, was given by English dermatologist, William Tilbury Fox.

1873 Tuberculous cavities in the lungs as a source of intestinal lesions were

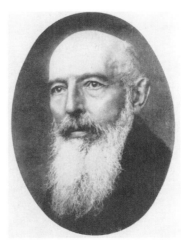

Gerhard Henrik Armauer Hansen

noted independently by Theodor Albrecht Edwin Klebs and F. Mosler of Germany. Klebs developed a fractional method of obtaining pure bacterial cultures in the same year.

1873 An early description of platelets in the blood was given by Sir William Osler, professor of medicine at Oxford, England.

1873 *Johannes Berger* born. A German psychiatrist who invented the encephalogram (1929) and used it in diagnosis of epilepsy.

1873 An infective dermatitis normally starting from a wound and remaining localized (erythema serpens) was described by London surgeon, William Morrant Baker.

1873 *J. Moritz Blumberg* born. A German surgeon and gynecologist who described rebound tenderness indicating peritoneal inflammation (Blumberg sign).

1873 A decrease in pulse volume during inspiration (pulsus paradoxus), and progressive bulbar palsy were described by German surgical professor, Adolf Kussmaul.

1873 *Georges Dreyer* born. An English pathologist who introduced a modified form of the Widal test for diagnosis of typhoid and paratyphoid (Dreyer test).

1873 *Eugene Lindsay Opie* born. A Virginia pathologist who suggested the presence of an antidiabetic substance in the islets of Langerhans of the pancreas (1903), while a

professor at the Johns Hopkins Hospital at Baltimore.

1873 One of the first descriptions of osteogenesis imperfecta (brittle bones due to defective ossification) was given by British dermatologist, Alfred Eddowes.

1873

Otto Loewi

Otto Loewi born. A German-born American pharmacologist who isolated the first neurotransmitter (1921), showing that a substance liberated from the stimulated vagus nerve ending, when perfused onto a second heart, was capable of slowing the heart beat.

1873 Henri Duret of France described the circulation of blood within the brain.

1873 *Otfried Foerster* born. A neurologist from Breslau who advocated intradural division of the posterior nerve roots as treatment for pain.

1873 *Francis Randall Hagner* born. A Washington urologist who designed an inflatable rubber bag placed in the urethra to arrest bleeding during prostatectomy, and an operation for acute epididymitis (Hagner operation).

1873   The Nuel space, between the outer rod of Corti and the adjacent row of hair cells, was described by Jean Pierre Nuel, professor of otology at Louvain in Belgium.

1873   *Max Huhner* born. A New York urologist from the Mount Sinai Hospital and originally from Germany, who devised the post-coital test for the motility of sperm, and studied male senility due to azospermia using testicular aspiration.

1873   The Volkmann canal in bones was described by German surgeon, Richard von Volkmann.

1873   *John Albertson Sampson* born. A gynecologist from Troy in the USA who described chocolate cysts of the ovary (Sampson cyst, 1921), and gave an account of pelvic lymphatics in relation to radical surgical treatment of cervical cancer (1904).

1873   *Alexis Carrel* born. A French-born surgeon who emigrated to America where he became the father of heart transplantation (1905), perfected end-to-end arterial anastomosis (1902), was the first to grow tumor tissue, and received the Nobel Prize in 1912.

1873   *Otfried O. Fellner* born. A German physician who studied reproductive endocrinology, hormonal contraception, and the function of the placenta.

1873   *Sir Andrew Balfour* born. A physician from Edinburgh who made important contributions to the study of tropical diseases, founded the Museum of Tropical Diseases, and was the first director of Wellcome Research Laboratories.

1874   *Auguste Rollier* born. A Swiss physician who advocated the use of increasing doses of sunlight in the treatment of tuberculosis (1913).

1874   The Schmidt clefts, found intersegmentally in the medullary sheath of peripheral nerves, were described by Henry Schmidt, a pathologist at the Charity Hospital in New Orleans.

1874   *Arthur Schüller* born. An Austrian physician who first developed skull X-rays for diagnosis of epilepsy.

1874   *Karl A. Hasselbalch* born. A Danish biochemist and physician who carried out pioneering work on blood pH, and with Nils Bohr and August Krogh, showed that the affinity of blood for oxygen varied with carbon dioxide pressure.

1874   Acetonemia as a cause of diabetic coma was recognized by German professor of surgery, Adolf Kussmaul.

1874   *Ernst Moro* born. An Austrian pediatrician in Vienna who described a startling reflex in infants producing an embracing attitude (Moro reflex).

1874   *Octave Crouzon* born. A French neurologist who carried out important work into hereditary dystrophies, described craniofacial dysostosis and hypertelorism due to autosomal dominant inheritance (Crouzon disease, 1912).

1874 *William George MacCallum* born. A Canadian-born pathologist who used calcium in treatment of tetany following parathyroidectomy, and first suggested the association between lesions of the islets of Langerhans and glycosuria.

1874 *Daniel Joseph McCarthy* born. A New York urologist who designed a panendoscope, prostatic electrotome, and several other instruments.

1874 The secretion theory for renal function was put forward by German professor of physiology, Rudolf Peter Heinrich Heidenhain.

1874 The giant motor cells in the fifth layer of the cerebral cortex, Betz cells were described by Russian anatomist, Vladimir Betz.

1874 *Alfred Gordon* born. A Philadelphia neurologist who described the extensor plantar response produced by squeezing the calf muscles (Gordon reflex) in cases of pyramidal tract lesions, and published an important study of the vaccinia and variola viruses (1925).

1874 *Alfred Baker Spalding* born. A San Francisco gynecologist who described an operation for uterine prolapse (1919).

1874 The infectious nature of lobar pneumonia was described by Aus-

trian physician, Theodor von Jürgensen.

1874 The conjunctival glands (Ciaccio glands) were described by Guiseppe Vincenzo Ciaccio, professor of comparative anatomy at Bologna in Italy.

1874 The brain center for olfactory function was recognized by Scottish neurologist, Sir David Ferrier.

1874

Antonio Egaz Moniz

Antonio Egaz Moniz born. A Portuguese neurologist who introduced a method of radiologically visualizing cerebral circulation by injecting radio-opaque sodium iodide into the carotid artery (1927), and performed the first frontal lobotomy (1935).

1874 *Nikolai Sergeivich Korotkov* born. A Russian physician who devised a method of measuring diastolic blood pressure by applying the stethoscope to the brachial artery during deflation of the cuff of the sphygmomanometer.

1874   *Georges Froin* born. A French physician who described inflammation of the meninges with obstruction of the spinal subarachnoid space associated with a coagulable state of the cerebrospinal fluid (Froin syndrome, 1903).

1874   *Alan Buchner Kanavel* born. A Kansas surgeon who described the Kanavel sign, a point of maximal tenderness in infections of the tendon sheath and found in the palm, proximal to the base of the little finger.

1874

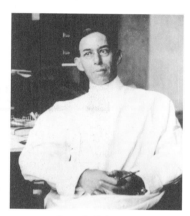

Joseph Erlanger

Joseph Erlanger born. An American physiologist at the Johns Hopkins Hospital and Nobel laureate (1944) who studied nerve conduction, and proved that the velocity of the impulse was proportional to the diameter of the nerve fiber.

1874   *Gustave Roussy* born. A French pathologist who demonstrated thalamic syndrome due to a lesion of the thalamus (1906).

1874   *August Schack Krogh* born. A Danish physiologist and Nobel

laureate (1920) who was a pioneer in study of the human capillary system, and demonstrated that capillaries are under nervous, hormonal and chemical control.

1874   *Frederick Parker Gay* born. An American pathologist who studied the cell count in cerebrospinal fluid in poliomyelitis.

1874   The serous space (Calorie bursa), inconsistently found between the arch of the aorta and the trachea, was described by Italian anatomist, Luigi Calorie.

1874

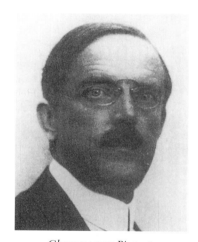

Clemens von Pirquet

Clemens Freiherr von Pirquet born. An Austrian pediatrician and immunologist who coined the term 'allergy' (1904), and devised the Pirquet test for diagnosis of tuberculosis (1907), where old tuberculin was applied through a needle scratch on the skin.

1874   *Jakob Erdheim* born. A Viennese physician who described parathyroid adenoma in relation to osteomalacia, pituitary disorders and aortic medionecrosis (1903).

1874 Internal cardiac massage for resuscitation was proposed by Moritz Schiff.

1874 Rows or chains of bacteria in pus were noted by Rickman John Godlee. Robert Koch named these bacteria streptococci in 1881.

1874 Application of electrodes to the human cortex to produce contralateral muscle contractions was demonstrated by American physician, Roberts Bartholow.

1874 A description of the basement membrane beneath the noncellular layer underlying the epithelium of the trachea, bronchi and alimentary tract was given by Georges Maurice Debove, a histopathologist from Paris.

1875 Varicella was proved to be an infectious disease by Steiner who inoculated volunteers with material taken from the vesicles of patients with the disease.

1875 The first description of Wernicke encephalopathy, acute superior hemorrhagic polioencephalitis, was given by French physician, Charles Jules Alphonse.

1875 *Cell Formation and Cell Division* was published by pioneer German botanist, Eduard Adolf Strasburger.

1875 *Otto Rossel* born. A physician from Switzerland who detected occult blood in feces using Barbados aloin and other reagents (Rossel test).

1875 Salicylic acid used in the treatment of pain relief in typhoid was first described and used by a physician from Switzerland, Carl Emil Buss.

1875 Ludwig Bandl described the line of demarcation between the thinned lower segment of the uterus and the contracted upper segment, found in obstructed labor (Bandl Ring).

1875 The American Neurological Association was founded.

1875 An account of the different types of atrial septal defect in pediatric cardiology was given by Karl Rokitansky of Czechoslovakia.

1875 *Alfred Fabian Hess* born. A New York physician who devised the Hess test to detect capillary fragility with the help of sphygmomanometer cuff to raise venous pressure.

1875 *Cecile Vogt* born. A French neurologist who carried out early work on neuroanatomy of the thalamus, hereditary pseudobulbar palsy, congenital chorea, and also mapped the brain.

1875 *Ernst Sauerbruch* born. A German cardiothoracic surgeon who invented the negative pressure chamber which allowed the chest to be opened without loss of respiration or collapsing of the lung, and who operated for cardiac aneurysm (1903).

1875 Rhythm of the failing heart on auscultation (gallop rhythm) was studied and explained by Pierre Carl Edouard Potain of Paris.

1875   A urinary bladder tumor was excised through the abdominal route by Austrian surgeon, Christian Albert Theodor Billroth.

1875   *Aleksei Ivanovitch Abrikosov* born. A Russian pathologist who described a tumor of striated muscle made of cell groups which resemble primitive myoblasts (Abrikosov tumor, 1926).

1875   Emma Call and Siegmund Exner of Vienna described degenerative cysts in ovarian granulosa cells (Call–Exner bodies).

1875   The first woman in America to perform major abdominal surgery and ovariotomy was Emiline Horton Cleveland, a professor of obstetrics at the Woman's Hospital, Philadelphia.

1875

Sir Henry Dale

Sir Henry Hallett Dale born. A British physician who won the Nobel Prize (1936) for his work on the transmission of nerve impulses, acetyl choline, norepinephrine, and the discovery of histamine.

1875   *Wilhelm Falta* born. An Austrian physician who studied endocrine and metabolic disorders, including diabetes mellitus, and wrote *The Diseases of the Bloodglands*.

1875   A testicular cyst (Malassez disease) was described by Paris physiologist, Louis Charles Malassez.

1875   *Hermann Schridde* born. A German pathologist who described hydrops fetalis (Schridde syndrome), and the thick hairs found on the temple and in the beard of cancerous or cachetic patients (Schridde cancer hair).

1875   Evidence for electrical activity in the brain of living animals (electroencephalography) was provided by Richard Caton, an English neurologist from Liverpool.

1875   Centrosomes in chromosomes were discovered and studied by German histologist, Walther Flemming.

1875   *Henry Kunrath Pancoast* born. A Philadelphia radiologist and pioneer in the use of radiotherapy, who described an epidermoid or adenocarcinoma of the lung involving the superior pulmonary sulcus (Pancoast tumor, 1932).

1875   Richard von Volkmann, a German surgeon, identified industrial tar and paraffin as carcinogens.

1875   The anti-inflammatory properties of salicylic acid were demonstrated by Franz Striker of Germany.

1875   *J. Calvé* born. A French orthopedic surgeon who described osteochondrosis of the vertebra (Calvé disease).

1875 *Frederick Tilney* born. The father of the New York School of Neurology whose work *The Brain from Ape to Man* is considered a classic on modern evolution, and wrote (with Henry Riley) *The form and functions of the central nervous system* in 1921.

1875 *Vladimir Petrovitch Filatov* born. A Russian surgeon who introduced the use of the pedicle flap in plastic surgery, and pioneered corneal transplant and tissue surgery.

1875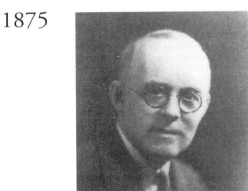

Arthur Coca

Arthur Fernandez Coca born. An American geneticist who described a form of genetic predisposition towards development of hypersensitivity to common environmental antigens, and named antibodies in the serum of atopic individuals atopic reaginins.

1875 The pathological features of congenital corrected transposition of the aorta and pulmonary artery were described by Czech professor, Karl Rokitansky.

1875 *John Auer* born. An American pharmacologist who described rod- or crystalline-shaped inclusions in myeloblastic leukemia due to faulty granule formation (Auer rods or bodies).

1875 *Carl Joseph Gauss* born. A German gynecologist who described unusual mobility of the uterus occurring in early pregnancy (Gauss sign).

1875 The ability of striated muscle to respond to increased stretch with a proportional increase in contraction (Starling law) was first described by Otto Frank, and his observation was later demonstrated in heart preparations by Ernest Starling.

1876 The Little area in the nasal septum was described by James Laurence Little, professor of surgery at Vermont.

1876 *C.S. Krishnaswami* born. An Indian physician who described the Whitmore bacillus (the causative organism of melidiosis) with Alfred Whitmore.

1876 The periodical appearance of the filarial parasite in blood of malaria patients, of diagnostic significance, was discovered by Sir Patrick Manson, while working in China.

1876 Stellate cells with phagocytic properties in the lining of the capillaries of the liver (Kupffer cells) were described by Karl Wilhelm von Kupffer, professor of anatomy at Königsberg.

1876 *John Timothy Geraghty* born. An American surgeon who developed the phenol sulphonaphthalein test of renal function (1910), described a new method of perineal prostatectomy.

1876 Adam Hammer of St Louis reported the first correctly diagnosed case of coronary artery occlusion in life.

1876 *Adolf Windaus* born. A German chemist famous for his work on the structure of cholesterol for which he received the Nobel Prize in 1928, and who also discovered that light activates ergosterol, converting it to vitamin D_2.

1876 *Sir Richard Robert Cruise* born. A London ophthalmologist who developed an operation for chronic glaucoma by making a corneoscleral wedge-shaped opening without irridectomy (Cruise operation).

1876 The Association of American Medical Colleges was founded.

1876 The first molars in congenital syphilis (Moon molars) were described by a dental surgeon from Guy's Hospital, London, Henry Moon.

1876 Hungarian dermatologist, Moritz Kaposi, described diabetic dermatitis.

1876 The Taylor apparatus, a steel support used in the treatment of Pott disease of the spine, was devised in New York by orthopedic surgeon, Charles Fayette Taylor.

1876 The Thomas splint for deformities of the hip, knee and ankle joints was devised by Hugh Owen Thomas, an English orthopedic surgeon from Liverpool.

1876 *Maurice Oppenheim* born. An Austrian dermatologist who wrote several books on venereal disease and skin disorders including necrobiosis lipoidica diabeticorum with American dermatologist, Eric Urbach (Oppenheim–Urbach disease).

1876 The anthrax bacillus was isolated by German bacteriologist Robert Koch, and he described a method of growing it in culture.

1876 *Maria Montessori* born. The first woman medical graduate from Rome, Italy who founded a system of self-education for children through skillfully directed play without formal classes.

1876 *Samuel Ernest Whitnall* born. A professor of anatomy from Manchester, although working in Canada, who described the Whitnall tubercle found on the zygomatic bone.

1876 *Localization and Functions of Cerebral Diseases*, an early neurological treatise, was published by Jean Martin Charcot of Paris.

1876 *George Coats* born. A Scottish ophthalmologist who wrote a classic treatise on thrombosis of the central vein of the retina, and described retinitis exudativa (Coats disease).

1876 *Constantin von Economo* born. An Austrian neurologist who identified and characterized epidemic encephalitis, and showed that this was caused by a virus.

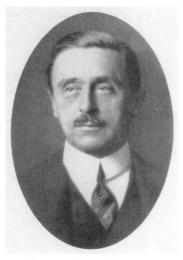

Constantin von Economo

1876 The discoloration and excoriation of the skin caused by scratching, secondary to human pediculosis (vagabond disease), was described by London physician, Edward Headlam Greenhow.

1876 *Paul Roemer* born. A German professor from Griefswald who prepared Roemer serum, an early antipneumococcal serum, and standardized the old tuberculin method.

1876 *Robert Barany* born. An otologist from Austria and Nobel laureate (1914) who was the first to study labyrinthine function of the ear, devised the Barany caloric rest for labyrinthine function (1906), and described Barany syndrome of unilateral deafness, vertigo and occipital headache (1918).

1876 *Alfred Ernest Barclay* born. A Manchester radiologist who described the Barclay niche, the protrusion

of barium into a duodenal ulcer crater.

1876 The inability to relax the muscles after contraction, occurring during early childhood (Thomsen disease), was first described by Ernest von Leyden and more comprehensively described later in the same year by Danish physician, Asmus Thomsen.

1876 The intercellular membrane in the ampulla of the semicircular canals was described by Urban Pritchard, an eminent London otorhinologist.

1876 *Otto Prausnitz* born. A British immunologist of German origin who transferred the fish hypersensitivity experienced by his partner Kürstner to his own skin using a hypodermic injection, and created sensitization on subsequent exposure to the sensitizing agent (Prausnitz–Kürstner reaction, 1921).

1876 *Maurice Favre* born. A French dermatologist who made important contributions to understanding of syphilis, describing lymphogranuloma inguinale in 1913.

1876 *Carl Gosta Abrahamson Forssell* born. A Swedish radiologist who pioneered radium treatment for cancer of the uterus, and described the Forssell sinus in the pyloric antrum.

1876 *Sir Gordon Morgan Holmes* born. A famous London clinical neurologist who described primary progressive cerebellar degeneration,

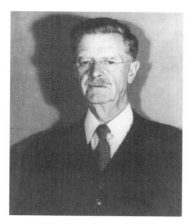

Sir Gordon Morgan Holmes

and gave an account of the function of the thalamus and its relationship to the cerebral cortex (1911).

1876 The intestinal parasitic roundworm that causes diarrhea (*Strongyloides stercoralis*) was described by Louis Normand in Cochin, China.

1876 *Marmaduke Stephen Mayou* born. A London ophthalmologist who described symmetrical changes in the macula in juvenile amaurotic idiocy (1904).

1876 *Some Effects of Lung Elasticity in Health and Disease* was published by Douglas Powell of the Middlesex and Brompton Hospitals.

1876 The Johns Hopkins University and Hospital in Baltimore was founded from the bequest of Johns Hopkins, a businessman from Maryland.

1876 Apoplexy caused by cerebral hemorrhage into the ventricles (Broadbent apoplexy) was described by English cardiologist and neurologist, Sir William Henry Broadbent.

1876 *John James Rickard Macleod* born. A Scottish professor of physiology who carried out important research on diabetes in Toronto, published *Physiology and Biochemistry in Modern Medicine* (1918), and shared the Nobel Prize for the discovery of insulin (1923).

1876 *Alexander Bittorf* born. A German pathologist who described the 'Bittorf sign' of pain in the distribution of the genitofemoral nerve due to lesions of the testis and ovary.

1876 *Stanislaus Joseph Mathias von Prowazek* born. A German microbiologist who found cell inclusion bodies in conjunctival cells in trachoma (1907), and postulated that they were collections of virus enveloped by material deposited from the infected cell.

1876 A treatise on rheumatism was published by a French dermatologist, Ernest Besnier, in which he described chronic arthrosynovitis (Besnier rheumatism).

1876 The Chvostek sign where facial muscles go into spasm on tapping the facial nerve, a diagnostic sign in tetany, was described by Austrian surgeon, Frantisek Chvostek.

1876 *Andre Latarget* born. A French professor of anatomy at Lyon who described the anterior gastric nerves which are used in selective vagotomy.

1876   *Fred Houdlett Albee* born. A surgeon from Maine who transplanted tissue from a tibia into the diseased spine of a patient with Pott disease (1906), and grafted living bone tissue for internal splints.

1876   The silver wire appearance of the thickened arteries during ophthalmoscopy was described by London neurologist, Sir William Richard Gowers.

1876

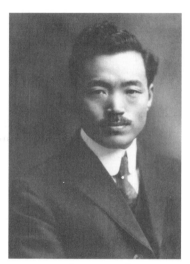

Hideyo Noguchi

Hideyo Noguchi born. A Japanese-born American bacteriologist who devised the Noguchi reaction, a diagnostic skin test and a modification of the Wasserman reaction using human instead of sheep corpuscles, and demonstrated the role of spirochetes in syphilis.

1876   The fungal disease of the skin, piedra, or black piedra, was noted and studied by Nicalou Ozorio in Columbia, South America.

1876   *John Swift Joly* born. A London urologist who devised an irrigating urethroscope, also used for cystoscopy, pioneered the use of radium for cancer treatment and devised the Dublin method of radiotherapy.

1876   The pyramidal tract, a part of the nervous system, was identified and named after Paul Emil Flechsig of Leipzig, Germany.

1876   The union of the spermatozoon and the ovum was described by German professor, Oscar Hertwig.

1876   The development of lesions along the lines of mechanical irritation of the skin, especially in cases of psoriasis (Koebner phenomenon), was described by a German dermatologist, Heinrich Koebner.

1876   Willow bark (from *Salix alba*), the source of salicylic acid and a folk remedy for fever and rheumatism for centuries, was introduced as treatment for acute rheumatism and rheumatic fever by John Thomas Maclagan.

1876   *Sir Thomas Peel* born. A London surgeon who described the operative removal of intrathoracic tumors through a sternal approach, and invented the Dunhill forceps used in thyroid surgery.

1876   *Ludwig Halberstaedtler* born. A German pathologist who described cytoplasmic inclusion bodies found in the epithelial cells of the conjunctiva in trachoma, with Polish zoologist, Stanislaw von Prowazek, (Prowazek–Halberstaedtler bodies).

1876   A description of metastasizing multinodular bronchial carcinoma was given by L. Malassez.

1876   The reflex nature of deglutition and its mechanism were described by Italian anatomist, Angelo Mosso.

1877   Isolation of indican from urine was done by Max Jaffe of Germany.

1877   Use of a wire thread to stimulate clot formation in an aneurysm was performed by Italian physician, Guido Baccelli.

1877   A description of angiokeratoma was given by English physician, E. Wynham Cottle.

1877   A photosensitive pigment in the retina (rhodopsin) was discovered by Italian anatomist, Franz Christian Boll.

1877   The first definite account of myasthenia gravis, caused by a disorder in neuromuscular function due to the presence of antibodies to acetylcholine receptors, was given by English physician, Samuel Wilks.

1877   Poikilocytosis, the term employed to denote changes in the shape and size of red blood cells in some cases of anemia, was coined by Heinrich Irenaeus Quincke, a German professor of medicine working in Bern, Switzerland.

1877   The first overseas branch of the British Medical Association was formed in Jamaica.

1877   A description of familial nephrogenic diabetes insipidus was given by London physician, Samuel

Jones Gee, in *Contributions to the History of Polydipsia*.

1877   Juvenile paresis was associated with congenital syphilis was described by Sir Thomas Clouston from Orkney, a superintendent at the Royal Morningside Asylum.

1877   A much improved hemacytometer was developed by London neurologist, Sir William Gowers.

1877   *Emil Looser* born. A Swiss surgeon from Zurich who described the Looser zones, seen on X-rays and mimicking fractures in osteomalacia.

1877   The role of chemicals in the transmission of nerve impulses, was suggested by German physiologist, Emil Heinrich Dubois-Reymond.

1877   Congenital mitral stenosis (Duroziez disease) was described by French physician, Louis Paul Duroziez.

1877   An early description of serum sickness was given by Austrian pediatrician and immunologist, Clemens von Pirquet.

1877   Hans Chiari of Germany provided the first case report of choriocarcinoma.

1877   *Béla Schick* born. A Hungarian pediatrician working in America, who gave the first description of serum disease, and developed the Schick test that determines a patient's vulnerability to diphtheria (1921).

1877   *Viktor Mucha* born. An Austrian dermatologist who worked on dark field illumination in diagnosing syphilis with Karl Landsteiner, and with German dermatologist Rudolph Habermann described pityriasis lichenoides et varioliformis acuta (Mucha–Habermann disease).

1877   Chloral hydrate was used as a premedication before giving chloroform, by French surgeon, Forne.

1877   Paul Ehrlich of Germany, who made great contributions to the field of hematology, used aniline dyes to stain white blood cells.

Paul Ehrlich

1877   The first nephrectomy for malignant disease of the kidney was carried out by Carl Johann August Langenbuch of Berlin, Germany.

1877   *Hans Sachs* born. A serologist from Heidelberg in Germany who devised a flocculation test for serodiagnosis (Sachs–Georgi test) with Walter Georgi in 1919.

1877   The ciliary glands (Sattler glands) were first described by a German ophthalmologist, Hubert Sattler.

1877   *George Grey Turner* born. A surgeon from Newcastle, England who reported successful resection of the thoracic esophagus, and described the Turner sign of local discoloration of the skin of the loin 2–3 days after an attack of acute pancreatitis.

1877   *Alexander Schmincke* born. A German pathologist who described lymphoepithelioma (Schminke tumor).

1877   A spasm of the levator palpebrae muscle of the eye in exophthalmic goiter (Abadie sign) was described by Charles A. Abadie, ophthalmologist, in Paris, France.

1877   *Louis Virgil Hamman* born. A Baltimore surgeon who described spontaneous mediastinal emphysema (Hamman disease), the Hamman sound in mediastinal emphysema, and the Hamman–Rich syndrome of diffuse pulmonary fibrosis.

1877   *Frederick Julius Gaenslen* born. A Milwaukee surgeon who described a method of subtrochanteric osteotomy for irreducible dislocation of the hip (1935).

1877   William Morrant Baker, a London surgeon, described a synovial cyst of the knee joint (Baker cyst).

1877   Luther Holden, a demonstrator in anatomy at St Bartholomew's Hospital, described the crease line caused by flexion of the hip (Holden line).

1877   *Georg Axhausen* born. A German orthopedic surgeon who pioneered bone grafts, and described osteochondritis.

1877

Theodore Avery

Theodore Oswald Avery born. A bacteriologist from Nova Scotia who pioneered molecular biology and immunochemistry, discovered type III antigen of pneumococcus, and demonstrated its antigenic functions in 1944.

1877   A classic case of rupture of an aneurysm at the bifurcation of the middle cerebral artery was reported by regius professor of medicine at Oxford, Sir William Osler

1877   *Sir Aldo Castellani* born. An eminent Italian bacteriologist who identified the trypanosome as the cause of sleeping sickness, and published over 200 papers on mycology.

1877   *Hal Downy* born. A Minneapolis hematologist who made important contributions to understanding leukemia, Gaucher disease, and lymphomas, and described atypical lymphocytes in infectious mononucleosis (Downy cells, 1936).

1877   *Jean G. Bachmann* born. An American physiologist who described longitudinally orientated atrial fibers which preferentially conduct impulses from the sino-atrial node from the right to left atrium (Bachmann bundle).

1877   *Emil Abderhalden* born. A German physiologist who described familial cystinosis (1903), and wrote a number of textbooks including *A Text on Methodology*.

1877   Angiokeratoma was originally described by English physician, E. Wyndham Cottle, and was later redescribed and named Mibelli disease.

1877   *Louis Gaston Labat* born. A Paris surgeon who devised a glass and metal device for locking the needle with a finger hold (Labat syringe), and perfected the method of infiltration of the nerve to produce nerve block for anesthesia.

1877   *The Manual of Diseases in Childhood* was published by Swiss pediatrician, Adolph d'Espine, with his classmate at the University of Geneva, C. Picot.

1877   *John Homans* born. An American surgeon from the Johns Hopkins Hospital who described pain elicited in the calf on dorsiflexion of the foot in cases of deep vein thrombosis of the leg (Homans sign).

1877   Osteotomy was pioneered in England by Henry Albert Reeves, a surgeon at the Orthopaedic Hospital, London.

1877   *Heinrich Otto Wieland* born. A German chemist who studied bile acids which aid digestion of lipids, and received the Nobel Prize for Chemistry (1927) for this work.

1877   A description of a rare bone disease, osteitis deformans, now known as ankylosing spondylitis, was given by British physician, Sir James Paget.

1877   *Spinal Disease and Spinal Curvature* was published by American orthopedic surgeon, Lewis Albert Sayre, who also invented the Sayre plaster bandage for Pott disease

1877   *Fritz Brenner* born. A German physician and pathologist who described a tumor of the ovary, usually benign, without endocrine activity (Brenner tumor, 1907).

1877   The electrically-lit cystoscope was devised by Berlin urologist, Max Nitze.

1878   *The Journal of Physiology* in England was founded by Michael Foster, professor of physiology at Cambridge.

1878   The fungus *Actinomyces israelii* was discovered by German urologist James Adolph Israel.

1878   *Lawrence Joseph Henderson* born. An American biochemist who developed nonograms to calculate pH values of blood, and showed that the affinity of blood for oxygen varied with the pressure of carbon dioxide.

1878   *Karl Connell* born. New York physician who described a band with two hooks (Connell harness) for fixing the face-piece of anesthetic apparatus to the head during anesthesia.

1878   The term 'enzyme' was used to denote a class of organic substances that activated a chemical change by German biochemist, Willy Kühne.

1878   *Francis H.A. Marshall* born. A British physician and a pioneer in reproductive physiology who studied the estrous cycle.

1878   *R. Bing* born. A French professor of neurology who described the extension of the big toe following stimulation of the dorsum of the foot in cases of pyramidal tract lesions (Bing sign).

1878   *Benjamin Lipschültz* born. An Austrian dermatologist who described a non-venereal ulcer of the vulva (Lipschültz ulcer), and eosinophilic nuclear inclusions in virally infected cells, e.g. herpes zoster or cytomegalovirus (Lipschültz body).

1878   The first hemoglobinometer, an instrument that compared blood color with a standard color, was devised by London neurologist, Sir William Richard Gowers.

1878   The part played by the diaphragm in respiration was described by George Minott Garland of New York.

1878   *Sir William Gordon-Taylor* born. A British surgeon who designed the one-stage hind-quarter operative amputation (1935).

1878   *Ernest Lowenstein* born. A Viennese pathologist who (with Danish bacteriologist, Orla Jensen), prepared the Lowenstein–Jensen medium to culture Mycobacterium tuberculosis.

1878   *Alwin Max Pappenheimer* born. A New York biochemist who described iron granules in erythrocytes in peripheral blood in hemolytic anemia (Pappenheimer bodies), devised a specific test for plasma cells (Pappenheimer stain), and introduced cod liver oil as treatment for rickets (1920).

1878   Summer prurigo, characterized by itching and the development of severe papules, was described by English surgeon, Jonathan Hutchinson (Hutchinson prurigo).

1878   The first attempt to use human donors for corneal transplants was made by Heinrich Sellerbeck of Germany.

1878   *Arthur Steindler* born. An American orthopedic surgeon who was a pioneer in biomechanics, and wrote *Orthopedic Operations*.

1878   *George Hoyt Whipple* born. An American pathologist and Nobel laureate (1934) who showed that iron was an important component of red blood cells (1925), and that eating liver could cure pernicious anemia and increase hemoglobin (1925).

1878   *Sergei Livovich Bogrow* born. A Russian anatomist who described the fibers running from the optic tract to the thalamus (Bogrow fibers).

1878   An American surgeon from Massachusetts, Henry Orlando Marcy, introduced antiseptic sutures in the surgical treatment of hernia.

1878   *Camille Biot* born. A French physician who described a variant of Cheyne-Stokes respiration seen in medullary compression of the brain (Biot sign).

1878   The basal ossicle between the phenoid and occital bones (Albrecht bone) was described by Hamburg anatomist, Karl Martin Paul Albrecht.

1878   A case of primary cancer of the ureter, established by microscopic diagnosis, was reported by a Swedish physician, P. Johann Wising.

1878   The nodes of Ranvier, regular interruptions in the medullary nerve fiber sheath, were described by Louis-Antoine Ranvier, a neurologist from Paris.

1878   William Smith Greenfield, a London surgeon, described giant cells in Hodgkin disease.

1878   *Oscar Klotz* born. A Canadian pioneer in the study of fatty acids and arteriosclerosis who published *Concerning the Pathology of some Arterial Diseases* (1925).

1878 Professor of anatomy at Bern, Christopher Theodor Aeby, described the muscle rectus labi proprius.

1878 The term 'myxedema' was introduced by English surgeon, William Miller Ord.

1878 Dermatitis exfoliativa infantum or staphylococcal scalded skin syndrome (Ritter disease) was described by Gottfried Ritter von Rittershaim.

1878 Arthur Hartmann devised an early version of the audiometer to measure hearing in humans.

1878 Meralgia parasthetica of the external cutaneous nerve of the thigh (Bernhardt disease) was described by German neurologist, Martin Max Bernhardt.

1878 Microscopy was advanced by adding the apochromatic objective and the oil immersion lens developed by German physicist, Ernst Abbé.

1878 *Hans Zinsser* born. A Harvard bacteriologist who worked on allergy, virus size, typhus and causes of rheumatic fever, differentiated epidemic from endemic ricketsial typhus, and wrote *Rats, Lice and History* (1935) on typhus fever.

1878 Intubation of the upper laryngeal orifice and trachea through the mouth inserted through the

Abbé technique for division of esophageal structure

mouth was performed by William MacEwen, a surgeon from Glasgow.

1878 Modern surgical treatment for cancer of the uterus through the vaginal route was introduced by Vincenz Czerny, professor of surgery at Heidelberg in Germany.

1878 *Frank Seymour Kidd* born. A London urologist who designed an operating cystoscope (Kidd cystoscope) with an electrode for diathermy of bladder tumors.

1878 The first case of an aneurysm eroding through the wall of the bronchus was presented by Douglas Powell of the Brompton Hospital.

1878 A maneuver to prevent pharyngeal obstruction by applying anterior traction at the ascending rami of the mandible during resuscitation was described by military surgeon, Johann von Esmarch of Göttingen. He wrote *Surgeon's Handbook on Treatment of Wounded in War*.

1878 The term 'karyokinensis' for certain typical changes in a cell during its division was coined by

W. Schleicher. Walther Flemming called the process 'mitosis' in 1880.

1879 Use of a three-way tap for pleural aspiration was introduced by F. Mosler.

1879 The role of intercostal muscles in respiration was established by American physiologists, Henry Newell Martin and Edward Mussey Hartwell.

1879 A special type of forceps for removal of adenoid growths from the nasopharynx was devised by German surgeon, Benjamin Loewenberg.

1879 Culture of streptococcus from a case of puerperal fever was done by Louis Pasteur. In 1881 he undertook the first public controlled trials on anthrax vaccine in animals.

1879 *Charles LeRoy Lowman* born. A graduate of the University of Southern California Medical School who founded the Orthopedic Hospital in Los Angeles (1922), and devised a bone holding instrument (Lowman clamp).

1879 *Jörgen Nilson Schaumann* born. A Swedish dermatologist from Stockholm who described the systematic nature of sarcoidosis in 1922 (Besnier–Boeck–Schaumann disease).

1879 Excision of the pyloric end of the stomach followed by axial anastomosis with the duodenum was described by Jules Émile Pean in Paris.

1879 The four small bodies beside the thyroid glands were described as accessory thyroid tissues by Swedish anatomist, Ivar Victor Sandström.

1879 *Arthur Sydney Blundell* born. A London orthopedic surgeon who described the Bankart procedure for separation of the anterior part of the glenoid labrum in recurring dislocations of the shoulder.

1879 Winckel disease, icterus, bloody urine and hemorrhage with a fatal outcome in neonates, was described by German gynecologist, Franz Karl Ludwig von Winckel.

1879 *Theodore John Dimitry* born. An ophthalmologist in New Orleans who described a method of evisceration of the eyeball, followed by insertion of an artificial ball before the sclera and conjunctiva were stitched over it.

1879 Nodules on the parietal and frontal bones of the skull in infants with congenital syphilis (Parrot nodes) were described by French physician, Jules Marie Parrot.

1879 A paralytic form of rabies was produced by Victor Galtier of Paris.

1879 A variable pressure adjustment to the locking device of the artery forceps was introduced by the British surgeon, Sir Thomas Spencer Wells.

1879 *Isford Isfred Hofbaur* born. An Austrian gynecologist who described histiocytes from the connective tissue of the chorionic villus

(Hofbaur cells), and used extract of the posterior pituitary in treatment of uterine inertia in labor.

1879 The surgical removal of a brain tumor involving the meninges was performed by Sir William MacEwen, a professor of surgery at the Glasgow Royal Infirmary.

1879 Maladie de Roger (Roger disease), a defect in the interventricular septum of the heart, was described by Henri Louis Roger, a surgeon in Paris.

1879 *Sir Fredrick Arthur Hurst* born. A physician at Guy's Hospital who wrote *The Sensibility of Alimentary Canal* and described dumping syndrome following gastroenterostomy.

1879 *Keith Lucas* born. An English neurophysiologist who described the all or none law, that a given stimulus evokes a maximum contraction or no contraction in the muscles, and also showed the same principle in motor nerve fibers.

1879 *Leo Buerger* born. A New York urologist who designed the Brown–Buerger cystoscope which aided irrigation of the bladder during cystoscopy, and described Buerger disease or thromboangiitis obliterans (arteriosclerosis, 1926).

1879 William Richard Gowers, the eminent London neurologist, published *Pseudo-hypertrophic Muscular Paralysis*, Gowers disease.

1879 Felix von Winiwarter described the obliteration of most of the arteries

of the leg due to a chronic proliferative process, later named endarteritis by Leo Buerger.

1879 *René Henri Leriche* born. A surgeon from Strasbourg who worked on surgery of the vascular system, pain and peripheral nerve injuries, and described impotence caused by thrombotic occlusion at the bifurcation of the aorta (Leriche syndrome, 1940).

1879 A fungus that attacks the skin, hair and nails (*Trichophyton concentricum*) was described by the father of tropical medicine in England, Patrick Manson, and later named by Raphael Blanchard.

1879 *Charles Rupert Stockard* born. An American physician who worked on the estrous cycle, embryonic development, and factors governing differentiation and regeneration.

1879 Prurigo nodularis (Hyde disease) was described by American physician, William Augustus Hardaway.

1879 Gonococcal bacteria were isolated by German bacteriologist, Albert Ludwig Siegmund Neisser.

1879 *Carlos Chagas* born. A Brazilian physician who discovered the protozoan, *Trypanosoma* and its insect vector causing trypanosomiasis (1909), the disease was later named after him.

1879 *Douglas Symmers* born. An American professor of pathology who described a disease with follicular lymphadenopathy and splenomegaly, later called Brill–Symmers disease.

1879 *Amedee Granger* born. A New Orleans radiologist who described the Granger line on the skull X-ray which represents the superior surface of the sphenoid bone where the optic groove lies.

1879 *Winifred Ashby* born. A British-born American pathologist who determined the lifespan of the red blood cell, and developed special techniques for estimating the survival of red cells (Ashby techniques).

Winifred Ashby

1879 *Hans Christian Jacobaeus* born. A Stockholm surgeon who used a modified cystoscope to perform cautery division of pleural adhesions, which led directly to the development of the thoracoscope and other similar instruments to view the interior of the body.

1879 *John Martin Wheeler* born. A New York ophthalmologist who described procedures for various eye conditions, including glaucoma and ectropion.

1879 The small cartilaginous rod attached to the vocal process of the arytenoid cartilage (Seiler cartilage), was described by American laryngologist of Swedish descent, Carl Seiler.

1879 *Walter Goldie Howarth* born. A London otorhinologist who devised an operation for frontal sinusitis where the anterior wall on the sinus was left intact to preserve the cosmetic appearance.

1879 *Eli Moschcowitz* born. A New York surgeon who studied the physiology of blood circulation, wrote *Hypertension of the Pulmonary Circulation* (1927), and pioneered psychosomatic medicine.

1879 *Carey F. Coombs* born. A British cardiologist and expert in rheumatic heart disease and coronary thrombosis, who described a short mid-diastolic mitral murmur heard in rheumatic fever, thought to be indicative of carditis (Carey-Coombs murmur).

1879 *Walther Spielmeyer* born. A German neurologist who studied juvenile amaurotic idiocy caused by lipid metabolism disturbance, and wrote an important book on microscopy of the nervous system.

1879 Duodenostomy was performed by German surgeon, Carl Johann August Langenbuch.

1879   *Josef Jadassohn* born. A dermatologist from Breslau who gave descriptions of maculo-papular erythrodermia (Jadassohn disease), the Jadassohn nevus, a plaque-like lesion of the skin which contains excess sebaceous glands, drug reactions of the skin, and patch tests for diagnosis and investigation.

1879   *Jules Tinel* born. A French neurologist from Rouen who described the tapping over the carpel tunnel causing paraesthesia over the median nerve distribution of the hand in carpel tunnel syndrome (Tinel sign).

1879   Angioma of the leptomeninges and ipsilateral portwine stain on the face in the region of trigeminal distribution (Sturge–Weber syndrome) was described by English Quaker physician, William Allen Sturge.

1879   Glyceryl trinitrate (nitroglycerin) was introduced as treatment for angina by William Murell of University College, London.

1879   *Francis Peyton Rous* born. A Baltimore oncologist and Nobel laureate (1966) who established the first blood banks, discovered a virus which induced a tumor capable of transmission from body to body (Rous sarcoma).

1879   Psittacosis (parrot fever) was described by Jacob Ritter in Switzerland, and the sources of many outbreaks were traced to consignments of diseased parrots.

1879   Obliteration of the lumen of most arteries of the leg by a chronic proliferative process (thromboangitis obliterans) was described by German physician, Felix von Winiwarter.

1880   The first operation for a perforated peptic ulcer was performed by German-born Polish professor of surgery, Johann von Mikulicz-Radecki.

1880   *Albert A. Epstein* born. An American physician who made important contributions to renal disease and diabetes, including a microchemical record for estimating sugar in the blood, and Epstein syndrome.

1880   *William Edwards Ladd* born. A Harvard pediatric surgeon who described the persistent peritoneal band (trans-duodenal band of Ladd) which caused intestinal obstruction (1932).

1880   British ophthalmologist Warren Tay described amaurotic family idiocy (Tay–Sachs disease) and its ocular manifestations.

1880   The term narcolepsy referring to recurrent, uncontrollable episodes of sleep was coined by French neurologist, Jean Baptiste Edouard Gelineau of Paris.

1880   An operation for radical excision of the tongue in a case of cancer was performed and devised by Swiss surgeon, Emil Theodor Kocher.

1880   *Marie Stopes* born. An English pioneer in contraception who opened the first birth control clinic, and wrote widely on the subject with works such as *Contraception: Its Theory, History and Practice* (1923).

1880 Adenoma sebaceum associated with mental deficiency and epilepsy was described by Desiré Magloire Bourneville of France (Bourneville disease).

1880 *Frank Howard Lahey* born. The founder of the Lahey Clinic in Massachusetts who trained in surgery at the Boston City Hospital then opened his clinic at 638 Beacon Street.

1880 The causative organism of enteric fever, *Salmonella typhi*, was discovered by Carl Joseph Eberth, professor of pathology at Halle in Germany.

1880 *Albert Sézary* born. A French dermatologist who described exfoliative erythroderma associated with the circulation of abnormal lymphocytes (Sézary syndrome).

1880 The paraurethral glands of the female (Skene glands) were described by Alexander Johnston Chalmers Skene, an American gynecologist of Scottish origin.

1880 *Diseases of the Nose and Throat* was published by eminent British otorhinologist, Sir Morell Mackenzie.

1880 Part of the wall of the right atrium which overlies the atrioventricular node (Koch triangle) was named after Berlin cardiologist and pathologist, Walter Karl Koch.

1880 *Joseph Kyrle* born. An Austrian professor of dermatology and syphilis who described a disease of the hair follicles due to keratin plugs, hyperkeratosis follicularis (Kyrle disease).

1880 *Edward Alfred Cockayne* born. An English physician who described dwarfism, microcephaly, retinal atrophy, mental retardation and progressive upper motor neuron dysfunction with autosomal recessive inheritance (Cockayne syndrome).

1880 A procedure for tying the fallopian tubes during a cesarean section in a patient with a contracted pelvis for the purpose of sterilization was recorded by S.S. Lungren of Toledo, Ohio.

1880 The Wölfler gland, an accessory thyroid gland, was described by German professor of surgery at Graz, Anton Wölfler.

1880 Charles Chamberland devised the pressure steam sterilizer, or autoclave, during research on methods of destroying bacteria.

1880 *Willis Cohoon Campbell* born. A Memphis orthopedic surgeon who advocated interpositional arthroplasty techniques for ankylosed joints and other diseases, and wrote *Operative Orthopedics* (1939).

1880 The first thyroidectomy for exophthalmic goiter was performed by a German surgeon, Ludwig Reich.

1880 Nitrous oxide was used to relieve labor pains by Stanislaw Klikovitch of Russia.

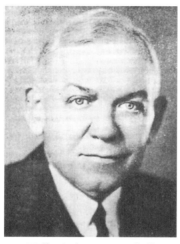

Willis Cohoon Campbell

1880   The outer cell mass of trophoblastic cells of the blastodermic vesicle (Rauber layer) were described by the German-born professor of anatomy from Estonia, August Antinous Rauber.

1880   Studies on the experimental demonstration of the role of grass pollens, and descriptions of the first pollen counts, were completed by Manchester physician, Charles Blackley.

1880   The protozoan, *Plasmodium*, that causes malaria was discovered by Charles Louis Alphonse Laveran, a French parasitologist, while a professor of pathological anatomy at the University of Rome, Italy.

1880   Suggested use of cocaine as a local anesthetic was made by Russian physician, Vasili Konstaninovitch Anrep.

1880   A procedure for nephrolithotomy, where the stone was removed through a lumbar incision, was performed by Sir Henry Morris of London.

1880   *Martin Haudek* born. A radiologist in Vienna who described the protrusion of contrast medium into the ulcer crater (Haudek sign) in cases of gastric ulcer.

1880   The sensory tactile nerve endings (Merkel corpuscles) were first described by Friedrich Sigmund Merkel, professor of anatomy at Göttingen.

1880   *Arthur C. Alport* born. A South African physician who described hereditary nephritis with nerve deafness and infrequently a mild platelet defect and cataracts (Alport syndrome, 1927).

1880   The peripheral neuritis of beriberi was described by Erwin Otto von Baelz.

1880   *Ernst Laqueur* born. A Dutch physician and urologist who was one of the discoverers of testosterone, and estrogenic activity in male urine.

1880   A survey by the Ophthalmological Society in England showed that 30% to 40% of blindness in all ages was due to ophthalmia neonatorum.

1880   The reflex involved in the act of deglutination was described by a German physiologist, Hugo Krönecker.

1880   *Jean Alexander Barré* born. A French professor of neurology at Strasbourg

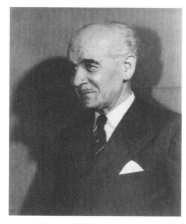

Jean Alexander Barré

who (with Y.C. Lieou) described Barré–Lieou syndrome (1928) in which occipital headache, tinnitus, vertigo and facial spasm occur as a result of sympathetic plexus around the spinal column in rheumatoid arthritis of the cervical spine.

1880 The mechanism of closure of empeyma was explained by A. M. Phelps of New York.

1881 Hepatotomy was introduced by Lawson Robert Tait of England.

1881 The earliest experimental work on lung resection (in rabbits) was done by M. H. Bloch in Danzig. He suggested the possibility of suturing the heart in cases of trauma.

1881 A pure form of hyoscine was isolated by German chemist, Albert Ladenburg.

1881 *Thomas Addis* born. A physician from Edinburgh who showed that normal plasma could correct the defect in hemophilia, made contributions on bile pigment metabo-

lism, and developed the Addis count for cells in urine (1925).

1881 The precursor of the red blood cell (reticulocyte) was identified by German bacteriologist and Nobel Prize winner, Paul Ehrlich, using his own staining method.

1881 William Chapman Jarvis, a laryngologist from New York, devised a wire snare (Jarvis snare) for removing polypi in the nose and throat.

1881 *William Edmund Cooke* born. An English pathologist who modified the Arneth count for white blood cells and renamed it the polymorphonuclear count.

1881 *Sir Thomas Lewis* born. An eminent British cardiologist and physiologist and a pioneer in the application of the electrocardio-graphic method for examination of the heart.

1881 A clinical method of measuring systolic blood pressure (sphygmomanometer) was devised by Samuel Siegfried Ritter von Basch of Vienna, Austria who applied external pressure to the artery and felt the pulse beyond the site of pressure (as used today).

1881 The *Aedes aegypti* mosquito was suggested to be the carrier of yellow fever by Carlos Finlay of Cuba.

1881 A description of progressive polyserositis, leading to ascites and pleural effusion, was given by German physician, Eugene Bamberger.

1881 The nucleus lateralis of the accessory nerve (Roller nucleus) was described by Christian Roller, a neuropsychiatrist from Strasbourg in France.

1881 *Hakaru Hashimoto* born. A Japanese physician who described organo-specific, auto-immune thyroiditis, and the lymphoid infiltration of the thyroid gland (1912).

1881 Siegmund Exner, professor of physiology at the University of Vienna, described the superficial tangential layer of the molecular cerebral cortex.

1881 Primitive nucleated blood cells (megaloblasts) were described by German bacteriologist, Paul Ehrlich.

1881 *Ernst Grafenberg* born. A Jewish gynecologist in Germany who pioneered the study of intrauterine contraception, studied the cyclic changes in pH of vaginal fluid, and devised a coiled silver wire as an intrauterine contraceptive device.

1881 *Allen Oldfather Whipple* born. A New York surgeon who carried out a pancreatoduodenectomy for cancer of the pancreas (1935).

1881 *Staphylococcus* was isolated by Alexander Ogston.

1881 The Fehling operation for treatment of prolapse of the uterus was devised by German gynecologist, Hermann Johannes Karl Fehling.

1881 *Enrique Finochietto* born. An Argentinean surgeon who devised the Finochietto tourniquet to arrest scalp hemorrhage, made of metal and controlled by a screw.

1881 Concato disease, polyserositis due to tuberculous inflammation of the serous membranes, was described by Italian physician, Luigi Maria Concato.

1881 *Sir Alexander Fleming* born. A Scottish bacteriologist who demonstrated the antimicrobial properties of lysozyme in tears and mucus (1922), and discovered that penicillium mold inhibited the growth of staphylococci (1928).

Penicillin fungus

1881 Volkmann contracture in the fingers and wrists following ischemia secondary to injury at the elbow or improper application of a tourniquet was described by German surgeon, Richard von Volkmann.

1881 A study of the mechanics and pattern of urine flow (urodynamics) was undertaken by the Italian physiologists, Angelo Mosso and Pellcani, who devised a manometer capable of recording the intravesical pressure at rest and during micturition.

1881 *Henri Gougerot* born. A Paris dermatologist who gave a complete description of sporotrichosis (with Charles Lucien de Beurmann in 1912), and wrote on sarcoidosis, lupus and cutaneous papillomatosis.

1881 *Walther Rudolph Hess* born. A Swiss physiologist and Nobel Prize winner (1949) who used electrodes to study brain functions.

1881 *Gathorne Robert Girdlestone* born. A British orthopedic surgeon and founder of the Central Council for Care of Cripples, after the Second World War, who developed the Girdlestone operation for arthrodesis of the hip.

1881 Theodor Billroth, a professor of surgery in Zurich and Vienna, performed the first successful partial gastric resection.

1881 *Epilepsy and other Chronic Convulsive Diseases* was published by William Richard Gowers, the eminent London neurologist.

1881 The sensory speech center in the posterior third of the gyrus temporalis superior (Wernicke area) was described by German neuropsychiatrist, Karl Wernicke.

1881 Small diplococci in the sputum of patients with lobar pneumonia were discovered by American bacteriologist, George Miller Sternberg.

1881 The protective effect of inoculating small doses of anthrax bacilli in animals which paved the way for active immunization was explained by Louis Pasteur.

1881 *Hans Reiter* born. A German physician from Leipzig who described urethritis, conjunctivitis and arthritis (Reiter disease) while working as an army surgeon during the First World War.

1881 Eugene Bamberger of Germany and Pierre Marie of Paris, described hypertrophic pulmonary osteoarthropathy (Bamberger–Marie disease).

1882 *William Edward Gallie* born. A Canadian professor of surgery who introduced fascial sutures for surgery of inguinal hernia (1927).

1882 *Erich Franz Eugen Bracht* born. A German pathologist and gynecologist who (with Hermann J. G. Wächter) described perivascular microabscesses in acute bacterial endocarditis (Bracht–Wächter bodies).

1882 In a classical account on mitosis, Walther Flemming described nuclear division involving the chromosomes in the cell.

1882 Recognition of tautomerism was influenced by the work of Nobel laureate (1905), Johann Friedrich Wilhelm Adolf von Baeyer, who studied condensation of phenols and aldehydes, and synthesized the dye, indigo.

1882 *Charles Foix* born. A French neurologist who described the Foix syndrome of ophthalmoplegia due to paralysis of the 3rd, 4th, 5th and 6th cranial nerves, secondary to pathology in the lateral wall of the cavernous sinus (1922).

1882 *Johanne Ostenfeld Christiansen* born. A Danish physician who discovered the part played by hemoglobin in the transport of carbon dioxide, and devised a method of preparing coagulated egg albumin for determining peptic activity.

1882   *Sir Paul Gordon Fildes* born. A London pathologist who established that females do not suffer from hemophilia, and devised a blood extract culture medium.

1882   *Vivian Bartley Green-Armitage* born. A London gynecologist who devised the Green-Armitage forceps for controlling hemorrhage from the uterus during cesarean section.

1882   The tubercle bacillus was isolated by German bacteriologist, Robert Koch, the first bacteria attributed to a human disease.

1882   Harrison Allen, an anatomist from Philadelphia, described the Allen fossa on the neck of the femur.

1882   *William Martin Flack* born. An English physiologist who discovered the sino-atrial node of the heart while working with Sir Arthur Keith.

1882   Richard von Volkmann of Germany described a primary epithelioma of the neck arising from branchiogenic cysts (branchiogenic carcinoma).

1882   The prolongation of the optic tract extending to the third nerve nuclei, the cerebellum and the pons (Stilling root) was described by Jakob Stilling, professor of ophthalmology in Strasburg.

1882   *Arthur James Ewins* born. An English chemist who isolated the neurotransmitter acetylcholine (1914), and whose work led to the development of the antibiotic, sulfapyridine, the first successful treatment for gonorrhea.

1882   *Sir Harold Delf Gillies* born. A plastic surgeon from New Zealand who described his operation for cleft palate (1921), and devised several surgical instruments named after him (Gillies forceps, Gillies needle-holder).

1882   The rare inherited disease, xeroderma pigmentosum, characterized by hypersensitivity to ultraviolet light and skin cancer, was described by Hungarian dermatologist, Moritz Kaposi.

1882   The first bed donation for antenatal care in Edinburgh was made by A.H. Freeland, assistant professor of midwifery at the University of Edinburgh.

1882   A classic description of von Recklinghausen disease, multiple tumors of the nerve with café-au-lait spots in the skin, known as neurofibromatosis, was given by professor of pathology in Königsberg, Friedrich Daniel von Recklinghausen.

1882   *David Percival Dalbreck Wilkie* born. An Edinburgh surgeon who described the supraduodenal artery (Wilkie artery), and stenosis of the same artery complicated by duodenal ulcer (Wilkie syndrome).

1882   The creation of a surgical fistula between the gallbladder and intestines (cholecystenterostomy) was suggested by Munich surgeon, Johann Nepomuk von Nussbaum.

1882 Eduard Heinrich Henoch, a German pioneer in pediatrics, published *Lectures on Diseases of Children, A Handbook for Physicians and Students.*

1882 Successful removal of the gallbladder was performed by German surgeon, Carl Johann August Langenbuch.

1882 Heinrich Quincke, a German professor of medicine who spent most of his working career in Switzerland, gave the first description of angioneurotic edema.

1882 *Robert Debré* born. A French pediatrician who wrote on measles, infectious edematous polyneuritis, muscle hypertrophy, pseudospasm of the pylorus, and sexual infantilism.

1882 *Herbert McLean Evans* born. An American physiologist who developed a diazo dye used to estimate blood volume and cardiac output (Evans blue).

1882 The occurrence of polycythemia in persons living at high altitude was observed by Paul Bert of France.

1882 Fatty infiltration of the heart was described by German physician, Ernst Viktor von Leyden.

1882 Determination of blood volume using carbon monoxide was undertaken by two French physicians, Charles Eugene Quinquad and Nestor Grehant.

1882 The first successful culture of gonococcus was made by German bacteriologist, Leo Leistikow.

1883 A test chart for astigmatism consisting of three parallel lines at various meridians devised by German oculist, Otto Heinrich Enoch Becker.

1883 Tremor of the hands as a sign of exophthalmic goiter was described by Pierre Marie of Paris.

1883 Routine examination of the eyes in school children was advocated by German ophthalmologist, Hermann L. Cohn.

1883 The first rib resection in London for empyema was performed by Arbuthnot Lane of Guy's Hospital.

1883 *Karl Friedrich August Lange* born. He developed the Lange test for cerebrospinal syphilis (1913).

1883 *Corynebacterium diphtheriae* was discovered by German bacteriologist, Theodor Albrecht Edwin Klebs.

1883 *William Waddell Duke* born. A Kansas pathologist who introduced a method of estimating bleeding time by making a needle puncture on the lobe of the ear and removing the blood every 30 seconds with blotting paper until it stopped.

1883 Beta-oxybutyric acid in urine was discovered by a German physical chemist, Ernest Stedelman.

1883 Barlow disease, or infantile scurvy, was described by Thomas Barlow of London.

1883 A translation of August Hirsch's *Handbuch der historisch-geographischen Pathologie*, was published in English.

1883 *Edward E. Lindeman* born. A New York surgeon who devised a direct method of transfusing blood through a two-way syringe (1913).

1883 *Otto Heinrich Warburg* born. A German biochemist and Nobel laureate (1931) who discovered the role of iron in oxidase enzymes leading to the discovery of the heme protein, and developed the gas manometer.

1883

Evarts Graham

Evarts Ambrose Graham born. A St Louis professor of surgery who developed cholecystography, performed the first pneumonectomy, and associated tobacco smoking with lung cancer.

1883 The retrorenal fascia (Zuckerkandl fascia) was described by Hungarian-born anatomist, Emil Zuckerkandl.

1883 *Bernard Aschner* born. An Austrian physician who discovered the oculo-cardiac reflex, created long-lived hypophysectomized dogs to study the pituitary, and wrote *Endocrine Disorders of Females* and *Constitutional Therapy*.

1883 Renal osteodystrophy in patients with chronic renal disease (renal rickets) was described by Richard Clement Lucas of Guy's Hospital in London.

1883 English physiologist, Sydney Ringer, described the influence of calcium on excitability and contraction of the heart muscles (calcium channel).

1883 The antithrombic substance present in the salivary glands of the leech (hirudin) was found to have anticoagulant properties by J. B. Haycraft.

1883 *Hugh MacLean* born. A professor of medicine at the University of London and director of the Medical Clinic at St Thomas' Hospital, who designed the urea concentration test for renal function (1920).

1883 Supraventricular tachycardia was shown to consist of a series of atrial extrasystoles by Austrian physician, Wilhelm Winternitz.

1883 Surgical treatments for thyroid disorders, which helped elucidate its function, were developed by Swiss-born surgeon and Nobel

Prize winner (1909), Emil Theodor Kocher.

1883   The Ranke angle in craniometry was described by Dutch anthropologist and physician, Hans Rudolphe Ranke.

1883   *George Nicholas Papanicolaou* born. An American anatomist and cytologist who introduced cytology into the diagnosis of cancer, investigated normal cyclical changes of the vaginal epithelium (1917), and described the role of the vaginal smear in cancer (1928).

1883   The role of chromosomes as carriers of heredity was recognized by German physiologist, Wilhelm Roux.

1883

Margaret Sanger

Margaret Higgins Sanger born. A pioneer of birth control in America who began her crusade on the prejudice against birth control with the book *Family Limitation*, and established the first contraceptive advice center in Brooklyn and the National Birth Control League.

1883   *Samuel Jones Crowe* born. An American otorhinologist who described compression of the internal jugular vein on the normal side, in cases of lateral sinus thrombosis, and a subsequent cause of engorgement of the retinal vessels (Crowe sign).

1883   *Ralph Milton Waters* born. A Wisconsin anesthetist who described a closed circuit method for cyclopropane anesthesia (1934).

1883   The Gram stain for bacteria was developed by Hans Christian Joachim Gram of Denmark, while working on methods for double-staining kidney sections.

1883   *Robert Bruce Young* born. An anatomist from Glasgow who studied the knee joint and described the trapezometacarpel ligament (Young ligament) between the 3rd and 4th metacarpals and the trapezium.

1883   Noonan syndrome, congenital heart defect, web neck and chest deformity with hypertelorism and mild mental retardation, was described by O. Kobylinski at the Estonian University at Dorpat.

1883   *Melvin Starkey Henderson* born. An orthopedic surgeon from Rochester, Minnesota who described the osteocartilagenous bodies in the joints (synovial chondromatosis, 1918).

1883   *James Strandberg* born. A Swedish dermatologist and professor in Stockholm who (with Ester E. Groenblad) described the skin abnormality pseudoxanthoma elasticum, with angioid streaks in the retina (Groenblad–Strandberg syndrome).

1883 *Klebsiella pneumoniae*, a genus of gram-negative bacillus was first isolated from a series of patients with pneumonia by Karl Freidlander and named Friedlander bacillus.

1883 *Sir Arthur William Mickle Ellis* born. A Canadian-born London physician who gave a classification of Bright disease based on clinical and histological features (1942).

1884 The infectious nature of herpes zoster was recognized by French physician, Louis Landouzy.

1884 Inspiratory distention due to bronchitis as a predisposing cause of emphysema was suggested by McVail of Glasgow.

1884 Esophageal manometry was performed in humans, to study esophageal motility, by German physiologist, Karl Hugo Krönecker and American physiologist, Samuel James Meltzer.

1884 The New York Cancer Hospital, the first hospital for cancer in the United States, was established, and later renamed the Memorial Hospital.

1884 A pure culture of *Salmonella typhi* was obtained by Georg Theodor Gaffky, a German bacteriologist from Hannover, who also demonstrated that it caused typhoid.

1884 *Montrose Thomas Burrows* born. A cancer specialist from America who demonstrated the method of growing tumor tissue in vitro, and described a substance called archusia which he believed was the source of cancer.

1884 The first accurate, clinical localization of a brain tumor (which was successfully removed) was made by English surgeons, Alexander Hughes Bennett, with Sir John Rickman Godlee.

1884 A case of hydropneumothorax was treated by French cardiologist, Pierre Carl Eduard Potain, by withdrawing the fluid and replacing it with air.

1884 *Carl Friedrich Meyer* born. A professor of microbiology at the University of California who introduced the generic term *Brucella* for bacteria which caused Malta fever, in honor of its discoverer Sir David Bruce.

1884 The zona radiata of the mammalian ovum was described by Theodor Ludwig Wilhelm Bischoff, professor of anatomy and embryologist at Heidelberg.

1884 Parthogenesis, or asexual reproduction, was demonstrated experimentally and named by Jacques Loeb, a French-born American scientist.

1884 Landouzy–Dejerine dystrophy, a hereditary form of facio-scapulo-humeral muscular dystrophy, transmitted by an autosomal dominant trait, was described by French neurologists, Louis Theophil Joseph Landouzy and Joseph Jules Dejerine.

1884 The causative organism in glanders, *Pfiefferella mallei*, was identified by Friedrich August Johannes Löffler.

1884 *Leo Mayer* born. An American orthopedic surgeon who was a pioneer in reconstructive tendon operations for polio, and carried out important studies on bone tumors.

1884 *Robert Foster Kennedy* born. An Irish neurologist who described shell shock as a form of hysteria, described Kennedy syndrome in *Epilepsy and the Convulsive State*, and wrote on brain tumors and their symptomatology.

1884 Cocaine was introduced as a local anesthetic in eye surgery by Karl Koller, at the recommendation of Sigmund Freud.

1884 The prevention of ophthalmia neonatorum using silver nitrate was proposed by Carl Sigmund Franz Crede, professor of obstetrics and gynecology at Leipzig, Germany.

1884 The origin and nature of hypernephroma (Grawitz tumor) was elucidated by German surgeon, Paul Albert Grawitz.

1884 The term dermatitis herpetiformis was introduced to describe a group of skin eruptions (Duhring disease) by American dermatologist, Louis Adolphus Duhring.

1884 *Hermann Rorschach* born. A Swiss neuropsychiatrist who devised the Rorschach test, a diagnostic procedure in mental disorders and personality tests using standardized ink blots.

1884 Surgery for displaced semilunar cartilage of the knee was first performed by Thomas Annandale from Newcastle-upon-Tyne.

1884 The terms haploid and diploid to describe halving and doubling of chromosome numbers were coined by German botanist, Eduard Adolf Strasburger.

1884 *Otto Fritz Meyerhof* born. An American biochemist and Nobel laureate (1922) who worked out the pathway of glucose metabolism in muscle, and proposed the theory related to metabolic changes in the cytoplasm of muscle during contraction.

1884 *Naughton Dunn* born. An English orthopedic surgeon who described an operation for paralytic foot in which the peroneal and tibialis posterior tendons were transferred to the achilles tendon.

1884 *Burrill Bernard Crohn* born. A New York physician who described a regional disease consisting of abdominal pain, diarrhea and a mass often in the lower quadrant (Crohn disease, or regional ileitis).

1884 Nervous dyspepsia associated with hyperchlorhydria (Rossbach disease) was described by a German physician, Michael Joseph Rossbach.

1884   Introduction of enteric coated pills by German dermatologist, Paul Gerson Unna.

1884   Use of the centrifuge for separating red and white cells was suggested by Swedish physician, Magnus Gustav Blix.

1884   Antipyrine was introduced into clinical practice as an antipyretic and analgesic by German physician, Wilhelme Filehene.

1884   The Memorial Sloan-Kettering Cancer Center at New York was incorporated and opened.

1885   The blood–brain barrier, that prevents the uptake of some substances by the brain, described by Paul Ehrlich.

1885   Thoracoplasty by resection of the ribs for treatment of tuberculosis was performed by Cèrenville of Laussane, Switzerland.

1885   The pharmacological properties of hyoscine were described by Philadelphia physician, Horatio Charles Wood.

1885   Rabies vaccine administered to humans by Louis Pasteur of France.

1885   *Sir Francis Martin Rouse Walshe* born. A British neurosurgeon who described the symptoms of acroparesthesia and neuritis of the hands caused by pressure from the scalenus anticus muscle in thoracic outlet syndrome.

1885   Cocaine was used for local anesthesia for dental extraction by American surgeon, William Halstead.

1885   James Leonard Corning of New York introduced spinal anesthesia.

1885   Scottish physician, Sir Thomas Richard Fraser, investigated kombe poison from Africa and demonstrated its therapeutic effect on dropsy.

1885   German bacteriologist, Theodore Escherich, gave the first account of the bacterium, *Escherichia coli*, infection in children.

1885

Vladimir Bekhterev

The superior vestibular nucleus in the cranial nerve was described by Russian neurologist, Vladimir Mikhailovitch Bekhterev.

1885   A specific condition involving peripheral atrophy of the optic nerve (Fuchs atrophy) was first described by German oculist, Ernest Fuchs.

1885   *Wilhelm Siegmund Frei* born. A German dermatologist who devised an intradermal skin test for lymphogranuloma inguinale (Frei test).

1885 The earliest recorded successful removal of a spinal tumor was reported by a Scottish surgeon, Sir William MacEwen.

1885 The posterior lateral tract (marginal tract) of the spinal cord, the Lissauer tract, was described by a neurologist from Breslau, Heinrich Lissauer.

1885 *Lemuel Whittington Gorham* born. An American physician from Albany, New York who studied the relationship between cardiac pain and coronary occlusion (1938).

1885 Daniel Elmer Salmon of Cornell University isolated American hog cholera bacillus while working with Theobald Smith at the US Bureau of Animal Industry.

1885 A characteristic pattern of fever in Hodgkin disease (Pel–Ebstein fever) was described by German physician Pieter Klazes Pel, and in 1887 by his compatriot, Wilhelm Ebstein.

1885 Ascending and descending branches of the dorsal spinal nerve roots (Nansen fibers) were described by Fridtjof Nansen, curator of the Bergen Museum and Arctic explorer.

1885 Exophthalmos, ptosis and paralysis of the area of the ulnar nerve following injury to the 8th cervical nerve and 1st thoracic root (Dejerine-Klumpke syndrome) was described by Augusta Dejerine-Klumpke of Paris.

1885 J. Ferran, a Spanish bacteriologist, made the first attempt at large-scale immunization against cholera during an outbreak of the disease in Spain.

1885 The occurrence of acid intoxication in renal failure (renal acidosis) was observed by Rudolf von Jaksch, a Czech physician from Prague.

1885 A rare form of familial intermittent paralysis in early childhood or adolescence, associated with a low serum potassium (periodic paralysis), was described by Karl Friedrich Otto Westphal of Berlin, Germany.

1885 The rubro-spinal tract of the spinal cord (Monakow bundle) was described by Russian neurologist at Zurich, Konstantin von Monakow.

1885 *George Richards Minot* born. A Boston physician and Nobel laureate (1934) who demonstrated that some anemias are caused by failure of bone marrow to produce enough red blood cells, and others are caused when blood cells are destroyed too rapidly, and established the value of a raw liver diet in treatment of pernicious anemias.

1885 The Ogston–Luc operation, involving incision at the edge of the orbit for frontal sinus disease, was devised by Scottish surgeon Alexander Ogston, and French surgeon Henry Luc.

1885 Downward displacement of the viscera (enteroptis) in association with neurasthenia (Glenard syndrome) was described by French physician, Frantz Glenard.

1885   *Josef Siegfried Thannhauser* born. A German physician who described the familial clustering of patients with xanthomas, hypercholesterolemia, and premature heart disease (familial hypercholesterolemia, 1938).

1885   Violent muscular jerks of the shoulders, extremities and face, beginning in childhood with explosive grunting or coprolalia (Tourette syndrome), were described by French neurologist, Georges Gilles de La Tourette.

1885   The anterior marginal bundle of the cerebellar tract (Löwenthal tract) was described by German physician, Wilhelm Löwenthal.

1885   *Adolf Edelman* born. An Austrian physician who was the first to describe anemia in chronic infections, in addition to devising a test for urobilin in urine (1915).

1885   *George Eli Bennett* born. An American orthopedic surgeon who worked through polio epidemics in the early 20th century, and established the first respirator unit for bulbar palsy.

1885   Cells responsible for bone growth and formation (osteoblasts) were described by Carl Gegenbaur, a comparative anatomist at the University of Würzberg in Germany.

1885   *Ludwig Haberlandt* born. An Austrian physician who searched for a heart hormone and developed hormonal contraception.

1885   A chronic relapsing condition of the colon (ulcerative colitis) was described by Sir William Allchin of London.

1885   *Friedrich Pauwels* born. A German orthopedic surgeon who worked on the biomechanical influences on the growth and behavior of bone and cartilage.

1886   *Elizabeth Kenny* born. A pioneer of nursing in Australia who established clinics for providing physical therapy to polio victims in several parts of the world, including Britain and America.

1886   Tumor of the synovial membrane (synovioma) was described by American surgeon from New York, Robert Fulton Weir.

1886   *William John Adie* born. An Australian-born English physician who worked at the National Hospital for Nervous Disease, gave an original description of narcolepsy, and Holmes–Adie syndrome of myotonic pupils and absent tendon reflexes (1931).

1886   The pneumococcus bacterium was isolated by Albert Fränkel of Germany.

1886   *Entameba histolytica* was isolated from a tropical abscess of the liver by Greek physician, Stephanos Kartulis.

1886   Operative treatment for hydronephrosis was performed by Friedrich Trendelenburg of Germany.

1886   A container for sterile solutions used for injections, the ampoule, was invented by a pharmacist, Stanislaus Limousin of Paris.

1886   Autosomal recessive disease in which bullous lesions of the skin occur from minor trauma (epidermolysis bullosa) was described by German professor of medicine, Johannes Goldscheider.

1886

Walter Dandy

Walter Edward Dandy born. An American neurosurgeon who devised a method of introducing air into cerebral vesicles, treated trigeminal neuralgia by resection of the trigeminal ganglion (1934), and described a form of hydrocephalus (Dandy–Walker syndrome, 1921.

1886   *Paul Schilder* born. An American psychiatrist who observed induration of cerebral substance due to slow inflammatory reaction (Schilder disease), and identified a subclass where extensive lesions of white matter occurred in both hemispheres (1921).

1886   *Archibald Vivien Hill* born. A physiologist from University College London and Nobel laureate (1922) who measured the heat produced in a contracting or recovering muscle related to lactic acid production, and provided an explanation of the transmission of nerve impulses (1926).

1886   Protection of pigeons from cholera infections by heat-killed cultures of chicken cholera bacilli was demonstrated by Theobald Smith.

1886   Jean-Martin Charcot and Pierre Marie of Paris described autosomal dominant inherited muscular atrophy due to neurological changes in the spinal cord and nerves (Charcot–Marie–Tooth–Hoffman syndrome).

1886   Seborrhoeic eczema (Unna dermatosis) was described by German dermatologist Paul Gerson Unna.

1886   William Richard Gowers, a London neurologist, published one of the most significant works of his era, *Diseases of the Nervous System*.

1886   A method of estimating creatinine in blood was devised by German biochemist, Max Jaffe.

1886   *G. Di Gugliemo* born. An Italian hematologist who described a form of anemia secondary to erythroleukemia (Di Gugliemo disease).

1886   *Paul Dudley White* born. A Harvard cardiologist who wrote a book on heart diseases (1931), and treated President Eisenhower for Wolf–Parkinson–White syndrome, due to an accessory conduction pathway which predisposes to cardiac arrhythmia, which he also described (1930).

1886 English physiologist, Leonard Charles Woolbridge showed that by injecting tissue thromboplastin intravenously into animals, their blood became incoagulable.

1886 Heat sterilization (which heralded the beginning of aseptic surgery) was introduced by Berlin surgeon, Ernst von Bergmann.

1886 *Charles Frederick Morris Saint* born. A South African physician at Groote Schuur Hospital who described the Saint triad, consisting of gallbladder disease, diverticulosis and hiatus hernia.

1886 *Harold Ensign Bennett Pardee* born. An American cardiologist who described the downward deflection of the T wave in ECG of coronary disease.

1886 The bacterial cause of erysipelas (Fehleisen streptococcus) was discovered by Friedrich Fehleisen, and was isolated two years later.

1886 A form of chronic synovitis of the knee joint seen in congenital syphilis (Clutton joints) was described by English surgeon, Henry Hugh Clutton.

1886 *Edward Calvin Kendall* born. An American biologist and Nobel laureate (1950) who headed the biochemistry section at the Mayo Foundation, and isolated thyroxin (1914), cortisone and other ste-

Edward Calvin Kendall

roids which he used in treatment of rheumatoid arthritis.

1886 *Lewis Hill Weed* born. An American neurologist who advanced the theory of cerebrospinal fluid circulation proposed by Gustav Retzius, and showed that the fluid was absorbed by arachnoid villi (1914).

1886 *Chester Jefferson Farmer* born. A Chicago chemist who developed microchemical assay methods for urea, creatinine and other substances.

1886 Minute particles in stained smears of vaccinial lesions (Buist–Paschen bodies) were observed by Scottish pathologist, John Brown Buist.

1886 Louis Pasteur and J. Joubert observed that bacterium produced a substance that killed other bacterium (antibiosis).

1886 Ballotement, a valuable sign for tumors of the kidney, was described by French pathologist, Jean Casimir Felix Guynon.

1886 A machine to give physiotherapy and apply manipulation to the body (Zander apparatus) was described by Swedish physician, Jonas Gustav Wilhelm Zander.

1886 Professor of histology at Graz, Austria, Otto Drasch, described the cuneiform cells in the mucous membrane of the trachea.

1886 An enlarged deformed kidney (Formad kidney) was observed in some cases of chronic alcoholism by American physician, Henry F. Formad.

1886 *Hamilton Hartridge* born. A London physiologist who devised the spectroscope (Hartridge reversion spectroscope) which gave two spectra of the same solution, and proposed the Hartridge cluster theory for color vision.

1886 *Sir Phillipe Samuel Bedson* born. A London bacteriologist who devised a laboratory diagnosis for lymphogranuloma venereum, through skin testing with an antigen (1936), and provided conclusive evidence for the etiological agent of psittacosis.

1886 One of the first human cases of actinomycosis was described by William Osler, a professor at Oxford, England.

1886 *Henry Albert Harris* born. A professor of anatomy at Cambridge who described the transverse lines near the epiphysis in the long bones.

1886 The first portable gas and oxygen machine was invented by London physician and pioneer in anesthetics, Sir Frederick William Hewitt.

1887 Irish surgeon, Charles Bent Ball, described a radical cure for abdominal hernia, the Ball operation.

1887 *Sir William Heneage Ogilvie* born. A London surgeon at Guy's Hospital who described functional obstruction of the large bowel in elderly patients (Ogilvie syndrome).

1887 Chronic relapsing pyrexia of Hodgkin disease (Ebstein fever) was described by Göttingen physician, Wilhelm Ebstein and Dutch physician, Pieter Klazes Pel.

1887 The cerebral manifestations and pathology of Tay–Sachs disease, amaurotic familial idiocy with ocular manifestations, were noted by New York physician, Bernard Parney Sachs.

1887 Infectious mononucleosis was described as glandular fever by Moscow pediatrician, Feodorovitch Filatov.

1887 *Alfred Washington Adson* born. A Minnesota neurosurgeon who was one of the first to use sympathectomy for the treatment of hypertension, cervical sympathectomy for Raynaud syndrome, and described the Adson sign of obliteration of the radial pulse when the head is turned to the affected side.

1887 The contact lens was introduced by Adolf Eugen Fick, a German physician in Zurich.

1887   The number of chromosomes was found to be constant for each cell in a given species by the Belgian cytologist, Edouard Joseph Louis Beneden.

1887   *Walter Schiller* born. An Austrian pathologist who devised the Schiller test for carcinoma, where the cervix is painted with Gram stain to detect unstainable areas of possible carcinoma.

1887   *Alfred Erich Frank* born. A German physician who identified diabetes insipidus as being due to a lesion of the posterior pituitary, and described non-thrombocytopenic purpura (Frank capillary toxicosis).

1887   *Julius Bauer* born. An Austrian physicist who wrote *Constitution and Disease*, and was one of the first to suggest multiple hormones within a single gland.

1887   A large aneurysm of the internal carotid artery eroding the sella and producing signs of bitemporal hemianopia was reported by Edinburgh surgeon, Byrom Bramwell.

1887   *Leopold Ruzicka* born. A Yugoslav chemist who became professor of chemistry at Utrecht, pioneered the study of sex hormones, and prepared testosterone artificially from cholesterol (1935).

1887   Charles Jacques Bouchard described toxemia resulting from the absorption of food products under the influence of bacteria.

1887   German physician, Max Bockhardt, described a superficial staphylococcal folliculitis occurring as a complication of skin diseases, including eczema and scabies (Bockhart impetigo).

1887   The area in the anterior wall of the vagina in contact with the base of the bladder and free of vaginal rugae was described by Karel Pawlik, a gynecologist from Prague, Czechoslovakia.

1887   Austrian pathologist, Anton Weichselbaum, isolated the causative organism of cerebrospinal fever, the meningococcus, from cerebrospinal fluid of patients with meningitis.

1887   *Eduard Gamper* born. An Austrian neurologist who described a reflex seen in children with severe brain damage and occasionally in normal premature babies (Gamper bowing reflex).

1887   Charles Barret Lockwood founded the Anatomical Society of Great Britain and Ireland.

1887   The secretory Paneth cells in the mucosa of the small intestine were independently described by M. Davidoff of St Petersburg and Joseph Paneth of Breslau.

1887   The Stohr cells in the pyloric gastric glands were named after Philipp Stohr, professor of anatomy at Würzberg who described them.

1887   Ephedrine was isolated from *Ephedra vulgaris* by Nagajosi Nagai.

1887   Alcohol injection for the treatment of neuralgia was introduced by

French physician, Jean Albert Pitres.

1887   Vittorio Marchi, an anatomist from Florence, Italy described the anterolateral descending tract of the spinal cord (Marchi tract).

1887   *Erwin Schroedinger* born. An Austrian physician and Nobel Prize winner who discovered quantum theory, the theory of heat, and wrote the famous work *What is Life?*

1887   A defect in the development of the hair follicles (Giovanni disease) was described by a Turin dermatologist, Sebastiano Giovanni.

1887   *Bernhard Dattner* born. A neurologist from the New York University Medical Center who designed a needle for aspirating cerebrospinal fluid, consisting of a fine inner needle within an outer moderate-bore needle for perforating the spinal dura mater.

1887   The infectious nature of acute anterior poliomyelitis was clinically described by Oscar Medin after studying a large breakout of this disease in Sweden.

1887   *Thomas Porter McMurray* born. The first professor of orthopedics in England who introduced sub-trochanteric osteotomy as treatment for osteoarthritis of the hip joint, and described the clinical test (McMurray test) for meniscal tear by rotating the knee.

1887   The American Orthopedic Association was founded.

1887   The color change in vulvovaginal mucosa as a sign of pregnancy (Chadwick sign) was described by Boston gynecologist, James Read Chadwick.

James Read Chadwick

1887   Circular suture for intestines were pioneered by New York surgeon, William Stewart Halstead.

1887   *Hermann Zondek* born. A German physician who elucidated endocrine function and hormone action, demonstrated the relationship between glands and organs, and wrote *Diseases of the Endocrine Glands.*

1887   *Detlev Wulf Bronk* born. An American neurophysiologist who studied the biophysical properties of motor nerve fibers (1927), and recorded the activity of single nerve motor units (1928).

1887   *Gustav Hoffer* born. An otorhinologist from Vienna who described the depressor nerve of the cardiac plexus, a branch of the superior laryngeal nerve.

1887 The forerunner of the electrocardiogram was measured, with a capillary electrometer, by Augustus Desire Waller, a physiologist at St Mary's Hospital, London.

1887 *Adrian Stokes* born. An American pathologist who found the specific virus of yellow fever, and died from it during his experimentation.

1887 *Robert Wartenberg* born. An American neurologist who described the Wartenberg sign, where the little finger is held up in ulnar paralysis.

1887 *William Cumming Rose* born. An American biochemist from Greenville, South Carolina who studied the role of amino acids and identified 10 that are indispensable for human nutrition.

1887 *Bernardo Alberto Houssay* born. An Argentinean physician and Nobel laureate (1947) who contributed to an understanding of feedback mechanisms in endocrinology, particularly in relation to insulin, with his work on the pituitary gland.

1887 The Roger sphygmomanometer, which used an aneroid manometer instead of mercury, was designed by New York physician, Oscar Harrison Roger.

1887 The bacterium in the spleen of patients dying from Mediterranean fever (brucellosis) was isolated by Sir David Bruce who named it *Micrococcus melitensis*.

1887 Mercury injections, in the form of diethyl mercury, were introduced as a treatment for syphilis by P. Hepp of Germany, but abandoned due to toxicity.

1887 An elective and successful operation for appendicitis was carried out by American surgeon, Thomas George Morton.

1887 March foot accompanied by pain and sometimes fracture of metatarsal bones due to prolonged marching was described by French physician, Jean Eugene Pauzat.

1887 An apparatus for artificial ventilation for opium poisoning was developed by George Fell at Buffalo, New York.

1887 An electric probe for detecting bullets and foreign metal bodies in humans was devised by American physician, John Harvey Girdner.

1887 The first record of abdominal distention in rickets was given by Richard C. Lucas, a surgeon at Guy's Hospital, London.

1888 The cortical visual center was discovered by Swedish pathologist, Salomon Eberhard Henschen.

1888 An obstetric bag to dilate the cervix was devised by French obstetrician, Camille L.A. Champetier de Ribes.

1888 The first successful removal of a brain tumor was carried out by American neurologist and surgeon, William Williams Keen.

1888 *Selman Abraham Waksman* born. An American biochemist and Nobel laureate (1952) who discovered streptomycin (recognizing its value in the treatment of tuberculosis), neomycin, and stretocin.

1888 L. Severini presented evidence that carbon dioxide produced vasodilation.

1888 The first clinical use of artificial pneumothorax in the treatment of tuberculosis was by Italian physician, Carlo Forlanini.

1888 August Gärtner discovered *Bacillus enteritidis* as a cause of meat poisoning and the bacterium was later renamed *Salmonella enteritidis*.

1888 The Graham Steell murmur, heard over the pulmonary artery in early diastole due to pulmonary hypertension resulting from mitral stenosis, was described by Graham Steell, a physician from the Manchester Royal Infirmary.

1888 Corneal grafting or plastic surgery of the cornea (keratoplasty) was introduced by Arthur von Hippel of Germany.

1888 *Russel Landram Haden* born. An American physician and hematologist who described an acid hematin method for estimating hemoglobin, and the peculiar target cell, with a bull's eye appearance.

1888 An early modern monographs on intracranial tumors was written by Byrom Bramwell, a physician to the Edinburgh Royal Infirmary.

1888 An important treatise on the surgical diseases of the bladder and prostate was published by Jean Casimir Felix Guyon, a professor in Paris and the founder of modern genitourinary surgery.

1888 The cells of the gastric secretory glands (parietal cells) were described by Prussian professor of physiology and histology, Rudolf Peter Heinrich Heidenhain.

1888 Theobald Smith, a bacteriologist from Harvard University discovered the tick to be the vector in Texas cattle fever.

1888 A tumor of the spinal cord was successfully removed by the father of neurosurgery in England, Sir Victor Horsley.

1888 *Sir Ivan Whiteside Magill* born. A consultant to the Brompton and Westminster Hospitals in London who devised an endotracheal tube used in anesthesia and resuscitation (Magill tube).

1888 Osteochondritis dissecans, a condition marked by the splitting of joint cartilage, especially in the knee and shoulder joints, was described by German surgeon, Franz König.

1888 *Robin Sanno Fahraeus* born. A German pathologist who studied the sedimentation properties of blood.

1888 Cancer of the pancreas was described by Swiss physician Louis Bard.

1888 Martinotti cells, a distinct cell type in the cerebral cortex, were described by Giovanni Martinotti, professor of anatomy at Bologna, Italy.

1888 An appendix before rupture was removed successfully by New York surgeon Henry Barton Sands.

1888 Non-tropical sprue due to gluten-induced enteropathy (celiac disease) was described by Samuel Jones Gee of St Bartholomew's Hospital.

1888 *Sigard Adolphus Knopf* born. A New York orthopedic surgeon who devised a pin for fixing fractures of the femoral neck.

1888 *Hans Christian Hagedorn* born. A Danish physician who started the first large-scale manufacture of insulin (with August Schack Krogh) by establishing the non-profit Nordisk Insulin Laboratory (1922).

1888 Giant gastric hypertrophy with hypoproteinemia, diarrhea and protein-losing enteropathy (Ménétrier disease) was described by French histopathologist, Pierre E. Ménétrier.

1888 *Clarence Cook Little* born. An American pioneer of cancer genetics who established the first inbred strain of mice, an essential stage in understanding drug action, transplantation, and treatment of cancer.

1888 The fibromuscular mass found between the coccyx and the anus in the perineum (Symington anococcygial body) was described by Scottish anatomist, Johnson Symington, professor of anatomy in Belfast.

1888 Congenital megacolon (Hirschsprung disease) was described by Danish pediatrician, Harald Hirschsprung.

1888 Outflow obstruction to the right ventricle, ventricular septal defect, right ventricular hypertrophy and dextroposition of the aorta (Fallot tetralogy) was described by Etienne Louis Arthur Fallot of France.

1888

Herbert Gasser

Herbert Spencer Gasser born. A Wisconsin physiologist, Nobel laureate (1944) and a director of the Rockefeller Institute for Medical Research, who studied the functional differentiation of nerve fibers.

1888 Treatment of neurotic diseases with persuasive therapy or psychotherapy was pioneered by Paul Charles Dubois, professor of neurotherapy in Bern.

1888 *Abraham Lewinshon* born. A graduate of Northwestern Medical School and a pioneer in pediatrics who wrote *Cerebrospinal Fluid in Health and Disease* (1919).

1888 *Kenji Takanagi* born. A Japanese orthopedic surgeon who pioneered intra-articular cinematography, and later used it in cases of spina bifida.

1889   Scottish physiologist, Alexander John MacWilliam, gave the first account of death caused by ventricular fibrillation.

1889   The temporal lobe as a center for olfactory and gustatory sensations was described by British neurologist, John Hughlings Jackson.

1889   A subcutaneous connective tissue disorder resulting from deposition of fat, giving rise to painful symptoms in postmenopausal women (Dercum syndrome) was described by Francis Xavier Dercum, a neurologist from Philadelphia.

1889   *John Alfred Ryle* born. A physician at Guy's Hospital in London who improved the stomach tube designed by Martin Rehfuss (1914), making it safer and more comfortable for the patient to swallow, and he also wrote *Gastric Function in Health and Disease* (1926).

1889   Acne varioliformis was described by the Norwegian pathologist, Caesar Peter Moeller Boeck.

1889   *Lord Edgar Douglas Adrian* born. A British pioneer in neurophysiology who did valuable work on the activity of the nervous system, later paving the way for the development of the electroencephalogram in clinical practice.

1889   The fibers of the optic tract (Bernheimer fibers) were described by Stephan Bernheimer, a professor of ophthalmology from Vienna.

1889   Diphtheria was shown to be due to the toxin and not the bacterium, by French bacteriologists, Pierre Roux and Alexander Emile Jean Yersin.

1889   The removal of several ribs to collapse the lung (thoracoplasty) was performed as treatment for empyema by Ernest George Ferdinand von Küstner.

1889   A classic description of infectious mononucleosis (Pfeiffer disease or drusenfieber) was given by Emil Pfeiffer of Germany.

1889   Carcinoma was transplanted into mammals by German pathologist, Arthur Nathan Hanau.

1889   The McBurney incision, whereby the abdominal wall is opened during appendectomy along the layer of muscle fibers rather than cutting across the fibers, was described by New York surgeon, Charles McBurney.

1889   *George Washington Corner* born. An anatomist from New York who discovered progesterone in the corpus luteum (1929) with fellow American physician, Willard Myson Allen.

1889   *Eli Kinnerley Marshall* born. An American pharmacologist at the Johns Hopkins Hospital, Baltimore who demonstrated the secretory function of the renal convoluted tubule using phenolsulfonephthalein.

1889   The first systematic experiments to show that pancreatectomy led to diabetes mellitus were carried out by Josef von Mering and Lithuanian professor in Breslau, Oskar Minkowski.

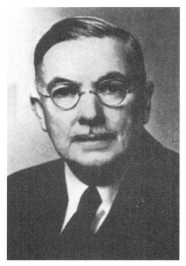

George Washington Corner

1889   *Barney D. Usher* born. An American dermatologist who researched the mechanisms of sweating and on the relationship of internal disease with eczema, and (with Francis E. Senear) described the association of pemphigus foliaceus with clinical and immunological features of lupus erythematosus (Senear–Usher syndrome).

1889   Paroxysmal atrial tachycardia was described by Léon Bouveret of Paris, who originally named it atrial tachycardia.

1889   Catgut was used for suturing intestines by New York surgeon, Robert Abbe.

1889   *Bernard Chavasse* born. A Liverpool ophthalmologist who developed myomectomy of the inferior oblique muscle (Chavasse operation).

1889   Bismuth was suggested as a treatment for syphilis by Paris physician, Felix Balzar.

1889

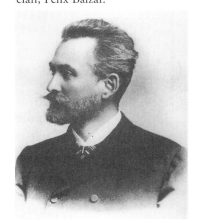

Gustav Walcher

The Walcher position in obstetrics with legs hanging down during delivery, was described by German gynecologist, Gustav Adolf Walcher.

1889   Telangiectasis, warty growths arranged in groups and thickening of the epidermis (angiokeratoma) was described by Italian dermatologist, Vittorio Mibelli (Mibelli disease).

1889   The efficacy of cod liver oil and crushed bone in treatment of rickets was experimentally demonstrated in England by Sir John Bland-Sutton.

1889   Rheumatoid arthritis in children between first and second dentition (Still–Chauffard syndrome) and pseudoxanthoma elasticum were described by French physician, Anatole Marie Emile Chauffard.

280

1889   *William Thomas Astbury* born. An English biochemist who demonstrated the diffraction pattern of DNA (1937), and classified proteins into the groups: keratin, myosin, elastin and collagen.

1889   *Paul Karrer* born. A Swiss biochemist born in Moscow and Nobel laureate (1937) who identified the structure of vitamin A, riboflavin (vitamin B_2), vitamin C, vitamin E, and vitamin K.

1889   The action of cocaine as a spinal anesthetic was discovered by German surgeon, August Karl Gustav Bier of Kiel.

1889   The site of maximum tenderness in the right iliac fossa in appendicitis (McBurney point) was described by New York surgeon, Charles McBurney.

1889   Osteoplastic resection of the skull (Wagner operation) was described by German surgeon, Wilhelm Wagner.

1889   Digital removal of necrotic tissue in a lung abscess was performed by T. Openchowski of Dorpat, Germany.

1889   An early description of multiple myeloma was given by Bohemian physician, Carl Hugo Huppert. His description preceded that of Kahler by a week.

1889   Surgical repair of traumatic diaphragmatic hernia was described by P. Postemski of Bologna.

1889   A laryngeal operation through the mouth was performed by Friedrich

Edward Rudolf Voltolini, an otorhinolaryngologist at Breslau.

1890   Quantitative relations between oxygen and hemoglobin were established by G. Hüffner, who showed that 1 gram of hemoglobin combined with 1.34 ml of oxygen.

1890   The Manchester operation for uterine prolapse, involving high amputation of the cervix and repair of the anterior and posterior vaginal walls, was devised by Archibald Donald of Manchester.

1890   The rare congenital condition amazia, (absence of the mammary gland) was highlighted by John William Ballantyne at the Edinburgh Obstetrical Society.

1890   The Hoffa method of operative treatment for congenital dislocation of the hip was designed by South-African born German surgeon, Albert Hoffa.

1890   Niels Ryberg Finsen, a Danish physician, demonstrated the bacterial effects of sunlight and developed a new method of treating lupus vulgaris with ultraviolet light.

1890   A tumor in the right temporosphenoidal area causing olfactory seizures was described by British neurologist, John Hughlings Jackson.

1890   Sebaceous adenoma, Pringle disease, was described by English dermatologist, John James Pringle.

1890   A staining method for *Actinomyces* was devised by mycologist, Eugen Bostroem.

1890   New York surgeon, Robert Abbe, devised a method of dilating esophageal stricture retrogradedly, by opening the stomach to receive a string saw through the buccal cavity.

1890   A slow progressive form of hereditary neuritis associated with kyphoscolisis, arthritis and ocular changes (Dejerine–Sottas syndrome) was described by French neurologists, Jules Sottas and Joseph Jules Dejerine.

1890   Diffuse hyperplasia of the skin with black pigmentation, or acanthosis nigricans, was described by Sigmund Pollitzer of Hamburg and Victor Janowsky.

1890   An acute rapidly progressive form of diabetes mellitus (Hirschfeld disease) was first described by German physician, Felix Hirschfeld.

1890   Tenderness localized in the right hypochondrium over the inflamed gallbladder in cholecystitis (Courvoisier sign), was described by Ludwig Georg Courvoisier, professor of surgery from Switzerland.

1890   The Penrose drain, a rubber tube with a gauze wick used in surgery, was devised by American gynecologist, Charles Bingham Penrose of Pennsylvania.

1890   Frontal lobotomy was performed on four mental patients at a Swiss mental hospital by G. Burckhard.

1890   Friedrich August Johannes Löffler noted flagella in bacteria which enabled motility.

1890   *Henry Patrick Wagener* born. An American ophthalmologist who described various grades of hypertension based on the funduscopic appearance of the retina.

1890   French scientist, Jacques Arsene d'Arsonval, showed that it was possible to use electricity to induce anesthesia (electrical anesthesia).

1890   Systematic exercises for tabetic ataxia were introduced by Heinrich S. Frenkel of the Freihoff Sanatorium in Switzerland, who advocated the use of extensive physiotherapy for neurological disease.

1890   Pulmonary osteoarthropathy was described in detail by Pierre Marie of Paris, France.

1890   *Hermann Joseph Müller* born. A New York geneticist and Nobel laureate (1946) who pioneered the study of mutation and created gene mutations following exposure to X-rays.

1890   The treatment of liver abscess by drainage through a needle was pioneered by John Rickman Godlee, a London surgeon at the Brompton Hospital.

1890   *John Leonard Kantor* born. A gastroenterologist at the Presbyterian Hospital in New York, who described the constriction of the terminal ileum in cases of Crohn disease.

1890   Themistokles Gluck of Germany recorded the first prosthetic replacement of a hip joint, and excise and replaced the knee, elbow, shoulder, wrist and hip joints at around the same time.

1890   Emil von Behring from Prussia, and Shibasaburo Kitasato, demonstrated the first successful clinical use of diphtheria antitoxin and proposed the word alexin (complement) for the substance.

1890   The intestinal disease amebic dysentery was studied and named by William Thomas Councilman of Harvard University.

1890   *Jacques Forestier* born. A French physician who introduced the treatment of rheumatoid arthritis with gold salts.

1890   Phonocardiography, a method of recording heart sounds, was introduced by Dutch physiologist Willem Einthoven and M. A. J. Geluk of Germany.

1890   Lupus vulgaris erythematoides, Leloir disease, was described by Henri Camille C. Leloir.

1890   The practice of correcting teeth irregularities (orthodontics) was developed by American, Edwin Hartley Angle of St Louis, who published *A System of Appliances for Correcting Irregularities of the Teeth.*

1890   *Sir Ronald Aylmer Fisher* born. A geneticist and statistician from London who carried out pioneering work on blood groups as genetic markers.

1890   Dutchman, Christian Eijkman, conclusively established beriberi as a deficiency disease.

1890   A differential rheotome to record the voluntary contractions of the muscle on a time related basis, was invented by German professor of physiology at Halle, Julius Bernstein.

1890   Microcytosis, characterized by the presence of small hemoglobin-containing erythrocytes or microcytes in the blood, were observed by Constant Vanlair and Jean Baptiste Voltaire Masius of Belgium.

1891   *Bernhard Zondek* born. A German-born Israeli gynecologist and endocrinologist who designed the first reliable pregnancy test with Selmar Aschheim (1928), and discovered gonadotrophins.

1891   *Roger Anderson* born. A surgeon from Seattle, Washington who devised the Anderson operation, a procedure for lengthening a tendon.

1891   Myxedema was treated successfully with injections of glycerin extract of sheep thyroid gland by George R. Murray of Newcastle-upon-Tyne, England.

1891   *Wilder Graves Penfield* born. An American-born Canadian neurosurgeon whose research at the Montreal Neurological Institute increased understanding of the higher functions of the brain and causes of diseases such as epilepsy.

1891   The structure and function of the placenta were accurately explained by Charles Sedgwick Minot, professor of comparative anatomy at Harvard.

1891 An attempt to treat Addison disease with glandular therapy was made by Sir William Osler at the Johns Hopkins Hospital Medical School in Baltimore.

1891 A rare form of familial epilepsy, myoclonus epilepsy, where clonic spasm of a group of muscles occurred in paroxysms (Unverricht disease) was described by German physician, Heinrich Unverricht.

1891 Strümpell disease, polioencephalomyelitis, was described by German neurologist, Ernst von Strümpell from Leipzig.

1891 A torn pericardium from a stab wound was successfully sutured by Henry C. Dalton of Washington University.

1891 Degenerative changes in the spinal cord associated with pernicious anemia (Putnam disease) was described independently by Charles Loomes Dana from Vermont and another American, James Jackson Putnam of Boston.

1891 The outpouching of the gallbladder near its junction with the cystic duct (Hartmann pouch) was described by Henri Albert Charles Antoine Hartmann, professor of surgery from Paris.

1891 Austrian and German pathologists, Hans Chiari and Julius Arnold described Arnold–Chiari syndrome, tongue-like abnormal protrusions of the cerebellum and medulla oblongata.

1891 Osmic acid was introduced to stain nerve tissue by Italian histologist, Vittorio Marchi.

1891 The consequence of removal of the cerebellum in higher mammals was studied by Luigi Luiciani.

1891 Paul Ehrlich, a German bacteriologist, differentiated between lymphocytic and myelogenous leukemia.

1891 *George Otto Lignac* born. A Dutch pathologist who contributed to the knowledge of skin pigmentation, cystine metabolic anomalies and their effects on the kidneys, and tumors, especially the effects of benzol as a leukemogenic agent.

1891 Avellis syndrome, unilateral paralysis of the larynx and soft palate, was described by German otorhinologist, Georg Avellis.

1891 *Frederic Eugene Basil Foley* born. American urologist who designed a pneumatic cold punch resectoscope for removal of the prostate through the urethra (1940), and a plastic operation for hydronephrosis caused by stricture at the ureteropelvic junction (1937).

1891 The abnormal position of the suprarenal glands in certain patients was described by German pathologist, Felix Jacob Marchand.

1891 An infant familial form of progressive spinal muscular atrophy (Werdnig–Hoffman syndrome), was described by Austrian neurologist, Guido Werdnig, with German neurologist, Johann Hoffman.

1891   Munich physiologist and pioneer in metabolic diseases, Max Rubner, measured metabolic changes in the body using it as a calorimeter, and described the specific dynamic action of food.

1891   A.C. Abbott at Johns Hopkins Hospital found a strain of *Staphylococcus aureus* which could withstand exposure to mercuric chloride.

1892   American physicist, Wilber Olin Atwater, devised a modern calorimeter with the capacity for measuring oxygen consumption, carbon dioxide elimination, and heat production.

1892   A form of traumatic spondylitis due to a fracture of the vertebra (Kümmell disease) was described by German surgeon, Hermann Kümmell.

1892   A method of water filtration to remove bacteria was introduced by German bacteriologist, Robert Koch.

1892   Maurice Arthus and Calixte Page showed the effectiveness of oxalates and citrate solutions as coagulants.

1892   A form of myotonia which develops in adult life following trauma or infection (Talma disease) was described by Sape Talma, a Dutch physician from Utrecht.

1892   *Hemophilus influenzae* was isolated by Richard Friedrich Johannes Pfeiffer, a Polish bacteriologist.

1892

Louis Vaquez

Osler–Vaquez disease, polycythemia associated with cyanosis, was described by French physician Louis Henri Vaquez in relation to people living at high altitudes who had congenital heart disease.

1892   *David Bloom* born. An American dermatologist who described an autosomal recessive disorder with sensitivity to sunlight, erythematous facial rash, short stature and increased risk of leukemia (Bloom syndrome).

1892   A form of dementia due and cerebral atrophy of the frontal and temporal lobes (Pick disease) was described as circumscribed cortical atrophy by Arnold Pick, a Czech psychiatrist at the University of Prague.

1892   Choleangitis, to denote inflammation of the lining membrane of the smallest bile ducts which cause jaundice, was used by Bernard Naunyn of Berlin.

1892   Solute concentrations of urine and blood were first compared to assess renal functions (osmolarity) by Heinrich Dreser of Germany.

1892   A process of reproduction by the fusion of two gametes during fertilization was described by August Friedrich Leopold Weismann of Jena.

1892   The causative organ of gas gangrene (*Clostridium welchii*) was identified by American pathologist, William Henry Welch.

1892   Döderlein bacillus in vaginal secretions in relation to puerperal fever was found by German gynecologist, Albert Siegmund Gustav Döderlein.

1892   Mikulicz syndrome, associated with hypertrophy of the salivary glands and xerostomia, was described by Polish surgeon, Johann von Mikulicz-Radecki.

1892   Gastroduodenostomy, excision of the stomach followed by a procedure of axial anastomosis with the duodenum, was performed by Mathieu Jaboulay of Paris.

1892   *Corneille Jean François Heymans* born. A French physiologist and Nobel laureate (1938) who developed experimental method for cross circulation, and proved that the aorta and carotid arteries had specialized cells which responded to changes in blood pressure and blood chemicals.

1892   Coccidiomycosis and the causative organism of mycosis fungoides was discovered in Buenos Aires, Argentina by Alejandro Posadas.

1892   *James Bertram Collip* born. A Canadian chemist who isolated a practical form of insulin for clinical use (1923), extracted parathormone from the parathyroid glands (1925), and identified hormones from the placenta.

James Collip

1892   An important early study on the gallstone was performed by Bernard Naunyn who published his findings in *Klinik der Cholelithiasis*, and later advocated drainage of the bile duct in cholecystotomy.

1892   Scrotal cancer due to chronic contact with tar and mineral oil was observed by London surgeon, H.T. Butlin.

1892   A hereditary form of edema of the legs (Milroy disease) was described by Nebraska professor of clinical medicine, William Forsyth Milroy.

1892 The American School of Osteopathy was founded in Kirksville by American osteopathic surgeon, Andrew Taylor Still, who is credited as founding this science.

1892 Acanthoma adenoides cystecum, a rare familial epidermoid carcinoma was described by English dermatologist, Henry Ambrose Grundy Brooke.

1892 The two-stage operation for carcinoma of the colon was devised by German surgeon, Oscar Thorvald Bloch.

1892 Periodic depression was suspected to be due to uric acid diathesis and Alexander Haig of London used lithium to treat it.

1892 *Sir Norman McAlister* born. An Australian ophthalmologist who noted increased risk of congenital heart disease and congenital cataracts in children of women who contracted rubella during their first trimester of pregnancy.

1892 Bladder cancer was first linked to a chemical compound involved in fuchsin manufacture by German surgeon, Ludwig Rehn.

1892 A reddish eruption on the soft palate in cases of rubella (Forchheimer sign) was described by American physician, Frederick Forchheimer.

1892 *Joseph Vincent Meigs* born. An American gynecologist who described ovarian tumor or neoplasm associated with ascites and pleural infection (Meigs syndrome), and the removal of the tumor which

usually resolves the pleural effusion.

1893 Use erysipelas and toxins in treatment of cancer was attempted by American surgeon, William B. Coley.

1893 The atrioventricular bundle of the conducting system of the heart, bundle of His, was described by Wilhelm His Jr, of Germany.

1893 A triad of defects in membranous bone, exophthalmos and polyuria (Hand–Schüller–Christian disease) were described by American pediatrician, Alfred Hand.

1893 German surgeon, Johannes Gad, studied the relationship of lactic acid to muscle contraction.

1893 A form of lymphosarcoma without leukemic features or involvement of the spleen (Kundrat disease) was described by Viennese pathologist, Hans Kundrat.

1893 American otorhinologist, George Walter Caldwell, described a radical antrostomy, later named the Caldwell–Luc operation.

1893 The islets of the olfactory cells in the hippocampal cortex were described by Spanish anatomist, Camillo Sanchez Caleja.

1893 A form of busitis of the achilles tendon (Albert disease) was described by Austrian surgeon, Eduard Albert.

1893 The cutaneous areas of the sensory nerve roots related to visceral organs were mapped by Sir Henry Head, a London neurologist.

1893 A skin condition commonly found in the tropics (prickly heat) was explained on the basis of retention cysts caused by blocking of sweat glands, by Sigmund Pollitzer of Hamburg.

1893 The yolk nucleus of the ovum was described by a professor of comparative embryology in France, (originally from Haiti), Edouard Gérard Balbiani.

1893 A series of lymphatic plexuses in the mucous membrane and skin of the anus (Quenu hemorrhoidal plexus) were described by Edouard Quenu, professor of surgical pathology in Paris.

1893 *Arnold Rice Rich* born. An Alabama pathologist at the Johns Hopkins Hospital who described the Hamman–Rich syndrome of diffuse interstitial pulmonary fibrosis leading to dyspnoea and clubbing (1944).

1893 *Edward Adelbert Doisy* born. An Illinois biochemist and Nobel Prize winner who worked on vitamin K structure, studied the hormonal mechanism of the estrous cycle, and extracted the first steroid hormone, estrone, from pregnant urine.

1893 *Lester Reynold Dragstedt* born. A Montana surgeon who devised a complete vagotomy and gastrojejunostomy as treatment for duodenal ulcer (Dragstedt operation).

1893 *Andrew Ivy* born. An American physiologist who described a test for skin bleeding time using multiple sites of skin puncture on the forearm (Ivy method or test), and in later life became associated with a controversial cancer treatment (Krebiozen).

1893 The accessory right lobe of the liver (Riedel lobe) was described by German professor of surgery, Bernhard Moritz Carl Ludwig Riedel of Jena.

1893 Chronic sclerosing osteitis or osteomyelitis, marked by small areas of necrosis but little suppuration, was described by Swiss surgeon, Carl Garré.

1893 The specialized band of cardiac connective tissue at the atrioventricular junction was identified and named the bundle of Kent by English physiologist, Albert Frank Stanley Kent.

1893 The introduction of the sphygmomanometer into clinical medicine by Samuel Siegfried von Basch of Vienna led to the recognition of essential hypertension.

1893 British physiologist, John Newport Langley, identified and named the postganglionic and preganglionic nerves.

1893 Hereditary cerebellar ataxia, a disease of late childhood involving lack of coordination, was described by Pierre Marie of Paris.

1893 The term fibrinolysis was used by French physician, Jules Albert Dastre, who observed the reduction in fibrin during phlebotomy in dogs.

1893 The British Nurses Association which was founded by Ethel Gorden Manson, matron at St Bartholomew's Hospital, and later received a royal charter to become the Royal College of Nursing.

1893 *Erich Urbach* born. A Czech biochemist, dermatologist and expert in venereal disease, who worked on the interaction of cutaneous disease with allergy and diet, on which he wrote several papers.

1893 Theodor Wilhelm Engelmann, professor of biology in Berlin, described the transparent homogeneous layer found on either side of the Krause membrane.

1893 Foundation of the first society of anesthetists in the world, the Society of Anaesthetists, by J. F. W. M Silk of the London Hospital, with Woodhouse Braine as its first president.

1893 Recognition of ancylostomiasis in America by the physician, Walter L. Blickhahn.

1893 Protozoal theory of cancer was proposed by G. H. Plummer. He proposed a parasitic theory of cancer in 1903.

1893 First description of anaplasia, where tumor cells show loss of differentiation and specific function, was given by David Paul von Hansemann, a German pathologist.

1894 The value of paracentesis of the pericardium to prevent cardiac tamponade was pointed out by S. Del Velcchio in Naples.

1894 The term fibrositis was coined by London neurologist, Sir William Gowers, to denote an unexplained state of diffuse muscle aches and pains.

1894 The Wyeth operation for amputation at the hip joint using elastic cords and needles to control bleeding was devised by New York surgeon, John Allan Wyeth.

1894 *Hamilton Bailey* born. A London surgeon who designed a suprapubic trocar for puncturing the urinary bladder.

1894 *Franklin McCue Hanger Jr*, born. A New York physician who devised the cephalin–cholesterol flocculation test for liver function (1938).

1894 *Claude Schaeffer Beck* born. A Pennsylvania pioneer in open heart

Claude Beck

massage in cardiac asystole, who described the Beck triad of low arterial pressure, high venous pressure and absent apex beat in cardiac tamponade.

1894 Latex or rubber gloves were introduced for aseptic surgery by American surgeon, William Halstead, who made bronze casts of his hand upon which the first surgical gloves were molded.

1894 The embolic theory for the spread of breast cancer was described by Roger Williams in his book, *Diseases of the Breast*.

1894 *Samuel W. Becker* born. An American dermatologist who described pigmented hairy epidermal naevus, which most commonly occurs in males and is often located on the shoulder (Becker naevus).

1894 Decortication of the lung as treatment for chronic empyema was introduced by French surgeon, Edmond Delorme.

1894 Measurement of cardiac output in animals was gauged by injecting, then analyzing the amount of dye that appeared in arterial blood in experiments conducted by Scottish surgeon, George Neil Stewart.

1894 A test for hearing (Gradenigo test) was devised by Italian otorhinologist, Giuseppe Gradenigo.

1894 Neuritis of the optic nerve accompanied by acute loss of vision, central scotoma, and convulsions (Devic optic neuritis) was described by French physician, M.E. Devic.

1894 The plague bacillus, *Pasteurella pestis* (or *Yersinia pestis*) was isolated from humans independently by Swiss bacteriologist Alexander Emile Jean Yersin and Shibasaburo Kitasato.

1894 *Otto Stader* born. A veterinarian from Pennsylvania who devised the Stader splint for treatment of fracture of the shaft of long bones.

1894 The first prosthetic shoulder joint replacement with an artificial joint of rubber and platinum was devised by Parisian surgeon, Jules Émile Pean.

1894 The sensory nature of the muscle spindle was demonstrated by Sir Charles Scott Sherrington, an English professor of physiology.

1894 Nasher fever, involving mucous membrane of the upper respiratory tract with toxic symptoms occurring mainly in India, was described by Fernandez at the Indian Medical Congress.

1894 Chromophil granules in the cytoplasm of nerve cells (Nissl bodies) were stained and described by Bavarian neurologist, Franz Nissl of Munich.

1894 The causative bacteria of angular conjunctivitis (Morax–Axenfeld bacillus) was discovered by German ophthalmologist, Theodor Axenfeld.

1894 Chicago surgeon, Frederic Fenger, devised the Fenger operation for relief of ureteral stricture causing hydronephrosis.

1894 The word extrasystole was coined by Theodore Wilhelm Engleman during his observations of extra heart beats in animals.

1894 *Thomas Fitzhugh* born. An American physician who (with Arthur H. Curtis) described pain in the right upper quadrant of the abdomen due to gonoccocal peritonitis (Fitzhugh–Curtis syndrome).

1894 A form of subcortical encephalopathy leading to a classic picture of dementia in the fifth and sixth decade of life (Binswanger disease) was described by a professor of psychiatry at Jena, Otto Ludwig Binswanger.

1894 Italian physician, Guido Banti, described a syndrome of splenomegaly and anemia leading to cirrhosis and ascites, known as Banti disease.

1894 British physiologists, Hugh Kerr Anderson and John Newport Langley used the term axon reflex to denote the reflex response of the urinary bladder to nerve stimulation.

1894 An operation to mobilize the undescended testis (orchiopexy) was performed by Charles Bell Robert Keetly of the West London Hospital.

1894 The White operation, castration for hypertrophy of the prostate, was devised by Philadelphia surgeon, J. William White.

1894 The term 'chordoma' was introduced by Swiss pathologist Moritz

Wilhelm Hugo Ribbert, who also suggested that a tumor originates from the embryonic remains of the notochord (1905).

1894 The association between cardiac abnormalities and Down syndrome was noted by London physician, Archibald Edward Garrod.

1894 Small vascular canals in the aqueduct of the cochlea (Sibenmann canals) were described by Swiss ophthalmologist, Friedrich Sibenmann.

1894 The causative agent of Madura foot was identified by Jean Hyacinthe Vincent and named *Streptomyces madurae*.

1895 Ipsilateral loss of sensation to pain and temperature due to vascular occlusion of inferior cerebellar artery (posterior inferior cerebellar artery syndrome) was described by Adolf Wallenberg of Berlin.

1895 The Masset test for the detection of bile pigments in urine, by adding sulfuric acid and potassium nitrate to give a distinctive green color, was devised by French physician, Alfred August Masset.

1895 A radical form of hysterectomy for cancer of the uterus (Clark operation) was described by American gynecologist, John Goodrich Clark of Baltimore.

1895 *Cryptococcus neoformans*, a fungus found in fruit juice that infects the nervous system, was described by F. Sanfelice of Italy.

1895 *Sir Lionel Ernest Howard Whitby* born. Professor of medicine at the University of Cambridge who proved the efficacy of sulfapyridine in the treatment of pneumococcal pneumonia (1938).

1895 The infraduodenal peritoneal recess (Poisson fossa) was described by French anatomist, Francis Poisson of Calais.

1895 Cryoscopic examination of urine was introduced by Hungarian physician, Alexander von Sandor Koranyi.

1895 Partial recovery of the facial nerve after suturing it to an accessory nerve was demonstrated by a neurologist at the Westminster Hospital, Sir James Purves Stewart, and London neurosurgeon Sir Charles Ballance.

1895 *Walter Freeman* born. A Philadelphia neurosurgeon who advocated prefrontal lobotomy in cases of specific mental diseases (1942).

1895 X-rays were discovered by German physicist and Nobel laureate (1901), Wilhelm Konrad Röntgen.

1895 Daniel David Palmer from Davenport, Iowa founded chiropractic medicine.

1895 Peritoneal dialysis was investigated by Dutch physiologist, Hartog Jakob Hamburger.

1895 George Oliver and Edward Sharpey-Schäfer from England demonstrated that extracts of the suprarenal gland, when injected intravenously, produced a contraction of the arteries and acceleration of the heart rate, thereby increasing blood pressure. The active substance was later named epinephrine.

1895 *Gerhard Domagk* born. A German biochemist and Nobel laureate (1939) who discovered the antibiotic, Protonsil, containing sulfanilide (1935), and introduced thiosemicarbazone for tuberculosis (1946).

1895 The Mackenrodt ligament, ligamentum transversum colli of the uterus, was described by Alwin Karl Mackenrodt, professor of gynecology in Berlin.

1895 Belgian physiologist, Jules Jean Baptiste Vincent, demonstrated that serum devoid of cells had bactericidal properties.

1895 The first successful hind-quarter operation, amputation of the lower limb including a part of the pelvis, was by French surgeon, Charles Girard.

1895 *Edward George Liddell* born. An English neurophysiologist who worked on tendon reflex activity and co-wrote *Reflex Activity of the Spinal Cord*.

1895 *Augustus Roi Felty* born. An American physician at the Johns Hopkins Hospital who described cases of rheumatoid arthritis with enlarged spleen and lymphatic glands, and a reduced white cell count.

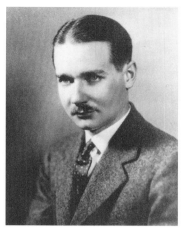

Augustus Roi Felty

1895 Treatment of inguinal hernia with overlapping sutures (Andrews operation) was undertaken by American surgeon, Edward Wyllys Andrews.

1895 A method of suprapubic enucleation of the prostate gland (Fuller operation) was described by New York surgeon, Eugene Fuller.

1895 Trendelenburg gait, caused by paralysis of the gluteal muscles causing waddling, was described by German surgeon, Friedrich Trendelenburg.

1895 A direct vision laryngoscope was invented by Alfred Kirstein, a Nuffield professor of anesthesia at Oxford.

1895 *Frederick Rowland George Heaf* born. A British physician from Cambridge University who devised a method for subcutaneous inoculation using atomized fluid injected under pressure (Heaf gun).

1895 An extensive text on electrophysiology was published by Wilhelm Biedermann, a pioneer in this field.

1895 The discovery that substances such as uranium salts emit radiation, was made by a French physicist and Nobel laureate (1903), Antoine Henri Becquerel, and the phenomenon later named radioactivity.

1895 *Erich Letterer* born. A German pathologist from Frankfurt who described a disorder of infancy with skin infiltrates, splenomegaly and bone tumors and affecting the reticuloendothelial system (Letterer–Siwe disease).

1895 *Herman Ludwig Blumgart* born. A pioneer in the use of isotopes in diagnostic medicine who introduced the use of radioactive substances in the evaluation of cardiac functions and velocity of blood flow.

1895 Pain in the tibial tuberosity of the ligamentum patellae (Schlatter disease) was described by Carl Schlatter, a Swiss surgeon from Zurich.

1895 Nephrostomy, for treatment of hydronephrosis, was popularized by Joachín Domínguez Albarrán, a genitourinary surgeon from Cuba and professor in Paris, France.

1895 Granulosa cell tumor was described by German pathologist, Clemens von Kahlden.

1895 Circulatory collapse in cerebrospinal meningitis (Waterhouse–Friderichsen syndrome) was originally described by Arthur Francis Voelcker.

1895 *André Frédéric Cournand* born. A French-born American pioneer of cardiac catheterization and Nobel Prize winner (1956).

André Cournand

1895 *Edward D. Churchill* born. An American thoracic surgeon who described segmental pneumonectomy and bronchiectasis, and increased respiratory rate due to distention of the pulmonary vascular bed (Churchill–Cope reflex).

1895 *Dickinson Woodruff Richards* born. An American cardiologist, pioneer in the application of the cardiac catheter to study blood pressure, oxygen tension and other physiological variables in health and disease and Nobel laureate (1956).

1895 An account of otosclerosis as a clinical entity was given by Adam Politzer of Vienna, Austria.

1895 Hemolytic disease of the newborn (erythroblastosis fetalis) was de-

scribed by the Scottish pioneer of antenatal care, John William Ballantyne, in *Deformities of the Foetus*.

1895 *J. Caffey* born. An American pediatrician who described infantile cortical hyperostosis, consisting of a persistent swelling of the mandible during infancy (1945).

1895 Granulosa cell tumor was described by German pathologist, Clemens von Kahlden.

1895 Vaginal cesarean section was performed by German gynecologist, Alfred Dührssen.

1895 The first suggestion of surgical relief for constrictive pericarditis was made by E Weill of France.

1895 The concept of iron deficiency anemia and its treatment with iron was advocated by German physician, Gustav von Bunge.

1895 Brazilian yaws (Breda disease) was described by Italian dermatologist, Achille Breda.

1896 Gonococcus as a possible cause of ulcerative endocarditis was pointed out by William Sydney Thayer of Baltimore and George Albert Blumer.

1896 Presentation of the first case of breast cancer treated by oophorectomy was given by George Thomas Beatson of Glasgow.

1896 *Bacterium paratyphosum* B was isolated by French physician, Emile Charles Achard.

1896   Amidopyrine was introduced into therapeutics by German physician, Wilhelm Filehne.

1896   Radiography in dentistry was introduced in America by William James Morton of New York.

1896   *Nicholas Bernstein* born. A Russian physiologist who discovered the concept of self-regulated motor systems and cybernetics, which arose from his study of the physiological mechanisms involved in human locomotion.

1896   Rocky Mountain spotted fever was found in the Montana and Idaho districts of America and was first described by Edward Ernest Maxey.

1896   The deadly bacteria *Bacillus botulinus* was described by Belgian bacteriologist, Emile Pierre Marie van Ermengem.

1896   *Henry L. Jaffe* born. An American orthopedic surgeon and bone pathologist who studied bones and the endocrine system, and wrote on bone tumors and metabolic and inflammatory diseases.

1896   Sir Frederick Still of Great Ormond Street Hospital in London wrote the pioneering work, *On a Form of Chronic Joint Disease in Children*, which included a description of Still disease (juvenile rheumatoid arthritis).

1896   A form of keratosis follicularis, marked by papules containing crusts which can be eliminated through squeezing (Darier disease) was described by French dermatologist, Jean Ferdinand Darier.

1896   Antivene, an antidote to snake venom, was prepared by French bacteriologist, Leon Calmette, at the Pasteur Institute in Lille.

1896   Miliary bodies on the mucous membrane of the lips and the oral cavity (Fordyce disease) were described by New York dermatologist, John Addison Fordyce.

1896   Renal decapsulation was performed by American comparative anatomist, R. Harrison, and revived by New York surgeon, George Michael Edebohls, seven years later.

1896   Primitive leukocytes in embryonic mesenchymal tissues (Saxer cells) were described by Fritz Saxer, a pathologist at Leipzig.

1896   Chronic inflammation of the thyroid leading to a hard mass in the gland (Riedel thyroiditis) was described by German professor of surgery, Bernhard Moritz Carl Ludwig Riedel.

1896   Patch tests in contact dermatitis were introduced by Swedish dermatologist, Josef Jadassohn.

1896   The development of cancer in the cervical stump following subtotal hysterectomy as a clinical entity was described by German gynecologist, Rudolf Chrobak.

1896   The amino acid, histamine, was isolated from sturgeon sperm by Albrecht Kossel, professor of physiology at Marburg and Nobel laureate.

1896 Jules François Babinski published a description of an abnormal extensor plantar response in pyramidal lesions (Babinski reflex), in his

Jules Babinski

Sur le Reflexe Cutane Plantaire dans Certaines Affections du Systeme Nervoux Central.

1896 A type of carcinoma of the ovary, often metastatic, and marked by areas of degeneration and signet-ring-like cells (Krukenberg tumor) was described by German pathologist, Friedrich Ernst Krukenberg.

1896 Rendu–Osler–Weber syndrome, characterized by multiple telengiectatic lesions of the face and upper gastrointestinal tract with a bleeding tendency, was originally described by Henri Rendu of Paris.

1896 End-to-end suture of the femoral artery was performed by a pioneer in vascular surgery, John Benjamin Murphy of Chicago.

1896 A diagnostic X-ray photograph in America was taken by Michael Idvorsky Pupin of Columbia University.

1896 The stomach bed, the organs on which the posterior section of the stomach rests, was described by Irish professor of anatomy, Ambrose Birmingham.

1896 A recessive trait leading to a defect in the binding of iodine by the thyroid gland (Pendred syndrome) was described by Vaughan Pendred in *The Lancet*.

1896 An analgesic mixture containing alcohol, cocaine, heroin and morphine (Brompton cocktail) was introduced for use in terminal cancer by H. Snow at Brompton Hospital.

1896 Ludwig Rehn of Frankfurt is generally credited as having performed the first successful cardiac surgery on a man with a stab wound through the heart.

1896 British physiologist, John Scott Haldane, noted carbon monoxide poisoning in the victims killed in a colliery explosion in south Wales.

1896 Leopold Freund observed the effect of X-rays on the skin in the treatment of ringworm infection.

1896 Acrocyanosis (Crocq disease) was named after Belgian physician and neurologist, Jean B. Crocq, who described it.

1896 The Schirmer test for tear formation using filter paper was designed by German ophthalmologist, Otto Wilhelm August Schirmer.

1896 Scottish surgeon, Sir Thomas George Beatson, advocated and performed surgical castration as treatment for advanced breast cancer in women.

1896 *José Valls* born. An Argentinean physician and orthopedic surgeon who pioneered regional lymph node biopsy for osteoarticular tuberculosis.

1896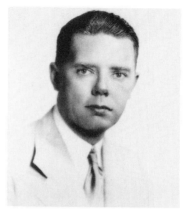

Cartoon depicting an early X-ray

German and French physicists, Wilhelm Röntgen and Antoine Becquerel, suggested the use of X-rays to prevent food decaying.

1896 A disease of the liver with ascites secondary to constrictive pericarditis (Pick cirrhosis) was described by Friedel Pick of Germany.

1896 The sign of pulmonary collapse at the left base in pericardial effusion was described by William Ewart, from the Hospital for Consumption and Diseases of the Chest in England.

1896 The scientific theory that changes in cerebral circulation were secondary to alterations in general circulation, was proposed by British physiologist, Sir Leonard Erskine Hill.

1896 The first report of the rupture of the intervertebral disc was given by Nobel laureate, Emil Theodor Kocher of Switzerland.

1896

Philip Hench

Philip Showalter Hench born. A Pittsburgh professor of medicine and Nobel laureate (1950) who noticed that conditions such as surgery, pregnancy and starvation which stimulated the adrenal cortex, also improved rheumatoid arthritis, and he noted the effect of cortisone on cases of this.

1896 The active agent in extract of thyroid gland, iodothyronine, was discovered by German chemist, Eugen Baumann.

1896 A disorder of collagen and elastic tissue (Marfan syndrome), characterized by slender long limbs, ectopia lentis, cardiovascular defects and hypermobility of the joints, was described by Parisian pediatrician, Antoine Bernard Jean Marfan.

1896 The insufflation method was used in a patient during surgery for partial resection of a lung was introduced by Theodore Tuffier and Louis Hallion of Paris.

1896 *Sir Hugh William Bell Cairns* born. An Australian neurologist who gave a clear description of hydrocephalus following obstruction of the flow of cerebrospinal fluid secondary to tuberculosis meningitis (1949).

1896 *Lee Foshay* born. A Cincinnati bacteriologist who devised a skin test for the diagnosis of tularemia, and prepared a serum for its treatment.

1897 John Beard of Edinburgh suggested that corpus luteum may be an inhibitor of ovulation during pregnancy, a diagnosis confirmed a year later by Auguste Prenant.

1897 The acne bacillus was first cultivated by French dermatologist, Raymond Sabouraud.

1897 Bernard Theodor Ludwig Claus Kronig and Theodor Paul introduced a quantitative study of disinfectants, and showed the disinfectant effects of acids and alkalis on bacteria.

1897 James William Brown established heart clinics for school children in Britain, and was a member of the editorial board of the British Heart Journal.

1897 *José Trueta* born. A Spanish surgeon who worked in Barcelona during the Civil War, developed the closed plaster method for treating wounds, and was one of the first to use penicillin for osteomyelitis.

1897 Ameloblast processes on the enamel cells of teeth (Tomes process) were described by Charles Tissimore Tomes, an anatomist and dentist at the London Hospital.

1897 The peritoneal pouch between the liver and gallbladder (Jacquemet recess) was described by French anatomist, Marcel Jacquemet.

1897 The American Association for Advancement of Osteopathy (later known as the American Osteopathic Association) was founded.

1897 *Ivar Palmer* born. A Swedish orthopedic surgeon who wrote a thesis on knee ligament injuries, including injuries of menisci, cruciate and other ligaments, and devised several instruments during the course of his work.

1897 The relationship of malaria to Anopheles mosquito bites was elucidated by the father of British tropical medicine, Sir Patrick Manson, who proposed the extracorporeal life cycle for the malarial parasite in the mosquito.

1897 *Manes Kartagener* born. A physician from Switzerland who described a hereditary disorder involving bronchiectasis with transposition of the viscera, Kartagener syndrome (1935).

1897 The Gastroenterological Association was founded.

1897   *Achile Mario Dogliotti* born. An Italian physician who introduced epidural anesthesia into obstetric practice, and performed the first surgical lesions of the pain temperature pathway (leminiscus lateralis) for pain control.

1897   A record of arrhythmia on paper was achieved by English cardiologist, Sir James Mackenzie, with his polygraph, which simultaneously recorded arterial and venous pulsations.

1897   *Charles Robert Harrington* born. A British physician who studied the thyroid gland, synthesized thyroxine, and worked on antihormones and immunochemistry.

1897   *Charles N. Armstrong* born. A British neurologist who successfully treated myxedema with extract of sheep thyroid.

1897   William Henry Howell of the Johns Hopkins University observed that blood pressure fell significantly during sleep (diurnal blood pressure).

1897   An antiserum for *Amanita phylloides* poisoning was developed by French bacteriologist, Leon Charles Albert Calmette.

1897   Muscular rigidity of the body produced by transection of the spinal cord through the upper part of the midbrain was described by Sir Charles Scott Sherrington of Oxford University, England.

1897   Arnold granules, (fragments of red blood vessels) were described by Julius Arnold, professor of anatomy at the University of Heidelberg.

1897   *Chi-Mao Meng* born. A Chinese orthopedic surgeon who devised an abduction osteotomy of the upper femur for old unreduced congenital hip displacements in adults.

1897   Chronic granulomatous lesions of the skin associated with bony lesions, and caused by the fungus *Blastomyces dermatidis* were described by American dermatologist, Thomas Casper Gilchrist.

1897

Tadeus Reichstein

Tadeus Reichstein born. A Polish scientist and Nobel Prize winner (1950) who synthesized ascorbic acid, isolated aldosterone, and worked on the isolation of cortisone.

1897   The absence of acid secretion in the stomach (achylia) was considered by F. Martius to be due to an inborn error of metabolism, and he suggested that gastritis was secondary to achylia rather than achylia being the cause of gastritis.

1897 A genus of flea (*Xenopsylla cheopis*) was shown to be a plague vector by Masanori Ogata.

1897 *John Franklin Enders* born. An American bacteriologist and Nobel laureate (1954) who cultivated the polio virus in human tissue, which led to the development of polio vaccine.

1897 The hydrodiascope, a device consisting of a small chamber filled with saline solution to be applied to the eye through the palpebral fissure, was invented by Ferdinand Siegrist of Switzerland.

1897 Johann August Löffler and Paul Frösch showed that foot-and-mouth disease in animals was caused by a filterable agent.

1897 *Piotre Kuzmich Anokhin* born. A Russian psychologist who proposed the concept of a self-regulatory system for the body (feedback mechanism).

1897 The infantile form of beriberi was described by Z. Hirota.

1897 Successful total gastrectomy for carcinoma of the stomach was carried out by the Swiss surgeon, Carl Bernhardt Schlatter.

1897 Alfred Bruck of Germany described multiple fractures, bone deformities and ankylosis of the joints (Bruck disease).

1897 The brachial plexus block was devised by George Washington Crile, by injecting the plexus with an anesthetic under direct vision.

1897 The cathode ray oscilloscope for recording variations of physical properties over a time period, was invented by a German physicist and Nobel laureate (1909), Ferdinand Braun.

1897 *Shigella shigae*, the bacillus of dysentery, was described by Kiyoshi Shiga, a Japanese microbiologist.

1897 A congenital anomaly of the heart, associated with an overriding aorta, patent interventricular septum and right ventricular hypertrophy (Eisenmenger syndrome) was described by German physician, Victor Eisenmenger.

1897 A foreign body, a pork bone, in the esophagus was removed by German laryngologist, Gustav Killian, using a bronchoscope.

1897 The first attempt to open into the labyrinth of the ear as treatment of otosclerosis was made by a German otologist, Adolf Passow.

1897 The first description of ovarian pregnancy was given by Dutch gynecologist, Benjamin Jan Kouwer.

1897 Johan Otto Leonhard Heubner, a German professor of pediatrics at Berlin and Leipzig, determined the caloric requirements of infants and introduced caloric feeding.

1898 Radiological demonstration of a gallstone was made by Austrian physician, A. Buxbaum.

1898   *Salmonella typhimurium* was isolated in patients with food poisoning by Herbert Edward Durham of England.

1898   The Roswell Park Memorial Hospital was established by Roswell Park at the University of Buffalo Medical School.

1898   The term 'cleidocranial dysostosis' was introduced by a French neurologist, Pierre Marie.

1898   Use of hen's egg for growing a virus was suggested by Monkton Copeman at the Milroy Lecture.

1898   *Bacterium paratyphosum* A was isolated by French physician, Norman Beechy Gwyn.

1898   The first suggestion of an inflatable balloon for treating achalasia cardia was made by J.C. Russel of Southport, England.

1898   The second attempt at internal cardiac massage in an arrested patient during surgery was made by T. Tuffier in Bern. The patient died of a pulmonary embolism.

1898   Reticular formations within the cytoplasm of the cell (Golgi bodies) were discovered by Camillo Golgi, professor of histology at Pavia.

1898   The superior nucleus of the vestibular nerve was described by Russian neurologist, Vladimir Bekhterev.

1898   Tinea nigra, caused by *Cladosporium mansoni* and characterized by blackness of the affected parts (also known as pityriasis nigra and microsporosis nigra), was described by Scottish microbiologist, Patrick Manson.

1898   A lecture to the American Medical Association on Surgery of the Lung was given by Irish–American surgeon, John Benjamin Murphy.

1898   *Yvunge Zotterman* born. A Swedish neurophysiologist who worked with Edward Douglas Adrian on recording and analyzing nerve impulses, and examined the thermal and pain sensations of the skin.

1898   Cells of the parathyroid glands (Welsh cells) were described by Scottish professor of pathology at Edinburgh, David Arthur Welsh.

1898   The earliest scientific monograph on diabetes, *Der Diabetes Mellitus*, was published by Bernard von Naunym, professor of clinical medicine in Strasburg.

1898   New York physician, Nathan Edwin Brill, described an illness similar in character to typhus found amongst immigrants from Europe (Brill disease).

1898   *Owen Harding Wangensteen* born. An American surgeon who devised a suction technique via a nasal catheter for management of intestinal obstruction, and described a technique for intestinal anastomosis (1940).

1898   A seroagglutination test for the tubercle bacillus was designed by Saturnin Arloing.

1898 *Alfred Wiskott* born. A German pediatrician who described a sex-linked recessive disorder characterized by recurrent infections, eczema, mild bleeding disorder and thrombocytopenia (Wiskott–Aldrich syndrome).

1898 French inventor, Jacques Arsene d'Arsonval, demonstrated that the contraction of muscles brought about by their intrinsic electrical activity could be reversed by applying an external current, suggesting a clinical use for electricity.

1898 Hayem–Widal disease, acquired hemolytic anemia, was described by Georges Hayem, and later described by French microbiologist, George Widal.

1898 The Wertheim radical pan-hysterectomy for cervical cancer was devised by an Austrian gynecologist, Ernest Wertheim.

1898 Budd–Chiari syndrome was originally described by Austrian pathologist, Hans Chiari.

1898 *The American Journal of Physiology* was founded.

1898 Chemical extraction of the active principle of the suprarenal gland (epinephrine) was done by John Jacob Abel of Johns Hopkins Medical School.

1898 *Lionel Sharples Penrose* born. An English geneticist who studied schizophrenia, carried out a major survey of the causes of mental illness, and noted increased maternal age as a cause of Down syndrome.

1898 *Clement A. Francis* born. An English otolaryngologist who published several papers on allergy and asthma, and described the Francis triad of asthma, nasal polyps and aspirin sensitivity.

1898 *William Howard Hailey* born. An Atlanta dermatologist who (with Hugh E. Hailey) described a familial benign pemphigus and autosomal lesion frequently involving the nape, or lateral aspects of the neck and axillae (Hailey–Hailey disease).

1898 *Enucleation of Uterine Fibroids* was published by a British gynecologist, William Alexander.

1898 The X-linked condition, Fabry disease, resulting in renal failure, corneal opacities and multiple skin lesions was described by German dermatologist, J. Fabry.

1898 A description of the clinical signs in pericarditis, including diastolic fixation of the apex, diastolic shock on palpation, and systolic retraction of the chest wall was given by English cardiologist, Sir William Broadbent.

1898 The first expanding dilator for treating esophageal stricture was developed by English physician, Josiah Cox Russel.

1898 *Helen Brooke Taussig* born. An Massachusetts pediatrician who pioneered surgical intervention for congenital heart disease and (with Frederick Taussig) performed the Blalock–Taussig shunt operation for Fallot tetralogy.

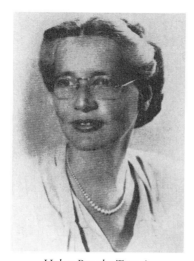

Helen Brooke Taussig

1898 Theobald Smith, professor of microbiology at Harvard, made the clear distinction between bovine and human tubercle bacilli.

1898 Direct bronchoscopy (tracheobronchoscopy) was performed by German laryngologist, Gustav Killian.

1898 Important clinical studies on gallstones were carried out by Bernard Naunyn of Berlin.

1898 *Arthur Maurice Fishberg* born. A New York physician who devised a concentration test for renal function.

1898 *Treponema vincentii*, a spirochete found in the throat of patients with Vincent angina, was identified by French bacteriologist, Henri Vincent.

1898 *Harold George Wolff* born. A professor of physiology at Cornell University who published a study of gastric function (1943), and

jointly published a treatise on pain with Stewart George Wolff (1946).

1898 The use of X-rays to study the movement of barium in the gastrointestinal tract was pioneered by Walter Bradford Cannon, of Harvard University.

1898 A method of obtaining urine samples from each kidney separately was described by Chicago surgeon, Malcolm La Salle Harris.

1898 The first attempt to classify neurons in the spinal and other ganglia was made by Alexander Stanislavovitch Dogiel, a neurologist and professor of histology at St Petersburg.

1899 *Austin Talley Moore* born. A surgeon from North Carolina who designed the Austin Moore prosthesis used as femoral head replacement in hip arthroplasty (1957).

1899 *Sir Frank Macfarlane Burnet* born. An Australian immunologist and

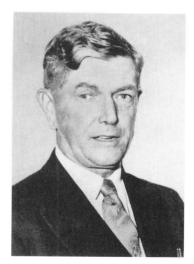

Sir Frank Macfarlane Burnet

Nobel laureate (1960) who perfected the technique of growing viruses in living chick embryos, and predicted the phenomenon of immunological tolerance.

1899 Ollier disease, consisting of non-ossified cartilage of the metaphysics and diaphyses of the long bones, was described by French surgeon, Léopold Louis Xavier Edouard Ollier.

1899 *Dame Annie Jean MacNamara* born. An Australian physician who discovered that there was more than one strain of the poliomyelitis virus which paved the way for the development of the Salk vaccine.

1899 The youngest human embryo of 13 days was described by a Hungarian gynecologist, Peters Hubert.

1899 H. Guilleminot used X-rays to assess the systolic and diastolic phases of the heart and aorta (angiocardiography).

1899 *Mary Hewitt Loveless* born. An American immunologist who investigated the differential nature of

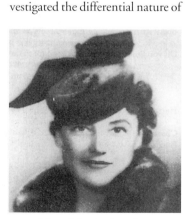

Mary Hewitt Loveless

serum skin sensitizing and blocking antibodies, discovering the association between blocking allergies, and hyposensitization in pollen allergy.

1899 The isoelectric point was first demonstrated by W.B. Harvey using denatured egg albumin which moved towards the cathode in acid solutions, and towards the anode in alkaline solutions.

1899 Janeway lesions, nodular hemorrhagic spots in the palms and soles of patients with subacute bacterial endocarditis, were described by New York physician, Edward Gamaliel Janeway.

1899 The American Hospital Association was given its present name after originally being called the Association of Hospital Superintendents.

1899 Themistokles Gluck, a German surgeon, devised an improved technique for laryngectomy.

1899 *Max Theiler* born. A South African-born American bacteriologist and Nobel laureate (1951) who worked on amebic dysentery and yellow fever, and attenuated the live yellow fever virus which led to the discovery of the 17D vaccine for this disease.

1899 *Henrik S.C. Sjögren* born. A Swedish ophthalmologist and neurologist who described a chronic autoimmune disease consisting of keratoconjuctivitis sicca and xerostomia with joint changes (Sjögren syndrome).

1899   A benign sarcoid syndrome (sarcoiditis) was described by Norwegian dermatologist, Caesar Peter Moeller Boeck.

1899   The Palmer School of Chiropractic Medicine was founded by Daniel David Palmer, who proposed the idea that diseases could be treated by the manipulation of the spine.

1899   Realignment of the patella for recurrent dislocation (Goldthwait operation) was described by Joel Ernest Goldthwait, an orthopedic surgeon from Massachusetts General Hospital.

1899   *Felix Turyn* born. A Polish physician from Warsaw who described pain in the gluteal region if the great toe is bent in cases of sciatica.

1899   The Ukrainian immunologist, bacteriologist and Nobel laureate, Elie Metchnikoff, observed an early substance similar to anti-lymphocyte globulin.

1899   Enlargement of the sella turcica (the pocket of the sphenoid bone on which the pituitary gland rests) on a skull X-ray in a case of acromegaly, was shown by Berlin neurologist, Herman Oppenheim.

1899   *Juda Hirsch Quastel* born. A British biochemist and a pioneer in biochemical aspects of brain disease, who developed liver function tests for schizophrenia, and worked on the role of glutamic acid in brain metabolism.

1899   *Sir Edward Charles Dodds* born. A professor at the Middlesex Hospital Medical School and later one of the youngest in London, who discovered the active synthetic estrogenic compound which he named stilbestrol (1938).

1899   *Hugo Roesler* born. An American cardiologist who described the rib erosion and aortic knob as radiological signs of aortic coarctation (1928), and who published *Clinical Röntgenology of the Cardiovascular System* (1937).

1899   Capillary blood vessels in the muscular fibers of the heart (Meigs capillaries) were first described by Arthur Vincent Meigs, a lecturer in histology at the University of Philadelphia.

1899   *Albert Claude* born. A Belgian-born American biologist and Nobel laureate (1974) who pioneered electron microscopy, and high-speed centrifugation for separating nucleus, mitochondria and microsomes.

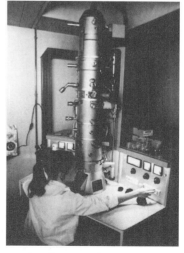

An electron microscope as pioneered by Albert Claude

1899   *Samuel Gordon Berkow* born. A New Jersey surgeon who proposed a table for estimating surface burn lesions.

1899   The denial of visual disturbance, Anton syndrome, was described by Austrian neurologist, G. Anton.

1899   The lipid theory of narcosis was proposed by Hans Horst Meyer of Berlin, to explain the action of narcotics through their solubility in lipids.

1899   *Charlotte Auerbach* born. A German-born British pioneer in the study of mutation who discovered chemical mutagenesis during studies on the effects of mustard gas, working alongside Hermann Müller.

1899   The first cure using X-rays for a basal cell carcinoma or rodent ulcer of the nose was developed by Thor Stenbeck of Sweden.

1899   A technique of artificial respiration with bellows (Fell–O'Dwyer technique) was adapted by New Orleans surgeon, Rudolf Matas.

1899   A book on embryonic tumor of the kidney (nephroblastoma, or Wilms tumor) was published by German professor of surgery, Max Wilms.

1899   The presence of beta-oxybutyric acid in diabetic ketoacidosis was demonstrated by Adolf Magnus-Levy.

1899   The impression on the pancreas made by the duodenum (Wiart notch) was described by French anatomist, Pierre Wiart.

1899   *Alfred Blalock* born. An American pioneer in surgery for congenital heart disease who introduced surgery of patent ductus arteriosus in children, and treated myasthenia gravis by performing thymectomy.

1899   William Charles Sullivan described fetal alcohol syndrome as a result of maternal alcohol ingestion.

1899   Intermediate thickness skin grafts (Ollier grafts) were described by French surgeon, Léopold Louis Ollier.

1899   Hans Eppinger, from Prague, isolated Actinomyces asteroides from a brain abscess.

1899   Harmful effects of prolonged high concentration oxygen therapy were pointed out by J. J. Lorrain-Smith.

1899   The first spinal anesthetic in the USA was given by Frederick Dudley Tait and Guido Caglieri in San Francisco. Their patient had a piece of bone excised from the tibia.

1900   Rodent ulcer or basal cell carcinoma (Krompecher tumor) was described by Hungarian pathologist, Edmund Krompecher.

1900   Fatal myocarditis associated with infiltration of the myocardium by leukocytes, lymphocytes, or multinucleate giant cells (Fiedler myocarditis) was described by Carl Ludwig Alfred Fiedler of Germany.

1900   Leishman–Donovan bodies (LD bodies), peculiar staining bodies found in the spleen of patients with Dum Dum fever, were noted by Scottish parasitologist, Sir William Boog Leishman.

1900 Sympathectomy for relief of pain due to vascular disease was performed by Mathieu Jaboulay of Paris.

1900 A German surgeon from Dresden, G. Kelling, used a cytoscope experimentally on dogs to examine the peritoneal cavity (laparoscopy).

1900 *Edgar V. Allen* born. An American physician who introduced coumarin anticoagulants to clinical practice, edited one of the first comprehensive textbooks on peripheral vascular disease, and devised the Allen test for peripheral vascular disease of the hand.

1900 *Sir Peter J. Kerley* born. A British radiologist from Cambridge who described the horizontal lines seen on a chest X-ray, in the lower zones of the lungs in cases of cardiac failure (Kerley lines).

1900 William James Mayo, of the Mayo family of American surgeons, devised a procedure of partial gastrectomy for carcinoma of the pyloric end of the stomach.

1900 *Manfred Joshua Sakel* born. A French physician who introduced insulin shock in the treatment of schizophrenia (1937).

1900 Philadelphia cytologist, Clarence Erwin McClung, described a half chromosome between early prophase and metaphase (chromatid).

1900 The first description of Ebstein anomaly in America was given by William George MacCallum, professor of pathology at the Johns Hopkins Hospital in Baltimore.

1900 *Bernard J. Alpers* born. An American neurologist who wrote books and papers on vertigo, dizziness and clinical neurology, and described progressive cerebral poliodystrophy (Alpers disease).

1900 Polish bacteriologist Jean Danysz grew a variant of *Bacillus anthracis*, capable of tolerating five times the normal inhibitory concentration of arsenic.

1900 Dystrophia adiposa genitalis was described in a young woman with a craniopharyngioma, by Paris neurologist, Joseph Babinski.

1900 *Sir Alan Sterling Parkes* born. An English physiologist who studied reproductive endocrinology, and published *The Internal Secretions of the Ovary* (1929).

1900 *Fuller Albright* born. The father of endocrinology in America who described bone change in kidney disease, osteomalacia of steatorrhea, vitamin D-resistant rickets, and the symptomatology of Parkinson disease on himself.

1900 The Wesbrook classification for diphtheria bacilli was proposed by American physician, Frank Fairchild Wesbrook of Minneapolis.

1900 Oppenheim disease, amyotonia congenita, was discovered and described by German neurologist, Herman Oppenheim.

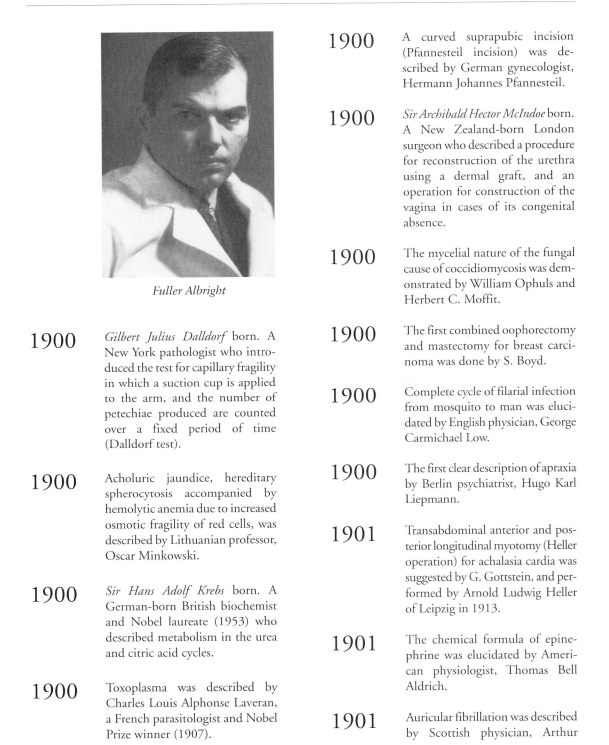

Fuller Albright

1900 *Gilbert Julius Dalldorf* born. A New York pathologist who introduced the test for capillary fragility in which a suction cup is applied to the arm, and the number of petechiae produced are counted over a fixed period of time (Dalldorf test).

1900 Acholuric jaundice, hereditary spherocytosis accompanied by hemolytic anemia due to increased osmotic fragility of red cells, was described by Lithuanian professor, Oscar Minkowski.

1900 *Sir Hans Adolf Krebs* born. A German-born British biochemist and Nobel laureate (1953) who described metabolism in the urea and citric acid cycles.

1900 Toxoplasma was described by Charles Louis Alphonse Laveran, a French parasitologist and Nobel Prize winner (1907).

1900 A curved suprapubic incision (Pfannesteil incision) was described by German gynecologist, Hermann Johannes Pfannesteil.

1900 *Sir Archibald Hector McIndoe* born. A New Zealand-born London surgeon who described a procedure for reconstruction of the urethra using a dermal graft, and an operation for construction of the vagina in cases of its congenital absence.

1900 The mycelial nature of the fungal cause of coccidiomycosis was demonstrated by William Ophuls and Herbert C. Moffit.

1900 The first combined oophorectomy and mastectomy for breast carcinoma was done by S. Boyd.

1900 Complete cycle of filarial infection from mosquito to man was elucidated by English physician, George Carmichael Low.

1900 The first clear description of apraxia by Berlin psychiatrist, Hugo Karl Liepmann.

1901 Transabdominal anterior and posterior longitudinal myotomy (Heller operation) for achalasia cardia was suggested by G. Gottstein, and performed by Arnold Ludwig Heller of Leipzig in 1913.

1901 The chemical formula of epinephrine was elucidated by American physiologist, Thomas Bell Aldrich.

1901 Auricular fibrillation was described by Scottish physician, Arthur

Roberton Cushny and American physician, Charles W. Edmunds, and published in 1906.

1901 Hunger pain in duodenal ulcer was described and named by Berkeley G.A. Moynihan of England.

1901 The descending posteriomedial part of the spinal tract was described by Scottish neurologist, Alexander Bruce.

1901 Hyperelasticity of the skin, bruising and joint extensibility due to faulty collagen synthesis (Ehlers–Danlos syndrome) was described by Danish dermatologist, Edvard Ehlers, and later by French physician, Henri A. Danlos.

Illustration of Ehlers–Danlos syndrome

1901 *Dorothy H. Andersen* born. An American pediatrician and pathologist who described cystic fibrosis of the pancreas (Andersen syndrome).

1901

Charles Brenton Huggins

Charles Brenton Huggins born. A Canadian-born US surgeon and Nobel laureate (1966) who pioneered hormone treatment of cancer, and investigated the physiology of the male urinogenital tract.

1901 German surgeon, Hermann Senator, described a syndrome of splenomegaly and anemia leading to cirrhosis and ascites (Banti–Senator syndrome).

1901 Phagocytosis was discovered by Russian embryologist, Elie Metchnikoff, who demonstrated the role of white cell in combating bacterial invasion.

1901 The anterior extremities of the inferior thyroarytenoid ligaments (Meyer cartilage) were described by Edmund Victor Meyer, a professor of laryngology at Berlin.

1901 *Raymond Greene* born. A British physician who used radioactive iodine in goiter, and made extensive studies of premenstrual tension.

1901 Sclerosis of the pulmonary artery, chronic cyanosis, dyspnea and bronchitis (Ayerza disease) was described by Argentinean physician, Abel Ayerza.

1901 A benign condition, with intermittent jaundice and normal liver functions, due to a defect in glucuronyl transferase (Gilbert disease) was described by French physician, Nicolas Augustin Gilbert.

1901 *Derek Denny-Brown* born. A neurologist from New Zealand who studied the reaction of a single motor neuron (1929), described bronchogenic carcinoma associated with degeneration of the dorsal ganglion cells and myopathy (Denny-Brown syndrome), and designed the cystogram (1933).

1901 Antenatal visits were started in America at the Boston Lying-in Hospital.

1901 Decortication of the lung in empyema (pleurectomy) to allow the lung to expand fully (Fowler operation) was use by New York surgeon, George Ryerson Fowler.

1901 The premature separation of normally implanted placenta with a fatal outcome, abruptio placenta, was described by Chicago obstetrician, Joseph Bolivar DeLee.

1901 *Irwin H. Page* born. An American cardiologist who described episodic hypertension characterized by tachycardia, nausea, sweating, vomiting and glycosuria (Page syndrome).

1901 The first fatal case of leucopenia was described by Philip King Brown and William Ophuls of America.

1901 *Richard Hollis Overholt* born. An American surgeon who carried out the first successful right pneumonectomy, used segmental resection for tuberculosis, and advocated the 'face down' position for thoracotomy to prevent sputum secretions from the diseased lung from moving into the contralateral lung.

1901 Extradural caudal injection was introduced by Jean-Athanase Sicard, a Paris neurologist.

1901 Radium was first used in treatment of tuberculous disease of the skin by French dermatologist, Henri Alexandre Danlos (with P. Bloch).

1901 German physicist, Wilhelm Konrad von Röntgen, received the first Nobel Prize for Physics.

1901 Jokichi Takamine of Japan crystallized the first pure epinephrine, while working in New Jersey.

1901 J. Schnitzler described abdominal angina as a form of spasmodic abdominal pain caused by mesenteric vascular insufficiency.

1901 Russian biologist, Ilya Ivanovitch Shigry, founded the first center for artificial insemination.

1901 *A Plea for a Pro-Maternity Hospital* was published by Scottish gynecologist, John William Ballantyne, a proponent of antenatal care.

1901 A progressive pigmentary disorder of the skin, often affecting the lower limbs (Schamberg disease), was described by Philadelphia dermatologist, Jay Frank Schamberg.

1901 A comprehensive review of hematology was published by Rud Limbeck of Vienna in *Clinical Pathology of Blood*.

1901 *A case of Tumor of the Hypophysis without Acromegaly*, dystrophia adiposa genitalis, or Fröhlich syndrome, was described by Viennese pharmacologist, Alfred Fröhlich.

1902 Jules François Babinski and Jean Nageotte described the Babinski–Nageotte syndrome, associated with hemianesthesia and crossed hemiplegia.

1902 The barbiturate, Veronal, was synthesized by German chemists, Emil Fischer and Josef von Mering, and named after the city of Verona.

1902 The Reed–Sternberg cell, a characteristic cell in Hodgkin disease, was described by Dorothy Reed of Johns Hopkins Hospital.

1902 The Sahli method to determine hemoglobin in blood was devised by Swiss physician, Herman Sahli.

1902 A chloroform inhaler, in which the concentration of vapor could be measured and its volume regulated, was described by A.G. Vernon Harcourt, a chemist at Christ Church, Oxford.

1902 Epinephrine was added to novocaine to prolong its effect by a Leipzig surgeon, Friedrich Wilhelm Braun.

1902 Radical testicular surgery involving the removal of the lumbar lymph nodes and spermatic vein was described by Philadelphia surgeon, John Bingham Roberts.

1902 Infectious eczematoid dermatitis (Engman disease) was described by American dermatologist, Martin Feeney Engman.

1902 English geneticist, William Bateson, popularized the work of Gregor Mendel in his *Mendel's Principles of Heredity*.

1902 The paravertebral triangle (Grocco triangle), where dullness occurs due to pleural effusion on the opposite side, was named after Italian physician, Pietro Grocco.

1902 The Wiesel paraganglion in the cardiac plexus of the nerves was described by Josef Wiesel, professor of medicine at Vienna.

1902 Brocq disease, a condition similar to lichen planus and psoriasis with lichenification, was described by Paris dermatologist, Anne Jean Louis Brocq.

1902 A form of narcosis during labor (twilight sleep) was introduced by German physician, Richard von Steinbuchel.

1902 *Gerhard Küntscher* born. A German surgeon at Kiel who devised the Küntscher nail for intramedullary fixation of fractures of the femur and tibia.

1902   *Barbara McClintock* born. An American geneticist from Connecticut and Nobel laureate (1983) who provided the ultimate proof for the chromosome theory of heredity.

1902   Archibald Edward Garrod, a physician from St Bartholomew's Hospital, studied inborn errors of metabolism and noted the heritable nature of some diseases such as alkaptonuria.

1902   Accessory, or X chromosomes, were suggested to be the determinants of gender by Clarence Erwin McClung, an American cytologist.

1902   The term 'anaphylaxis' was coined by professor of physiology, Robert Charles Richet.

1902   *Louis K. Diamond* born. An American physician who switched from hematology to pediatrics at the Children's Hospital, Boston, where he instigated new chemotherapeutic techniques in the treatment of childhood leukemia.

1902   *Johannes Zoon* born. A Dutch dermatologist who described a benign condition of the foreskin causing irritation and some fixation with discoloration, and cured by circumcision.

1902   End-to-end arterial anastomosis using triple thread sutures was perfected by the father of organ transplantation from America, Alexis Carrel.

1902   English pathologist, Joseph Everett Dutton, described the first case of human trypanosomiasis (Dutton disease).

1902   Swelling of the pneumococcal bacterial capsule when treated with its antiserum (Quellung reaction) was observed by Fred Neufield of Berlin.

1902   Radical vaginal hysterectomy for uterine carcinoma was introduced by Viennese gynecologist Friedrich Schauta (Schauta operation).

1902   The heterozygote was described and named by William Bateson.

1902   Prolonged gestation leading to postmaturity, (Ballantyne–Rung syndrome) was described by Scottish midwife and gynecologist, John William Ballantyne.

1902   *Arne Wilhelm Kaurin Tiselius* born. A Swedish chemist from Stockholm and Nobel laureate (1948) who isolated several viruses, and separated and identified amino acids, sugars and other molecules ion exchange chromatography.

1902   Surgical shock was comprehensively researched by American surgeon and physiologist, George Washington Crile.

1902   The concepts of genotype and phenotype were introduced by a Danish professor of genetics at Copenhagen, Wilhelm Ludwig Johanssen.

1902   The effect of an electric current on the tissues causing a change in concentration of electrolytes in the membranes (Nernst theory) was put forward by German physicists, Walther H. Nernst and E.H. Riesenfeld.

1902 Multiple tumors in African children (Burkitt lymphoma) were observed and recorded by medical missionary, Sir Albert Cook, in the *Journal of Tropical Medicine*.

1902 The amino acid, hydroxyproline, was isolated from gelatin by German chemist, Emil Fischer.

1902 The first successful transdiaphragmatic cardiac massage, combined with artificial respiration following cardiac arrest during operation, was performed by British physiologists, Ernest Starling and William Arbuthnot Lane.

1902 Isolation of bovine tubercle bacilli from tuberculous children was done by American physician, Mazÿck Porcher Ràvenel.

1902 The term myotonica atrophica was introduced by Russian physician, Gregori Ivanovich Rossolimo.

1902 Esophagoscope equipped with incandescent lighting was developed by New York physician, Max Einhorn.

1902 Foundation of the Imperial Cancer Research Fund in the UK.

1903 Virus as a cause of cancer was independently proposed by A. Borrel and Chandra Bose.

1903 The term 'antivirus' was introduced by French physician, Alexandre Besredka.

1903 Peroxidase enzyme was discovered by a German biologist, A. Bach.

1903 The first description of infantile acrodynia was given by German pediatrician, Paul Selter.

1903 The development of ventricular aneurysm in relation to myocardial infarction was established by D.G. Hall of Edinburgh.

1903 The first description of diffuse pneumonic form of primary carcinoma of the lung was described by J.H. Musser.

1903 A bone wax made of iodoform and oil for filling bone defects was introduced by Austrian surgeon, Albert von Mosetig-Moorhof.

1903 Biopsy of bone marrow in humans for diagnostic purposes was suggested by German physician, Alfred Wolff.

1903 Experimental production of arteriosclerosis by repeated injections of epinephrine was introduced by French physician, Otto Josuè.

1903 One of the first departments of radiotherapy for cancer was established at the Cancer Hospital in London under the direction of J.D. Pollock.

1903 French physiologist, Nicholas Arthus, used repeated subcutaneous injections of horse serum into rabbits causing sensitization.

1903 *Howard Carman Moloy* born. A New York gynecologist who proposed a valuable classification for

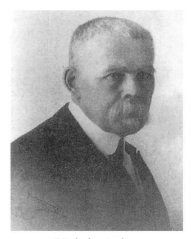

Nicholas Arthus

the female pelvis with William Edgar Caldwell (1933).

1903   *Frédéric Woringer* born. A French dermatologist who specialized in histopathological changes in various skin conditions, and described (with P. Kolopp) Pagetoid reticulosis, or Woringer–Kolopp disease.

1903   A demonstration that sarcoma can be transmitted through 40 generations of rats was given by Danish veterinary pathologist, Carl Oluf Jensen.

1903   The slit lamp for study of the living eye was invented by Swedish ophthalmologist, Alvar Gullstrand.

1903   A congenital condition of thick and hard bones due to the failure of resorption of intercellular ground substance (osteopetrosis) was described by German radiologist, Heinrich Ernst Albers-Schönberg.

1903   *Maurice Friedman* born. An American physiologist and physician who

modified the Ascheim–Zondek pregnancy test, using rabbits instead of mice (Friedman test, 1931).

1903   *Sir Russel Claude Brock* born. A British pioneer of thoracic surgery who performed the first cardio-esophageal resection for carcinoma of the cardia (1942), and described Brock syndrome.

1903   Bonnier syndrome, vertigo, trigeminal neuralgia and locomotor weakness due to lesions of the vestibular apparatus and 5th nerve nucleus, was described by Paris physician, Pierre Bonnier.

1903   *John Heysham Gibbon* born. An American cardiovascular surgeon who used the heart–lung bypass machine on animals (1939), and employed the first pump oxygenator in humans during cardiac surgery (1954).

1903   *George Wells Beadle* born. An American geneticist and Nobel laureate (1958) who developed the concept that specific genes control specific enzymes.

1903   Mönckeberg arteriosclerosis, caused by calcification of the medial layer of the arteries, was described by German pathologist at Bonn, Johann Georg Mönckeberg .

1903   The ultramicroscope was invented by Austrian chemist and Nobel Prize winner (1925), Richard Adolf Zsigmondy.

1903   *Haldan Keffer Hartline* born. An American physiologist and Nobel laureate (1967) from Johns

314

Hopkins Medical School, who pioneered neurophysiology of vision.

1903 Deep X-ray therapy for cancer was used by German surgeon, Georg Clemens Perthes.

1903 Painful tibial tuberosity in adolescence (Osgood–Schlatter disease) was described independently by American orthopedic surgeon, Robert Osgood, and Swiss surgeon, Carl Schlatter.

1903 The earliest study on the physiology of apnea in humans was done by Italian physiologist, Angelo Mosso.

1903 Extensive work on syphilis was carried out by Austrian pathologist, Hans Chiari.

1903 *Norman Rupert Barrett* born. An Australian surgeon who reported a case of successful surgical repair of a ruptured esophagus (1950), and who described reflux esophagitis two years later.

1903 Radioactivity was discovered by joint French Nobel laureates, Pierre and Marie Curie.

1903 *Sir John Carew Eccles* born. An Australian neurophysiologist and Nobel laureate (1963) who proposed that synaptic transmission in the nervous system was an electric rather than a chemical phenomenon, and demonstrated control of the nervous system by inhibitory synapses.

Sir John Carew Eccles

1903 Marchiafava–Bignami syndrome, consisting of tremor, convulsions and coma related to alcohol intake, was described by Ettore Marchiafava and Amico Bignami of Italy.

1903 Widespread deposition of cystine crystals were described in children who had died of Fanconi syndrome by Swiss physiologist, Emil Aberhalden.

1903 Karl Landsteiner and Julius Donath demonstrated that paroxysmal hemoglobinuria was an autoimmune disease.

1903 Measurement of time-related electrical changes in tissues was simplified with the invention of the string galvanometer by Dutch physiologist, Willem Einthoven.

1903 *Sidney Farber* born. An American pathologist, cancer specialist and fund raiser who worked on childhood leukemia and described disseminated lipogranulomatosis (Farber disease).

1903 The first clear description of infantile acrodynia, a disease marked by swelling and reddy-bluish discoloration of the feet and hands, was given by German pediatrician, Paul Selter (pink disease or trophodermatoneurosis).

1903 Inflammation of the spinal canal (arachnoiditis) was described in a patient as meningitis circumscripta spinalis by William Gibson Spiller, J.H. Musser and Edward Martin.

1903 French neurologist, R. Cestan and physician, L.J. Chenais, described ipsilateral paralysis of the vocal cords and soft palate (Cestan–Chenais syndrome).

1903 Bulb-type nerve endings were described by St Petersburg neurologist, Alexander Stanislavovic Dogiel.

1903 Parathyroid adenoma was described by Jakob Erdheim from Austria.

1903 *Gregory Goodwin Pincus* born. An American physiologist who pioneered the study of steroid hormones, and developed the contraceptive pill (1951), demonstrating its efficacy and determining the correct amounts of progesterone to be used (1954).

1903 *Erik Waaler* born. A Norwegian pathologist who (with Harry M. Rose) developed the Rose–Waller test for rheumatoid factor, using its ability to agglutinate red cells.

Gregory Goodwin Pincus

1904 *Guy F. Marrian* born. A British physician who isolated estriol from human pregnant urine, and studied steroid biochemistry and sex hormones.

1904 The polymorphs were differentiated into five different groups according to their nuclear configuration by German physician, Joseph Arneth.

1904 Findings that the brains of infants dying from jaundice were yellow at autopsy were described by Christian Georg Schmorl, who noted that certain areas of the brain, such as the basal ganglia, were more intensely colored, and he named the condition kernicterus.

1904 Paul Ehrlich, a German bacteriologist, produced the first man-made chemotherapeutic agent, trypan red, which cured mice infected with trypanosomiasis.

1904 Rheumatic disorders were studied by American physician, Joel Ernest

Goldthwait, who classified arthritis into villous, infectious, atrophic and hypertrophic.

1904 A genus of tick which causes relapsing fever by transmitting the spirochete, *Borrelia recurrentis*, was identified independently by two groups; Ross and Milne in Uganda, and Everett Dutton and Todd in the Congo.

1904 *Robert Degos* born. A French dermatologist who described fatal cutaneo-intestinal syndrome, characterized by the association of skin papules due to vasculitis, and multiple infarcts of the gastrointestinal tract (Degos disease).

1904 *Lester Smith* born. An English biochemist who worked on dietary requirement for vitamin A, developed the first commercial production of penicillin, and isolated vitamin B_{12}.

1904 August Kohler made possible detailed examination of bacterial structure by introducing ultraviolet light for microphotographic study.

1904 *Werner Theodor Otto Forssmann* born. A cardiographer and Nobel laureate (1954) from Germany who performed cardiac catheterization in animals, and catheterized himself through a vein using a ureteral catheter, confirming the position of the catheter in the right auricle by X-ray.

1904 The Gradenigo syndrome, acute otitis media followed by abducens nerve or internal rectus palsy, was described by Giuseppe Gradenigo, an Italian otorhinologist.

1904 Bacteriotropins were discovered by Fred Neufield and William Rampau.

1904 The S-shaped oxygen dissociation curve of hemoglobin was described by Danish physician, Christian Bohr.

1904 *Sir George White Pickering* born. A professor of medicine at Oxford who studied hypertension, noted the protein nature of renin and its role in hypertension, and reported a case of internal carotid artery reconstructive surgery.

1904 The characteristic lesion in rheumatic carditis, Aschoff body, was described by a German pathologist, Karl Albert Ludwig Aschoff.

1904 A positive pressure chamber for breathing, which displaced the negative-pressure cabinet, was developed by Ludolph Brauer.

1904 The term hypernephroma was introduced by German pathologist, Otto Lubarsch.

1904 Berlin psychiatrist, Hugo Karl Liepmann, discovered that, in right-handed persons, there is a dominance of the left cortical hemisphere.

1904 The structure of histamine was determined by German physiologist, Hermann Pauly.

1904 Shortness and curvature of the terminal phalanges in the little

317

fingers (Siegert sign) in mongolism or Down syndrome was described by German pediatrician, Ferdinand Siegert.

1904 Elliptocytosis in human red cells was described by American physician, Melvin Dresbach.

1905 Pharmacologist, W.E. Dixon of Cambridge, showed that the sensory fibers are less resistant than motor fibers to local infiltration by an anesthetic (Dixon law).

1905 The term artificial hibernation was coined by S. Simpson and P.T. Herring. They showed that cooling below 28 °C could act as general anesthetic.

1905 Diagnosis of primary carcinoma of the lung using X-rays was made by German physician, Max Otten.

1905 Presentation of the first large series of 99 patients with breast carcinoma, treated by oophorectomy, was made by a surgeon to the London Hospital, Hugh Lett at the Royal Medical and Chirurgical Society.

1905 Fracture of the medial condyle of the femur (Stieda fracture) was described by German surgeon, Alfred Stieda.

1905 The Long Island Society of Anesthetists, the first society of anesthetists in the United States, was founded by G.A.F. Erdmann, and later became the New York Society of Anesthetists.

1905

Ulf Svante von Euler

Ulf Svante von Euler born. A Swedish pharmacologist and Nobel laureate (1970) who observed raised levels of catecholamines in patients with pheochromocytoma, and isolated and studied prostaglandin, and noradrenaline.

1905 *Robert Edward Gross* born. An American cardiothoracic surgeon who performed the first successful surgical closure of a patent ductus arteriosus (1938), operated on a patient with coarctation (1945), and devised surgical techniques for treating atrial septal defect (1952).

1905 Vasovesiculography, to visualize the male reproductive organs on X-ray, was devised by Chicago surgeon, William Thomas Belfield.

1905 The structure and function of specific areas of the cerebral cortex were elucidated by Australian pathologist, Alfred Campbell.

1905 The relationship between sex organs and suprarenal glands was defined by William Bullock and James Harry Sequira.

1905 British physiologists, William Maddocks Bayliss and Ernest Henry Starling obtained a substance from the intestinal mucous

318

membrane which had a remote action on the pancreas, which they named 'secretin'.

1905 The fungus and causative agent of histoplasmosis (*Histoplasma capsula-tum*) was described by American, Samuel T. Darling.

1905 *Guido Dagnini* born. An Italian neurologist and cardiologist who described how percussion of the radial aspect of the back of the hand causes adduction and extension where there is hyperflexia or a pyramidal tract lesion (Dagnini reflex).

1905 The term 'parasympathetic nervous system' was introduced by John Newport Langley, a neurophysiologist from Newbury, England, who also coined the terms 'preganglionic' and 'postganglionic'.

1905 *George Herbert Hitchings* born. An American biochemist and Nobel laureate (1988) who discovered the folic acid antagonist 2-aminopurine (1948), the anti-malarial pyrimethamine (1952), the anti-leukemia drug 6-mercatopurine, and the immunosuppressants azathioprine and zidovudine.

1905 The London School of Tropical Medicine was established as part of the University of London, then amalgamated with the School of Hygiene to become the London School of Hygiene and Tropical Medicine in 1925.

1905 *Peter F.M. Bishop* born. A British endocrinologist and gynecologist who pioneered female reproductive endocrinology, and investigated the actions of secretins.

1905 Moritz Wilhelm Hugo Ribbert, a histopathologist in Zurich, initiated the theory of the embryonal origin of cancer.

1905 *Severo Ochoa* born. A Spanish-born American geneticist and Nobel laureate (1959) who isolated two enzymes from the Krebs cycle, determined a number of genetic codons, and studied protein synthesis and initiating factors in the binding of N-formyl-methionine.

1905 Arrhenoblastoma, a tumor of the ovary containing convoluted tubules and resembling the seminiferous tubules of the testis, was described by E.P. Pick of Berlin.

1905 The Raabe test to detect albumin in urine using trichloroacetic acid was devised by German physician, Gustav Raabe.

1905 Scientific evidence for communicability of polio was provided by Otto Ivar Wickman during an epidemic in Sweden.

1905 The syphilis spirochete, *Treponema pallidum*, was discovered by Fritz Richard Schaudinn, who worked as a protozoologist at the Institute of Tropical Diseases in Hamburg, Germany.

1905 An hereditary form of childhood macular degeneration, Best disease, was described by Franz Best, a German physician.

1905   The term 'azotemia' was coined by French microbiologist, Georges Fernand Isidore Widal, to denote a syndrome that resulted from retention of nitrogenous materials, normally eliminated by the kidneys

1905   Globular nuclear remnants in the erythrocytes from peripheral blood (Howell–Jolly bodies), were originally described by William Henry Howell of Johns Hopkins Hospital, Baltimore.

1905   London physiologist John Sydney Edkins suggested a hormonal theory for gastric secretion.

1905   *Hans Heller* born. An Austrian endocrinologist who studied water metabolism and neurohypophysial hormones.

1905   *Conrad Hal Waddington* born. An English embryologist and pioneer in genetic engineering who studied the effects of chemical messengers on embryonic development, and examined the effects of genes and environment.

1905   The first heart transplantation, in a dog, was reported by French-born American biologist, Alexis Carrel.

1905   Block of thoracic ganglia of the sympathetic chain by paravertebral injection of drugs (thoracic sympathetic block) was performed by Hugo Sellheim.

1905   Studies on serum sickness were carried out by Austrian immunologist, Clemens von Pirquet, who defined 'allergy' as a situation where there was 'changed reactivity' regardless of resulting immunity or hypersensitivity.

1906   A description of the proprioceptors, highly specialized somatic sensory end organs of the muscles, tendons and joints, was given by Sir Charles Scott Sherrington, an English professor of physiology.

1906   *Luis Frederico Leloir* born. A French-born Argentinean biochemist and Nobel laureate (1970) who worked on diabetes and the adrenals, noted the proteolytic action of renin from kidneys leading to production of angiotensin, and discovered glucose-1-phosphate kinase.

1906   The causative organism of whooping cough, *Bordetella pertussis*, was discovered by Belgian Nobel Prize winner, Jules Jean Bordet, and French bacteriologist, Octave Gengou.

1906   *Karl August Folkers* born. An American biochemist and pioneer in the study of vitamin structure and function, who synthesized vitamin B_6, used vitamin B_{12} in treatment of pernicious anemia and elucidated the structure of streptomycin.

1906   The causative organism of yaws, *Treponema pertenue*, was discovered by Marquis Aldo Castellani.

1906   The first recording of a fetal electrocardiogram was produced by M. Cremer of Germany.

1906 William Sampson Handley from the Royal College of Surgeons and a pioneer in surgery for cancer of the breast, wrote *Cancer of the Breast and its Operative Treatment.*

1906 Rough and smooth dysentery bacilli and their relevance to antigenic properties was noted by Joseph Arkwright, a bacteriologist at the Lister Institute.

1906 Eduard Conrad Zirm successfully transplanted a cornea.

1906 Nitrogen was used in the production of artificial pneumothorax for the treatment of tuberculosis by German physician, Ludolph Brauer.

1906 The atrioventricular node of the conducting system of the heart (Tawara node) was discovered by Japanese anatomist, Sunao Tawara.

1906 *Ernst August Friedrich Ruska* born. A German scientist from Heidelberg who invented the electron microscope (1931), and shared the Nobel Prize for Physics in 1986.

1906 *Yan-Qing Ye* born. A Chinese orthopedic surgeon who researched bone metabolism and microstructure, and undertook surgery on fracture dislocation of the spine with cord injury.

1906 The Ochsner sphincter in the duodenum, below the opening of the bile duct, was described by a professor of surgery at the University of Illinois, Albert John Ochsner.

1906 *Max Delbruck* born. A German biophysicist, Nobel laureate (1969), and pioneer in genetics of the phage who discovered that viruses can exchange genetic material to create new viruses (1964).

1906 The importance of amino acids in digestion and metabolism was shown by Otto Knut Olof Folin, a Swedish-born professor of biochemistry at Harvard.

1906 *Albert Bruce Sabin* born. A Polish–American microbiologist who researched vaccines against Japanese B encephalitis and dengue fever, and developed the live attenuated oral vaccine for polio (1957).

1906

Harry Rose

Harry M. Rose born. An American microbiologist who developed ferritin-conjugated antibodies for electron microscope studies, and the Rose–Waller test for rheumatoid factor using the properties of agglutinated red blood cells.

1906 Radiological visualization of the renal tract (pyelography) was introduced by Alexander von Lichtenberg of Germany.

1906 Treatment of sea sickness with atropine sulfate and strychnine was developed by American naval surgeon, Conrad Alfred Girard.

1906   The rotating Bárány chair for studying nystagmus, and the Bárány caloric test for labyrinthine function were named after Robert Bárány of Vienna.

1906   *Benjamin Castleman* born. An American pathologist who described an unusual solitary tumor, probably a lymphoma, which on resection may not recur (Castleman tumor).

1906   English ophthalmologist, Claude Worth, developed the amblyoscope, a stereoscopic instrument designed to train the eye to overcome squint.

1906   *George Wald* born. A New York biochemist and Nobel laureate (1967) who worked on visual purple in the retina and its conversion on illumination to vitamin A, and established the relationship between night blindness and vitamin A deficiency.

1906   The diagnostic symptoms of supraspinatous tendon rupture were described by Boston orthopedic surgeon, Ernest Amory Codman who also pioneered the application of X-rays to orthopedics in *The Use of X-rays in the Diagnosis of Bone Disease*.

1906   The formation of acid in diabetic coma (acidosis) was noted and named by Bernard Naunyn of Berlin.

1906   The importance of the lymphatics in the spread of mammary carcinoma was first stressed by English surgeon, William Sampson Handley.

1906   The Pathological Society of Great Britain and Ireland was founded at the University of Manchester.

1906   Passive hypersensitivity was demonstrated to be transferable by Richard Otto of Berlin, Germany.

1906   Anterior spinal fusion in the treatment of Pott disease and Pott paraplegia was employed by Russell Aubra Hibbs of Kentucky and Fred Houdlett Albee of Maine.

1906   *Hirsh Wolf Sulkowitch* born. A Boston physician who devised the Sulkowitch test for detecting calcium in urine.

1906   Thalamic syndrome, consisting of paroxysms of contralateral pain, ataxia and choreoathetoid movements due to thrombosis or lesions of the thalamogeniculate artery, was described by Joseph Jules Dejerine and Gustav Roussey of Paris.

1906   Recurrent attacks resembling petit mal but not epileptiform in nature (pyknoepilepsy) were described by German physician, Max Friedmann.

1906   German bacteriologist, August Paul Wasserman, developed the complementation test for syphilis.

1906   A serum against meningococcal infections was developed by German physician, Georg Jochmann.

1906   The pharmacological effects of cholinesterase inhibitors was demonstrated by A.H. Hunt and H. Lehman.

1906 Suxamethonium halides were prepared by R. Hunt and R. Taveau.

1906 Paravertebral somatic block was introduced by H. Sellheim and further developed by A. Läwen in 1911.

1906 New York surgeon, N.W. Green devised a mechanical ventilator which inflated and deflated the lung through a tracheal cannula.

1906 The invention of a inflatable rubber bag to control bleeding after suprapubic prostatectomy was undertaken by American surgeon, James Emmons Briggs.

1906 Berlin psychiatrist, Hugo Karl Liepmann, demonstrated that hallucinations can be induced by artificial means during his study of alcoholic delirium.

1907 A precipitin reaction test for hydatid disease was devised by two French physiologists, Charles Auguste Fleig and Marcel Lisbonne.

1907 The term 'chemotherapy' was introduced by Paul Ehrlich.

1907 Suprasymphysial transperitoneal cesarean section was introduced by German gynecologist, Fritz Frank.

1907 The effectiveness of diphtheria toxin in guinea pigs was demonstrated by Theobald Smith, professor of microbiology at Harvard University.

1907 The first description of adrenal sarcoma with metastasis to skull (Hutchison tumor) was given by Robert Grieve Hutchison.

1907 Spinal anesthesia was introduced into Britain by A.E. Barker of University College, London, with his classic paper in the *British Medical Journal*.

1907 The Brenner tumor, a peculiar benign neoplasm of the ovary, was described as oophoroma folliculare by Fritz Brenner of Germany.

1907 A branch of the ramus anterior of the acoustic nerve (Voit nerve) was described by German embryologist and professor of anatomy, Max Voit.

1907

Daniel Bovet

Daniel Bovet born. An Italian pharmacologist and Nobel laureate (1957) who founded a laboratory for chemotherapeutics in Rome, discovered the first antihistamine compound (1936), and studied drugs which block the action of epinephrine and noprepinephrine.

1907 The normal cyclical changes in the endometrium, previously thought to be due to inflammation, were described by two Viennese gynecologists, Ludwig Adler and Fritz Hitschmann.

1907 *Jerome William Conn* born. A Michigan physician whose major interests were the physiology and pathology of human metabolism and nutrition, and who described Conn syndrome of excess secretion of aldosterone leading to hypertension.

1907 A classic work on thoracic outlet syndrome, and the first cervical rib as a cause of pressure symptoms, was written by William Williams Keen of America.

1907 Acholuric familial jaundice (Minkowski–Chauffard syndrome) was described by French physician, Anatole Marie Emile Chauffard.

1907 *Hans Selye* born. A Canadian physician who developed the general adaptation syndrome concept, and wrote *Textbook of Endocrinology*.

Hans Selye

1907 *Edward John Bowlby* born. An English pioneer in the effects of maternal deprivation on the mental health and development of children.

1907 The lateral nucleus of the cuneatus was described by Russian physician, Leonid Wassiljewitsch Blumenau.

1907 The Royal Society of Medicine was formed from the Royal Medico-Chirugical Society of London, and the Medical Society of London.

1907 *Harold Rae Cox* born. An American bacteriologist who prepared a typhus vaccine (Cox vaccine) from yolk-sac culture of rickettsial species (1940).

1907 The first case of complete disappearance of polymorphonuclear leukocytes (agranulocytosis) from the blood was given by Werner Shultz.

1907 *Paul Hamilton Wood* born. One of England's greatest cardiologists who studied congenital cardiology and atrial septal defect, and published *Diseases of the Heart and Circulation* (1950).

1907 Digitalis in treatment of auricular fibrillation was used by English cardiologist, Sir James Mackenzie, who also described the functional pathology of cardiac tissue.

1907 Whipple disease, deposit of fats and fatty acids in the intestinal lymphatic tissues (intestinal lipodystrophy) was described by New York physiologist, George Hoyt Whipple.

1907   Hypertrophic cardiomyopathy, or hypertrophic obstructive cardiomyopathy, was described by Alexander Schmincke of Germany.

1907   A tuberculin skin test was introduced by German microbiologist, Clemens von Pirquet.

1907   Inclusion bodies in conjuntival cells in trachoma were observed by German microbiologist, Stanislaus Joseph von Prowazek, who postulated that they were collections of virus enveloped by material deposited from the infected cell.

1907   Bronchoscopy was used in the management of asthma by Franz Novotny.

1907   The Stone operation for ununited fracture of the tibia was described by Boston surgeon, James Savage Stone.

1907   Maurice Nicolle of the Pasteur Institute demonstrated the phenomenon of passive anaphylaxis.

1907   Histamine was synthesized by Adolf Windhaus.

1907   Alzheimer disease, a form of presenile dementia, was described and studied by German psychiatrist Alois Alzheimer of Munich.

1907   Chronic subdural hematoma was described in detail by Sir Charles Edward Ballance, a neurosurgeon in London.

1907   *Horace Winchell Magoun* born. An American pioneer in neuroendocrinology whose early research was on the structure and function of the hypothalamus in relation to sleep, eating and body temperature.

1907   A book on endoscopy, including tracheobronchoscopy, was written by American laryngologist, Chevalier Jackson, who also removed an endobronchial tumor using a bronchoscope.

1907   Knee and other joint transplantation from cadavers as treatment for advanced joint disease, was first performed by Eric Lexer, a surgeon from Königsberg, Germany, and a pioneer in plastic surgery.

1907   The American Association for Cancer Research was established by a group of leading pathologists including James Ewing.

1907   Osler–Rendu–Weber syndrome, hemorrhagic telengiectasis, was described by Sir William Osler.

1907   Iridencleisis for relief of glaucoma was introduced by French ophthalmologist, Sören Holth.

1908   *Myron Prinzmetal* born. A cardiologist from Buffalo who described unstable angina, with transient ischemic changes in ECG due to spasm of the coronary arteries (Prinzmetal angina).

Illustration of early ECG

325

1908 S. Saltykow emphasized the presence of high levels of cholesterol in the diet as a cause of atherosclerosis.

1908 Osteochondritis deformans juvenilis, consisting of femoral osteochondrosis leading to tenderness and muscular spasm of the hip (Legg–Calvé–Perthes disease) was described by Harvard orthopedic surgeon, Arthur Thornton Legg.

1908 *Herman Richner* born. A Swiss dermatologist who described (with fellow countryman Ernst Hanhart) hyperkeratosis of the palms and soles from childhood with pseudoherpetic keratitis and mental retardation (Richner–Hanhart syndrome).

1908 Cutaneous nodules in subacute bacterial endocarditis (Osler nodes) were described by Sir William Osler, regius professor of medicine in Oxford, England.

1908 Aseptic necrosis of the navicular bone (Köhler disease) was described by German radiologist, Alban Köhler.

1908 Paul Ehrlich, a German bacteriologist, and Russian embryologist, Elie Metchnikoff, shared the Nobel Prize for Physiology or Medicine for their contributions to immunity and serum therapy.

1908 *Murray Llewellyn Barr* born. A Canadian physician who discovered extra chromatin in the X chromosome and named it the 'Barr body.

Murray Barr

1908 *Michael Ellis Bakey* born. An American cardiovascular surgeon who developed a surgical cardiovascular center of international repute.

1908 The Rothera test to detect acetone in the urine was devised by Australian biochemist, Arthur Cecil Hamel Rothera.

1908 Abdominoperineal resection of the rectum for rectal carcinoma, Miles operation, was devised by English surgeon, William Ernest Miles.

1908 The suspensory ligament of the axilla, Campbell ligament, was described by Brooklyn professor of surgery, William Francis Campbell.

1908 The first attempt at pulmonary embolectomy was made by German surgeon, Friedrich Trendelenburg.

1908 Karl Abraham founded the Berlin Psychoanalytic Society.

1908 *David G. Cogan* born. An American neuro-ophthalmologist who described Cogan syndrome of vertigo, tinnitus, progressive bilateral deafness, pain in the eyes and photophobia, blurred vision, and a congenital form of 3rd nerve apraxia.

1908 Generalized arteritis of the medium size and larger arteries, Takayasu syndrome, was described by Mikito Takayasu of Japan.

1908

Victor Horsley

A stereotactic apparatus for accurate location of electrodes in the brain was produced by Sir Victor Alexander Haden Horsley, the founder of British neurosurgery.

1908 Elbow joint transplantation in ankylosis was pioneered by Russian surgeon, Peter Ivanovitch Buchmann.

1908 French physicians, Edouard Brissaud and Jean A. Siccard, described facial spasm and contralateral paralysis of the limbs (Brissaud–Siccard syndrome).

1908 The American Society for Pharmacology and Experimental Therapeutics was founded.

1908 The Lanz line, joining two anterior superior iliac spines, was described by Swiss surgeon, Otto Lanz.

1908 Neuralgia of the lower half of the face, nasal congestion and rhinorrhoea secondary to a lesion in the pterygo-palatine ganglion was described by Greenfield Sleuder of New York.

1908 The first transmission of polio to monkeys, through inoculation of brain tissue filtrate taken from a fatal case of poliomyelitis, was made by Carl Landsteiner and E. Popper.

1908 The first description of multinodular localized carcinoma of the lung (at autopsy) was given by M. Löhlein.

1908 Slowing of heart rate on applying pressure to the eyeball (Aschner reflex) was described by Bernhard Aschner of Austria.

1908 A description of a human embryo of 14 days was given by Thomas Hastie Bryce, an anatomist in Glasgow.

1908 The first description of *Salmonella paratyphi* was given by German bacteriologists, Erich A. Heubner and Paul T. Uhlenhuth.

1908 A description of an ether–air inhaler was given by Louis Ombredanne, a French pediatric surgeon.

1909   The first demonstration of anaphy-lactogenic properties of preformed antigen–antibody complexes was given by E. Frieberger.

1909   The term 'chromatolysis' was introduced by Georges Marinesco, a neurologist at Bucharest.

1909   Rickettsiae were identified as a cause of typhus by French physician Charles J.H. Nicolle.

1909   Tonic rigidity in cases of active hyperventilation was demonstrated by H.M. Vernon. J.B. Collip and P.L. Backus, in 1920, studied the phenomenon and named it 'tetany'.

1909   Sclerocorneal trepanning for relief of glaucoma was introduced by English ophthalmologist, Robert Henry Elliot.

1909   Arsphenamine or salvarsan was discovered by Paul Ehrlich and Japanese bacteriologist, Sahachiro Hata (in 1912).

1909   The Institut Curie, for cancer research, was founded at Paris in honor of Marie Curie.

1909   Radiographic visualization of the lachrymal duct with bismuth was described by James Ewing of the Cornell University Medical College in New York..

1909   Arthur Francis Bainbridge, an English physiologist and bacteriologist, classified various strains of *Salmonella*.

1909   *Rita Levi-Montalcini* born. An Italian neurologist and Nobel Prize winner (1986) who carried out studies on in vitro nerve growth, and discovered nerve growth factor.

Rita Levi-Montalcini

1909   Some of the first detailed studies of the urinary passages were written by Cuban-born French professor of medicine, Joaquin Dominguez Albarrán.

1909   One of the first surgeons to be awarded a Nobel Prize was a professor of surgery from Bern, Switzerland, Theodore Kocher, for his work on goiter.

1909   The causative agent of American trypanosomiasis, Chagas disease, was discovered by a physician at the Osvaldo Cruz Institute in Rio de Janeiro, Carlos Chagas.

1909   William Carpenter McCarthy of the Mayo Clinic carried out work on the cytology of gastric ulcers and proposed that chronic gastric ulcers were potentially cancerous.

1909 Crude oxytocin was first used in labor by English obstetrician from Liverpool, William Blair Bell.

1909 Membrane potential was proposed by the German chemist and Nobel Prize winner (1909), Wilhelm Ostwald

1909 Waldenstrom syndrome, aseptic necrosis of the epiphysis of the femoral head, was described by Stockholm surgeon, Henning Waldenstrom.

1909 Chloroform and ether were first used as intravenous anesthetics by L. Burkhardt.

1909 Carl Julius Rothberger and Heinrich Winterberg, independently demonstrated atrial fibrillation in humans.

1909 The first account of myotonia dystrophica (Curshmann–Batten–Steinert syndrome), consisting of frontal baldness, testicular atrophy, dystrophy of sternomastoid muscles and myotonia of lingual muscles, was described by F.E. Batten of London.

1909 The Hartmann operation, removal of the upper rectum or sigmoid for cancer, together with closure of the rectal stump and establishment of colostomy, was described by French surgeon, Henri Hartmann.

1909 Irrigation and observation of the bladder was made possible with the Brown–Buerger cystoscope, devised by Leo Buerger.

1909 The bacterium responsible for Peruvian Oroya fever (*Bartonella bacciliformis*) was found in red blood cells by a South American physician from Peru, Alberto L. Barton.

1909 A diagnostic test for meningitis (Brudzinski sign) was described by Polish physician, J. Brudzinski.

1909 A full and accurate description of prurigo nodularis was given by American dermatologist, James Nevin Hyde.

1909 A form of sarcoidosis involving the parotid glands (Heerfordt syndrome) was described by Danish ophthalmologist, Christian Fredrick Heerfordt.

1909 Degeneration of the macula lutea and optic nerve, associated with ataxia, was described by C. Behr of Germany and named Behr disease.

1909 Injection of a local anesthetic into a vein of a limb, using a tourniquet, was introduced by August Karl Gustav Bier of Kiel.

1909 A diagnostic serological test for echinococcus (Weinberg test) was described by Paris physician, Michel Weinberg.

1909 *Eldon J. Gardner* born. An American geneticist who described the hereditary autosomal dominant condition associated with colonic polyposis and increased risk of carcinoma (Gardner syndrome, 1951).

1909 *Walsh McDermott* born. An American physician and founder of the Institute of Medicine of the

National Academy of Science, who introduced pyrazinamide in combination with isoniazid as first-line treatment for tuberculosis.

1909 The modern era of anesthesia began with the introduction of endotracheal anesthesia by Samuel James Meltzer and John Auer of the Rockefeller Institute, New York.

1909 Successful removal of the pituitary in an acromegalic patient was done by Harvey Cushing of the Johns Hopkins Hospital in Baltimore.

1910 A fungus that attacks the skin, hair and nails (*Epidermophyton rubrum*) was described by Marquis Aldo Castellani, during his work in Sri Lanka.

1910 The leukotoxic action of benzene was demonstrated by L. Selling of Johns Hopkins Hospital which led to its use in the treatment of leukemia.

1910 A modified Wasserman test for syphilis (Emery test) was devised by English physician, D. Walter Emery.

1910 The electrocardiographic changes of bundle branch block were described by Viennese physician, Hans Eppinger.

1910 The suggestion that secretions of the pancreas depended on a reflex between duodenal mucosa and vagus was made by Russian Nobel Prize winner, Ivan Petrovich Pavlov.

1910 *Jacques Lucien Monod* born. A French biochemist and Nobel laureate (1968) who proposed the operon theory of gene regulation and the concept of messenger RNA.

1910 A modern approach to the pathogenesis and causation of duodenal ulcer was made by Berkeley George Moynihan of Leeds.

1910 Etienne Lombard, a French physician, devised a test for simulated unilateral deafness (Lombard test).

1910 Fat at the apex of the heart, causing confusion with enlargement of the heart on chest X-ray (Schwarz sign), was described by a German radiologist, Gottwald Schwarz.

1910 A book on the importance of the adrenal glands and the role of internal secretions was published by German physician, Arthur Biedl.

1910 *Streptococcus viridans* was isolated from the blood of patients with bacterial endocarditis by a German professor of medicine at Hamburg, Hugo Schottmüller.

1910 The formula to determine the concentrating power of the kidney, using urea and blood ratios and known as the Ambard coefficient, was proposed by physiologist Leo Ambard in Strasbourg.

1910 The pathology of leprosy was described by German dermatologist, Paul Gerson Unna.

1910   The active principle of ergot in rye was identified by Sir Henry Hallett Dale, an English physician and Nobel laureate.

1910   *Sven Löfgren* born. A Swedish physician who described erythema nodosum, hilar lymphadenopathy and acute iritis seen in sarcoidosis (Löfgren syndrome).

1910   Bernhard Aschner demonstrated the presence of a substance in the anterior pituitary gland that influenced growth (growth hormone).

1910   John Jacob Abel of Johns Hopkins University used leeches to prevent the clotting of blood during his experiments on artificial kidneys.

1910   Right heart failure caused by bulging of a hypertrophied interventricular septum in hypertension, was described by Hippolyte Bernheim.

1910   The phenol sulfonaphthalein test to estimate renal functions was devised by Leonard George Rowntree, director of the Philadelphia Medical Institute, and another American, John Timothy Geraghty.

1910   Subcutaneous injection of a controlled amount of tuberculin for diagnosis of tuberculosis was introduced by French physician, Charles Mantoux.

1910   Sickle-cell anemia was first described by James Bryan Herrick of America.

1910   The term 'neurinoma' was introduced by Uruguayan pathologist, José Verocay in Prague, to describe a type of fibroma derived from the endoneurium or the neurilemma.

1910   Kalman Pandy, a Hungarian psychiatrist, devised a method of detecting an increase in globulin in cerebrospinal fluid (CSF).

1910   American pathologist, James Homer Wright, devised the Wright stain for megakarocytes and platelets.

1910   British orthopedic surgeon, Dilwyn Evans, described lateral wedge tarsectomy as treatment of clubfoot.

1910   The first demand intermittent-flow gas and oxygen machine for anesthesia was introduced by Elmer Isaac McKesson of Toledo, Ohio.

1910   Use of a modified cystoscope to view the interior of the thorax (thoracoscopy) was introduced by H.C. Jacobaeus in Stockholm.

1910   Arterial patch graft in vascular surgery was introduced by Alexis Carrel.

1910   The resemblance between the effect of histamine and anaphylaxis was pointed out by Sir Henry Dale and Sir Patrick Playfair Laidlaw of Cambridge.

1910   The relationship between the pituitary and the reproductive system was pointed out by American otorhinologist, Samuel Jones

Crowe, Harvey W. Cushing and J. Homens.

1910 Idiopathic paroxysmal myoglobinuria was described in a 12-year-old boy by F. Meyer-Betz.

1910 Surgical relief for constrictive pericarditis was carried out by M.P. Hallopeau at the Necker Hospital, Paris.

1910 Gigantism due to pituitary secretion was described by French physician, Pierre Emile Launois and M. Cleret.

1910 Cyclodialysis for glaucoma, formation of communication between suprachoroidal space and the anterior chamber of the eye was introduced by German ophthalmologist, Leopold Heine.

1910 Anti-pneumococcal serum was prepared by German bacteriologists, Fred Neufeld and Ludwig Haendel.

1911 Transmission of fowl sarcoma by an agent from the tumor cells was demonstrated by P. Rous.

1911 Division of the phrenic nerve in the neck to relax the lower lobe of the lung as treatment in tuberculosis was suggested by Stuertz of Cologne.

1911 The first accurate description of the chemical content of cerebrospinal fluid was given by French neurologist, William Mestrezat.

1911 Successful transmission of measles to monkeys was achieved by

American pathologists, Joseph Goldberger and J.F. Anderson.

1911 Use of the capon-comb test was introduced by French physician, Antoine Pezard, for evaluation of androgens.

1911 Demonstration of the heterophile antigen by John Forssmann, a Swedish pathologist.

1911 The lactogenic property of neural-lobe extract of the pituitary was demonstrated by Isaac Ott and J.C. Scott.

1911 Use of a syringe and glass container lined with paraffin wax to prevent clotting during blood transfusion was introduced by A.H. Curtis and V.C. David in Chicago.

1911 The first thoracoplasty was done by German cardiothoracic surgeon Ernst Ferdinand Sauerbruch of Berlin. He provided successful surgical relief for constrictive pericarditis in 1913. He carried out the first successful resection of ventricular aneurysm in 1930.

1911 The H+ ion was identified as a major stimulus to respiration by H. Winterstein.

1911 The National Society for Cancer Relief was founded by Douglas Macmillan following the death of his father through cancer.

1911 A method of maintaining excised animal organs alive by providing physiological surroundings was introduced by French-born American biologist, Alexis Carrel.

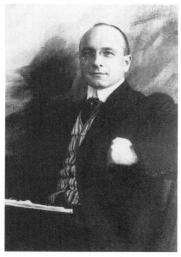

Alexis Carrel

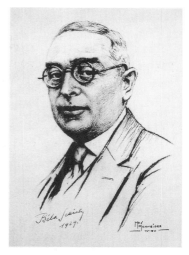

Béla Schick

1911   *Niels Kai Jerne* born. A Danish immunologist and Nobel laureate (1984) who studied the maturation of the immune system and developed the network theory of idiotypic regulation of lymphocytes and antibodies.

1911   A magenta-colored smooth tongue devoid of papillae as a feature of riboflavin deficiency (ariboflavinosis) was observed by English physician, Hugh S. Stannus.

1911   Alberto Ascoli devised the thermoprecipitin reaction for diagnosis of anthrax.

1911   A skin test for determining susceptibility to diphtheria (Schick test) was devised by Béla Schick, a Hungarian pediatrician working in New York.

1911   Part of the hemoglobin molecule (heme) was synthesized by American biochemist, David Shemin from New York.

1911   The Coffey operation, in which ureters are transplanted into the colon, was designed by surgeon from Portland, Oregon, Robert Calvin Coffey.

1911   The first move towards the British government taking responsibility for the health of the nation was made with the enactment of the National Health Insurance Act.

1911   A virus which induced a tumor in chickens, capable of being transmitted to other closely-related chickens (Rous sarcoma) was discovered by American pathologist, Francis Peyton Rous.

1911   The first attempt to protect from hay fever by injecting an extract of pollen (desensitization) was made by Leonard Noon and John Freeman.

1911   Self-administration techniques for nitrous oxide in obstetrics were demonstrated and reported by

American surgeon, A.E. Guedel while working in Indianapolis.

1911 The term 'schizophrenia' for dementia praecox was introduced by Eugene Bleuler, professor of psychiatry at Burgholzi Hospital.

1911 *Denis Parsons Burkitt* born. An Irish pioneer in chemotherapy for cancer who gave his name to Burkitt lymphoma, after working on multiple tumors in the jaws of African children.

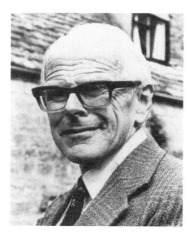

Denis Parsons Burkitt

1911 Direct measurements of heat evolved during contraction of a muscle were made by British Nobel Prize winner, Archibald Vivian Hill.

1911 An increase in epinephrine output during emotional stress resulting in palpitations and sweating (Cannon syndrome) was described by an American physiologist, Walter Bradford Cannon.

1911 *Willem Johan Kolff* born. A Dutch-born American physician and pio-

neer of the artificial kidney who constructed the first rotating drum artificial kidney, in wartime Holland, and developed the artificial kidney and a heart–lung machine after moving to America.

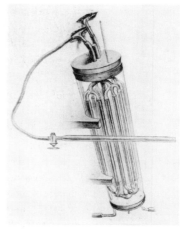

Kolff's original dialysis machine

1911 Jean Clunet of France demonstrated the experimental production of malignant tumors using X-rays.

1911 The role of hormonal factors in the female reproductive cycle was recognized by Viennese surgeon, Eugen Steinach.

1911 A crude gastroscope, consisting of a tube which a patient could swallow, was devised by London physician, William Hill.

1911 Bárány syndrome, described by Robert Bárány in 1918, was first noted by Alfred Bing as cystic serous meningitis of the posterior fossa.

1911 The fibers of the scalenus anterior which passed through the cervical pleura were described by John Stuart Dickey, an anatomist from Belfast working in Ontario.

1911 A bag for collecting expired air for respiratory function studies (Douglas bag) was devised by English respiratory physiologist, Claude Gordon Douglas.

1911 Proof that chloroform can cause death (from ventricular fibrillation) in light anesthesia was provided by Goodman Levy.

1911 'Crossing-over', a process of exchange of corresponding segments between chromatids of homologous chromosomes, by breakage or reunion during pairing, was described by American geneticist, Thomas Hunt Morgan.

1911 Findings that showed how extirpation of the corpora lutea in guinea pigs accelerated the next ovulation, while extirpation of other parts of the ovary had no such effect, were recorded by American pathologist, Leo Loeb.

1911 Noradrenaline was discovered by George Barger and Henry Dale at Edinburgh University and the National Institute for Medical Research.

1911 American physician, Joel Ernest Goldthwait, wrote on treatment of lumbar disc prolapse by operation, and also invented a procedure for recurrent dislocation of the patella.

1911 Premature separation of a normally implanted placenta, accompanied by albuminuria, azotemia and shock (Couvelaire syndrome) was described by French obstetrician, Alexandre Couvelaire.

1911 Neoarsphenamime, which is effective in treatment of relapsing fever, syphilis and trypanosomiasis, was produced by German bacteriologist, Paul Ehrlich.

1911 *André Bazex* born. A French professor of dermatology at Toulouse who described acrokeratosis paraneoplastica (Bazex syndrome).

1911 *Sir Bernard Katz* born. A German-born British neurophysiologist and Nobel laureate (1970) who worked on the chemical mechanism of neurotransmission, particularly acetylcholine.

1911 One of the first and most detailed descriptions of paroxysmal nocturnal hemoglobinuria (Marchiafava–Micheli syndrome) was given by Italian physician, Ettore Marchiafava.

1911 *Sir John Charnley* born. An eminent British orthopedic surgeon who pioneered artificial hip joints, first using Teflon without success, then gaining better results using polythene (Charnley prosthesis).

1912 *Konrad Emil Bloch* born. A German-born American biochemist and Nobel laureate (1964) who carried out work on fatty acids and cholesterol which led to an understanding of the formation of ketones and cholesterol.

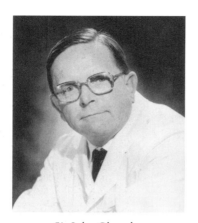

Sir John Charnley

1912 The first comprehensive treatise on hand surgery was published by American surgeon, Allen Buckner Kanavel.

1912 The vascularity of malignant gliomas was shown by English physician, Howard Henry Tooth.

1912 *Harry Fitch Klinefelter* born. A professor of medicine from the Johns Hopkins Hospital who described Klinefelter syndrome (also known as XXY), consisting of gynecomastia, azoospermia with increased levels of follicle stimulating hormone in male (1942).

1912 The myenteric reflex which effects the propulsion of food or a foreign body in the intestines was described by American physiologist, Walter Bradford Cannon.

1912 French gynecologist, Antoine Basset, described a form of radical vulvectomy as treatment of carcinoma of the vulva (Basset operation).

1912 The Ramstedt operation for relief of congenital pyloric stenosis was de-

vised by German surgeon, Conrad Ramstedt.

1912 Oguchi syndrome, characterized by night blindness and grayish appearance of the fundus, was observed in Japan by ophthalmologist, Chuta Oguchi.

1912 Hepatolenticular degeneration due to abnormality of copper metabolism (Wilson disease) was described by British neurologist, Samuel Alexander Kinnier Wilson.

1912 A skin sensitivity test (Casoni test) was devised for diagnosis of hydatid disease by Italian physician, Tomaso Casoni.

1912 German organic chemist, Heinrich Otto Wieland, demonstrated that bile acids were steroids, based on the structure of cholesterol.

1912 The importance of unmyelinated nerve fibers in the dorsal roots was recognized by Chicago neurologist, Stephen Walter Ranson.

1912 A theory to explain electrical properties of muscle was proposed by German professor of physiology at Halle, Julius Bernstein.

1912 A successful pulmonary embolectomy of the femoral artery was performed by Einar Samuel Henrick Key of Germany.

1912 Ipsilateral paralysis of the 3rd and 4th nerves with contralateral hemianesthesia due to compression of the arterial supply to the inferior nucleus ruber by mesencephalic lesions (Claude syndrome) was described by Henri C. J. Claude.

1912 William Meredith Boothby of the Mayo Clinic and Boston surgeon, Frederic Jay Cotton, used the Cotton-Boothby apparatus for nitrous oxide–oxygen–ether anesthesia.

1912 The first publication on use of phenobarbitone in treatment of epilepsy was written by a German physician, Alfred Hauptmann.

1912 *On the Growth of Bone* was published by Scottish surgeon, Sir William MacEwen, who developed the idea of grafting one piece of bone to take the place of another.

1912 *George Emil Palade* born. A Romanian cell biologist and Nobel laureate (1974) who developed cell fractionation methods, and described the cell organelles: mitochondria, endoplasmic reticulum, ribosomes and the Golgi apparatus.

1912 English geneticist, William Bateson and Sir Clifford Allibut, created a scientific forum for birth control.

1912 *Julius Axelrod* born. An American pharmacologist who discovered catechol-O-methyl transferase, which regulates the production of norepinephrine.

1912 Incomplete development, fusion or absence of the first cervical vertebra (Klippel–Feil syndrome) was described by French neurologists, Maurice Klippel and Andre Feil in Paris.

Julius Axelrod

1912 Melioidosis, a glanders-like disease, was described by surgeons, Alfred Whitmore and C.S. Krishnaswami, who carried out their studies in India.

1912 *Albert H. Coons* born. An American immunologist who devised the Coons fluorescent antibody method.

1912 An important treatise on lead poisoning was written by Thomas Morison Legge of England with K.W. Goadby, *Lead Poisoning and Lead Absorption*.

1912 The features of acute coronary thrombosis were described by Chicago physician, J.B. Herrick.

1912 Spasm and rigidity of intercostal muscles due to inflammation of the pleura or lung (Pottenger sign) was described by an American from St Louis, Francis Marion Pottenger.

1912 Regulation of temperature was one of the first functions of the hypothalamus discovered by V.R. Isenschmidt and Ludolph von Krehl.

1912 The findings of Austrian chemist, Richard Adolf Zsigmondy, aided analysis of proteins in cerebrospinal fluid (CSF).

1912 The autoimmune condition of lymphoid infiltration of the thyroid gland (Hashimoto thyroiditis), was described by the Japanese surgeon, Hakaru Hashimoto.

1912 Henry Peter George Bayon demonstrated experimental production of cancer by injection of tar.

1912 *Primary Malignant Growths of the Lungs and Bronchi*, written by Isaac Adler, encouraged further study on carcinoma of the lung.

1912 Thymectomy was performed as treatment for myasthenia by Ernst Ferdinand Sauerbach of Germany.

1912 Spasm of the upper esophagus (Plummer–Vinson syndrome) was described by Henry Stanley Plummer, a professor at the Mayo Clinic in the United States, who differentiated it from carcinoma.

1912 Torald Hermann Sollmann and Edgar Dewight Brown of Minnesota described the carotid sinus depressor reflex.

1912 German physician, A. Laewen of Zwickau, used curare during surgery to produce muscle relaxation.

1912 William Roberts of Manchester Royal Infirmary, and the pharma-

ceutical chemist, Benger, developed digestive enzyme products (Benger food).

1912 A supraclavicular technique for brachial plexus block was devised by German surgeon, D. Kulenkampf, who experimented with the method on himself.

1912 Intra-arterial anesthesia using a pneumatic cuff was introduced by J. Goyanes of Spain.

1912

H.H. Janeway

An apparatus for intermittent endotracheal insufflation for anesthesia was devised by H.H. Janeway. He introduced the first patient-triggered ventilator in 1913.

1912 The study of movements of the stomach by inserting a balloon through a fistula was introduced by American physiologist, Anton Julius Carlson.

1912 The first use of subcutaneous injections of soluble salts of emetine as treatment for amebiasis was by

Sir Leonard Rogers, a London pathologist.

1912 The first modern dissection lobectomy was carried out by Morriston Davies of University College Hospital, London.

1913 Application of rubber bellows in blood transfusion was introduced by A.R. Kimpton and J.H. Brown. Their method was widely used during World War I.

1913 The oxygen dissociation curve of hemoglobin was described by Joseph Barcroft and E.P. Poulton.

1913 Transthyroid pharyngotomy for carcinoma of the hypopharynx was described by Wilfred Trotter.

1913 The first attempt at surgical correction of tracheoesophageal fistula in two infants was made by H.M. Richter. Both infants died of respiratory complications.

1913 The term 'lipid nephrosis' was first used by German physician, Fritz Munk.

1913 A successful removal of a pineal tumor was performed by German neurologist, Herman Oppenheim and Berlin surgeon, Fedor Krause.

1913 A rectal oil–ether mixture was introduced by James Tayloe Gwathmey of New York, who in the following year published his classic textbook *Anesthesia*.

1913 Ivor Christian Bang of Germany devised the microchemical method of estimation of blood glucose.

1913 A classic description of traumatic lipemia and fatty embolism of the lung, was given by American physician, Aldred Scott Warthin.

1913 Mammography, used to detect breast cancer, was developed by German surgeon, A. Salomen.

1913 The abdominal operation for carcinoma of the uterus was introduced by German surgeon, Wilhelm Alexander Freund.

1913 Thomas Janeway described heart failure as a manifestation of hypertensive vascular disease.

1913 Starvation as a method of lowering blood sugar in treatment for diabetes (Allen starvation) was proposed by Frederick Madison Allen, a Boston diabetologist.

1913 The reticuloendothelial system was described by German pathologist, Ludwig Aschoff.

1913 Lymphogranuloma venereum (Favre disease) was described by Maurice Favre, a professor of pathological anatomy in Lyons, who also proposed a classification of reticuloendothelial diseases.

1913 Maude Slye of Chicago began cancer experimentation that showed malignancy to be a dominant trait and susceptibility a recessive gene trait.

1913 The concept of representing the electrical forces of the heart by recording the vector forces from the surface of the body (vectorcardiography) was proposed by Dutch physiologist, Willem Einthoven.

1913 The Lange test for cerebrospinal fluid, using gold chloride to detect various forms of cerebrospinal syphilis, was devised by Carl Friedrich August Lange of Berlin.

1913 New York urologist, Max Huhner, estimated the motility and the number of spermatozoa during postcoital examination..

1913 An early case history for Simmonds disease (hypopituitarism resulting from atrophy of the anterior pituitary lobe) was published by Leon Konrad Glinski of Poland.

1913 Work on histocompatibility was carried out by Clarence Cook Little of Mount Desert Island, Maine, and led to significant advances in transplantation medicine and the study of cancer.

1913 Paris surgeon, Eugéne Louis Doyen performed a valvotomy for stenosis of the pulmonary valve.

1913 American orthopedic surgeon John B. Murphy pioneered modern arthroplasty for ankolyzed joints.

1913 The methodology for extraction of pollen, and identification of allergenic protein were provided by Scottish physician, William Dunbar.

1913 *Stephen William Kuffler* born. An American neurobiologist, born in Hungary, who studied mechanisms of synaptic transmission, retinal physiology, and electro physiology of glial cells.

1913 Primary anastomosis of the esophagus was suggested as treatment for congenital atresia by H.M. Richter.

1913 A string galvanometer to record the electrical activity of the brain was introduced by Russian physiologist, Pravdich Neminsky.

1913 The British Medical Association (BMA) was founded.

1913 Emil Hatschek designed an apparatus to measure viscosity of blood.

1913 Abnormality of the sex chromosome during meiosis (non-disjunction) was discovered by Colin Blackman Bridges.

1913 *Geoffrey W. Harris* born. A British physician who studied pituitary secretion and its interaction with the brain, and showed the brain is a target organ for ovarian hormones.

1913 *Roger Wolcott Sperry* born. An American neuroscientist and Nobel laureate (1981) who helped establish the way in which nerve cells are wired into the central nervous system, and pioneered split-brain experiments.

1913 Successful resection of thoracic esophagus for carcinoma was performed by a New York surgeon, Franz Torek.

1913 *Patrick Christopher Steptoe* born. An English gynecologist who began his work on in vitro fertilization with British physiologist, Robert Edwards, and achieved the first 'test-tube baby' (1978).

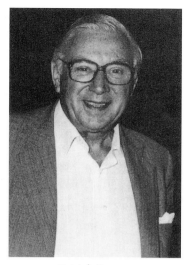

Patrick Steptoe

1913 The peritoneal band extending from the mesocolon to the duodenojejunal flexure (Pringle band) was described by Dublin surgeon, Seton Sydney Pringle.

1913 Monocytic leukemia was described by Hamburg physicians, Hassan Reschad and V. Schilling-Torgau.

1913 The American College of Surgeons was founded.

1913 *Chenopodium* was used as an antihelmintic in ancylostomiasis by German physicians, Wilhelm August Paul Schuffner and Herman Vervoort.

1913 The fenestration operation for otosclerosis was suggested by George John Jenkins of London.

1913 The first comprehensive description of venereal lymphogranuloma was given by French physicians, Joseph Nicolas, J. Durand and

Maurice Favre, and is also known as fourth venereal disease, or Nicolas–Durand–Favre disease.

1913 The American Society for Control of Cancer was established by American pathologist, James Ewing and associates, who also helped to start the *Journal of Cancer Research*.

1914 Mumps, a disease known since ancient times, was found to be caused by a filterable agent by British bacteriologist, Mervyn Henry Gordon.

1914 Sodium citrate was added to blood to prevent coagulation independently by Louis Agote and Albert Hustin.

1914 *Max Ferdinand Perutz* born. An Austrian biochemist and Nobel laureate (1962) who determined the amino acids in hemoglobin, and the alpha-helical structure of myoglobin.

1914 Wilhelm Gennerich, a German dermatologist, introduced treatment of neurosyphilis by intraspinal injections of arsphenamine and designed a special device for forcing the salvarsanized cerebrospinal fluid into the brain.

1914 Experimental studies on renal transplantation were carried out by Alexis Carrel, an American biologist and pioneer in transplantation.

1914 The method of assessing the patency of the fallopian tubes (salpingography) was devised by William Cary Hollenback of America.

1914   *Horace Gilbert Smithey* born. An American cardiac surgeon who worked on a surgical treatment for aortic stenosis, and suffered and died from it before finding a cure.

1914   Active extract of the thyroid, thyroxin, was isolated by Edward Calvin Kendall of Detroit, Michigan, who named it while he was researching at the Mayo Institute.

1914   Sensory aphasic syndrome accompanied by apraxia and alexia, in lesions of the left parietal lobe, was described by French neurologist, Joseph Jules Dejerine.

1914   Barium enema as a diagnostic test in radiology was introduced, thereby increasing recognition of colonic diverticular disease.

1914   English physiologist, Arthur Francis Bainbridge, discovered that cardiac inhibition produced vagal tone, and that accelerator nerves caused cardiac excitation.

1914   *Loren Larsen* born. An American orthopedic surgeon who described Larsen syndrome of skeletal dysplasia with stunting of stature, associated with joint laxity, congenital dislocation of elbows, knees and hips, shortened spatulate digits and depression of the nasal bridge.

1914   *Infection and Resistance* was written by New York bacteriologist and immunologist, Hans Zinsser, who worked on allergy, virus size, typhus and causes of rheumatic fevers.

1914   Lipoidosis with anemia, mental retardation, retinal degeneration, hepatosplenomegaly and skin pigmentation (Niemann–Pick disease) was described by Albert Niemann, a Berlin pediatrician.

1914   Antidiphtheria serum, produced from the blood of infected horses, was employed for active immunization against diphtheria by William Hallock Park.

1914   The National Institute for the Blind was established in England which developed William Moon's embossed reading system based on Roman capitals.

1914   *Jack Pepys* born. An American microbiologist who identified the causative organism of farmer's lung (*Micropolyspora faeni*), and made major contributions to understanding the etiology and pathogenesis of allergic alveolitis, occupational asthma, and allergic bronchopulmonary aspergillosis.

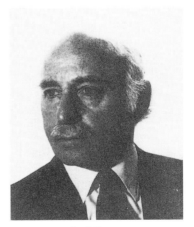

Jack Pepys

342

1914   The symptoms and complications arising from sinusitis were described by English physician, Sir St Clair Thompson.

1914   New York neurologist, James Ramsay Hunt, suggested the visualization of the carotid artery in patients presenting cerebral symptoms (carotid angiography).

1914   *Geriatrics: The Disease of Old Age and their Treatment* was published by Nascher, the father of this specialty in America.

1914   *Sir Allan Lloyd Hodgkin* born. A British physiologist and Nobel laureate (1963) who conducted research into nerve impulses, and described the mechanism by which nerves conduct electrical impulses.

1914   Study of digestion by withdrawal of a test meal from the stomach was made possible with the invention of the stomach tube designed by Martin Emil Rehfuss.

1914   Experimental proof that rubella (German measles) is caused by a virus was provided by Alfred Fabian Hess of Germany.

1914   The viral etiology of the common cold was demonstrated by German bacteriologist, Walther Kruse.

1914   A method by which blood is removed from the body, followed by separation into cells and plasma, before returning the cells to the body (plasmaphaeresis) was demonstrated in animals by American biochemist, John Jacob Abel.

1914   *Frederick C. Bartter* born. An American physician best-known for his description of Bartter syndrome, diminished sodium resorption of the kidney leading to hypokalemic alkalosis.

1914   William Buchanan Wherry, an American bacteriologist, isolated the causative organism of tularemia.

1914   Auto-blood transfusion was successfully used by Thies in cases of severe hemorrhage from ruptured ectopic pregnancy and ruptured spleen.

1914   The pathway of cerebrospinal fluid was studied by American anatomist, Lewis Hill Weed.

1914   Bronchography was discovered when Weingartner of Berlin noticed the appearance of bronchi when bismuth, used for study of the esophagus, accidentally spilled over into the lungs.

1915   The clinical importance of routine bacteriological study of sputum was established by J.A. Luetscher.

1915   Use of an intravenous dye for determination of blood and plasma volume was introduced by Leonard G. Rowntree, Norman M. Keith, and John T. Geraghty.

1915   Pneumonolysis was carried out by Swedish surgeon, Hans Christian Jacobaeus, in which he used galvanocautery to divide pleural adhesions.

1915 British physiologist, Sir William Maddock Bayliss' classic *Principles of General Physiology* was published.

1915 Achalasia, the failure of smooth sphincters to relax at the gastroesophageal junction, was named by Sir Frederick Arthur Hurst.

1915 The causative agent of Weil disease, *Leptospira icterohemorrhagia*, was identified independently by Ryukichi Inado and Yutaka Ido of Japan.

1915 The American College of Physicians was founded.

1915 *Thomas Huckle Weller* born. An American virologist from Michigan and Nobel laureate (1954) who worked on *Schistosoma* and poliomyelitis cell cultivation, and on chickenpox and shingles viruses.

1915 Antacid therapy for peptic ulcer with frequent milk feeds and compounds such as magnesium hydroxide, was popularized by American physician, Bertram Welton Sippy.

1915 *Mortality from Cancer Throughout the World* was written by American, Frederick Ludwig Hoffman, one of the first cancer statisticians.

1915 X-rays were shown to suppress antibody response (total body irradiation) by American pathologist, Ludwig Hektoen.

1915 Canadian bacteriologist, Felix D'Herelle, discovered the bacteriophage.

1915 An individual containing both male and female genetic elements (gynandromorph) was described and named by R. Goldschmidt.

1915 The now obsolete test for hemolysis (Weil test), based on the observation that erythrocytes of syphilitic patients are resistant to the hemolysing effect of cobra venom, and was devised by New York physician, Richard Weil.

1915 Lewis Hall described the pathway and circulation of cerebrospinal fluid (CSF).

1915 Norman Macdonnell Keith introduced a method of estimating plasma and blood volume by injecting dye.

1915 James Haig-Ferguson, an obstetrician from the Royal Hospital in Dublin, started the first antenatal clinic.

1915 The rise of phosphate levels in blood of patients with renal failure (hyperphosphatemia) was observed by Greenwald.

1915 Sonar or ultrasound was developed by a French scientist, Paul Langevin, for ships to detect icebergs.

1916 *Frederick Chapman Robbins* born. An American physiologist, pediatrician and Nobel laureate (1954) from Alabama who succeeded in cultivating the poliomyelitis virus, an important step in the development of polio vaccine.

1916 The nature and origin of connective tissue was explained by French neurologist, Jean Nageotte.

1916   G.V. Black and F.S. McKay described mottled teeth due to endemic fluorosis in Colorado.

1916   Polish bacteriologist, Arthur Felix, devised an agglutinin reaction for diagnosis of typhus.

1916   Discoloration of the skin around the umbilicus in cases of ruptured ectopic pregnancy (Cullen sign) was described by Canadian-born American gynecologist, Thomas Stephen Cullen.

1916   Reiter disease, characterized by urethritis, conjunctivitis, and arthritis, was described by bacteriologist, Hans Reiter of the German Medical Corps.

1916   A prototype of the modern X-ray vacuum tube (Coolridge tube) was invented by American physicist, William David Coolridge, who replaced the cold aluminum cathode by a hot tungsten cathode.

1916   A rise of uric acid in the blood which precedes the rise of urea in renal failure, was noted by Victor Carlyl Myers.

1916   A warm ether insufflation apparatus was introduced by Sir Francis E. Shipway of Guy's Hospital, London.

1916   *Maurice Hugh Frederick Wilkins* born. A New Zealand-born British physicist and Nobel laureate (1962) known for his work on DNA X-ray crystallography.

1916   An acute ascending form of demyelinating motor neuropathy (Guillain–Barré syndrome) was described by French neurologists, Georges Guillain and Jean Alexander Barré.

1916   Fever, stomatitis and mucocutaneous eruption (Stevens–Johnson syndrome) was first described by Robert Rendu of Paris.

1916   A congenital condition of atrial septal defect associated with mitral stenosis (Lutembacher syndrome) was described by René Lutembacher of Paris.

1916   Unilateral paralysis of the 9th, 10th, 11th and 12th cranial nerves following lesions in the retroparotid space (Villaret syndrome) was described by Maurice Villaret of Paris.

1916   A block in the flow of cerebrospinal fluid during lumbar puncture by applying pressure on the jugular vein (Queckenstedt test) was devised by German physician, Hans Heinrich Queckenstedt.

1916   *Jean-Baptiste Dausset* born. A French physiologist and Nobel Prize winner (1980) whose work led to the discovery of the major histocompatibility complex, and who developed tissue typing.

Jean-Baptiste Dausset

1916   Use of trypsin for preparing cells for transfer from plasma clot cultures of virus was developed by P. Rous and F.S. Jones.

1916   A modern method of trephining the skull for inflammation of the brain was introduced by American surgeon, Harris Peyton Mosher.

1917   Adrenaline-like properties of ephedrine were described by H. Amatsu and S. Kubota of Japan.

1917   The first description of epidemic encephalitis lethargica, a month before Economo's description, was given by French physician, Jean Renè Cruchet.

1917   A review of 500 cases of gunshot wounds of the chest was made by George Gask, professor of surgery at St Bartholomew's Hospital.

1917   Acriflavin was introduced as an antiseptic by Carl Hamilton Browning.

1917   *Sir Andrew Fielding Huxley* born. An English neurophysiologist and Nobel laureate (1963) who deduced a physico-chemical explanation for conduction of impulses in nerve fibers, and worked on muscle contraction and relaxation, proposing the sliding filament theory.

1917   *Robert Burns Woodward* born. An American organic chemist and Nobel laureate (1965) who worked on the antimalarial drug, quinine (1950), and synthesized cortisone, cholesterol, lysergic acid, reserpine, vitamin B_{12} and colchicine.

1917   Paroxysmal intense pain in the anus and the internal sphincter and of unknown etiology (Thaysen syndrome) was described by Alexander MacLennan, a lecturer in surgery at Glasgow University.

1917   Creation of a controlled vacuum by means of an air pump for suction of the lens was made possible with an instrument designed by Jose Ignacio Barraquer of Barcelona.

1917   The first clear account of galactosemia was given by Friedrich Goppert of Berlin.

1917   A rare form of Parkinsonism due to degeneration of the globus pallidus, which occurs before the third decade, was described by James Ramsay Hunt, a neurologist from the University of Columbia.

1917   The hereditary disease due to a disturbance of mucopolysaccharide metabolism (gargoylism or Hurler syndrome) was described in two brothers by Canadian professor of medicine, Charles Hunter.

1917   A special head stethoscope to monitor fetal heart sounds while both hands were free to examine the mother or deliver the child was designed by Chicago obstetrician, David Sweeny Hills.

1917   Radium treatment for cancer of the uterus was developed by Swedish radiologist, Carl Gustav Abrahamson Forssell.

1917   The British Orthopaedic Association was founded.

1917

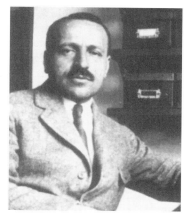

George Papanicolaou

A study of exfoliative cytology related to normal cyclical changes of the vaginal epithelium was made by American cytologist, Nicholas George Papanicolaou, leading to mass screening for cervical cancer.

1917 Fouchet reagent, to test for the presence of bilirubin in urine, was prepared by French chemist and physician, Andre Fouchet.

1917 *Robert Anderson Aldrich* born. An American pediatrician who described a sex-linked disease with increased susceptibility to infections, dermatitis and thrombocytopenia (Wiskott–Aldrich syndrome), and worked on heme synthesis and inborn errors of metabolism.

1917 The beneficial effects of treating general syphilitic paresis by inoculation with malaria were demonstrated by Austrian psychiatrist, Julius Wagner–Jauregg.

1917 The Krukenberg amputation, a method used to allow the stump to retain some function, was described by a German orthopedic surgeon, Hermann Krukenberg.

1917 Inattention to objects in one half of the visual field with inability to recognize these objects (Riddoch syndrome) was described by a neurologist from Scotland, George Riddoch.

1917 The standard color-blindness test was devised by Japanese ophthalmologist, Shinobu Isihara of Tokyo.

1918 *Arthur Kornberg* born. An American biochemist from New York and Nobel laureate (1959) who discovered DNA polymerase, and showed that DNA required a template and base-pairing to produce helical strands.

1918 Hereditary hemorrhagic thrombasthenia (Glanzmann syndrome) was described by Swiss pediatrician, Eduard Glanzmann.

1918 Bone holding forceps (Farr forceps) were devised by American surgeon, Robert Emmet Farr.

1918 *Gertrude Belle Elion* born. An American biochemist and Nobel laureate (1988) who worked on the synthesis of compounds that inhibited DNA synthesis, particularly pyrimidines, with potential as anti-cancer therapy, and developed acyclovir.

1918 Cold agglutinins were observed in the serum of patients suffering from 'an unusual form of bronchopneumonia' by Baltimore physician, Mildred Clark Clough and R.M. Richter of Johns Hopkins Hospital.

1918   *Frederick Sanger* born. An English biochemist and double Nobel laureate (1958 and 1980) who unraveled the complete sequence of amino acids in insulin, provided a sequence of amino acids for a protein, and carried out work on the structure of DNA and RNA.

1918   A method of introducing air into the ventricles of the brain to visualize it on X-rays was devised by a neurosurgeon at Johns Hopkins Hospital, Baltimore, Walter Edward Dandy.

1918   An operative method for femoral hernia (Dowden operation) was devised by Edinburgh surgeon, John Wheeler Dowden.

1918   *Clarence Walton Lillehei* born. An American pioneer of open-heart surgery who was born and trained in medicine in Minnesota where he spent most of his career.

1918   Deficiency of iodine was shown to be the principal cause of goiter by David Marine from Cleveland Ohio and Jean François Coindet.

1918   The heart's changes occurring in myxodema were recorded by German physician in Israel, Hermann Zondek.

1918   An isomer of quinine was used by Dutch physician, Karel Frederik Wenckebach for treatment of atrial fibrillation.

1918   Japanese professor Kenji Takanagi from Tokyo University devised a modified cystoscope.

1918   *Entamoeba histolytica* was obtained in pure culture by English bacteriologist, D. Ward Cutler.

1918   W.T. Longcope and F.M. Rackemann demonstrated the morphological lesions of serum sickness to be a result of antigen–antibody reactions.

1918   Effectiveness of quinine in treatment of auricular fibrillation was demonstrated by German physician, Walter Frey.

1918   Use of preserved blood and establishment of blood banks was proposed by American physician, Oswald Hope Robertson.

1919   The first demonstration, although accidental, of transfer of immediate hypersensitivity between humans was made by M.A. Ramirez.

1919   *Bacterium paratyphosum* C was isolated by Swiss physician, Ludwig Hirschfeld.

1919   The causative organism of Rocky Mountain Spotted Fever was named *Dermancentronicus rickettsi* by American pathologist, Simeon Burt Wolbach.

1919   An early method of surgical treatment for uterine prolapse was devised by an American obstetrician and gynecologist, Alfred Baker Spalding.

1919   While studying thromboplastic substances, William Henry Howell of Johns Hopkins Hospital, isolated heparin from the liver, brain and heart.

1919 Neuroglia (the supporting structure of the nerve tissue) was differentiated into microglia and oligodenroglia using silver stain by Spanish histologist, Pio del Rio Hortega of the National Institute for Cancer in Madrid.

1919 A mastoidectomy was performed in England by English neurosurgeon, Sir Charles Alfred Ballance, who wrote *Essays on the Surgery of the Temporal Bone.*

1919 Ovarian endometriosis was described by D.B. Casler at Johns Hopkins Hospital.

1919 Goodpasture syndrome, associated with acute nephritis and hemoptysis, was described in an 18-year-old male by American virologist, Ernest William Goodpasture.

1919 *Leslie Zieve* born. An American hepatologist who is best remembered for his description of transient hemolytic anemia associated with hyperlipoproteinemia, jaundice and liver disease.

1919 *Sir Godfrey Newbold Hounsfield* born. An English engineer who invented the CAT (computerized tomography) scanner, and shared the Nobel Prize with Allan Cormack in 1979.

1919 *John F. Criggler* born. An American pediatrician who (with Victor A. Najjar) described jaundice due to the inability to conjugate bilirubin with glucuronic acid (Criggler–Najjar syndrome).

1919 Experimental rejuvenation with testicular transplant was reported by a French physiologist of Russian origin, Serge Voronoff.

1919 Werner syndrome, characterized by polydactyly, absence of thumbs and tibia and reduced knee movements was described by P. Werner.

1919 *Joseph Edward Murray* born. An American surgeon, Nobel laureate (1990) and pioneer in renal transplantation who performed the first renal transplant between identical twins (1954) and non-identical twins (1961).

1919 Oncology was established as a specialty in America by James Ewing, professor of oncology at Cornell University Medical College, New York, with the publication of his work, *Neoplastic Diseases.*

1920 Athetosis, emotional lability, and rhythmic oscillation of the limbs due to a lesion in the corpus striatum (Vogt syndrome) were described by French physician, Cécile Vogt and German neurologist Oskar Vogt.

1920 A detailed account of the endothelial tumor of the shaft of long bones (Ewing sarcoma) was given by James Ewing, professor of oncology at the Cornell University Medical College in New York.

1920 Isador Clinton Rubin used tubal insufflation to treat sterility resulting from occlusion of the fallopian tubes.

1920 *Charles Heidelberger* born. A professor of oncology at Wisconsin who pioneered research on anticancer agents and introduced flurouracil as a tumor inhibitory compound (1957).

1920 Endotracheal anesthesia was developed by Ivan Whiteside Magill and E. Stanley Rowbotham of London.

1920 *The Journal of Neurology and Psychopathology* was founded by a British–American neurologist, Samuel Alexander Kinnier Wilson of the National Hospital, Queen's Square, London.

1920 A technique of tying and dividing the fallopian tubes for sterilization was devised by Ralph Hayward Pomeroy, a New York obstetrician.

1920 *Baruj Benacerraf* born. A Venezuelan-born American immunologist and Nobel laureate (1980) who studied immunological responses to diseased cells and organ transplantation.

1920 *François Jacob* born. A French biochemist who shared the Nobel Prize (1965) for his work on gene regulation and the formulation of the operon theory.

1920 Bacterium became generic term for most intestinal bacteria in the reports of the American Committee headed by Charles Edward Amory Winslow.

1920 Tumors were classified into four groups with regard to malignancy, on the basis of the undifferentiated state of the cells, by American pathologist, Albert C. Broders.

1920 A test for function of the kidneys (urea concentration test) was devised by Hugh MacLean and Owen Lambart de Wesselow.

1920 The earliest synthetic organic mercurial diuretics (mercupurin, mercuhydrin) were introduced and remained in use for almost two decades.

1920 Neural connections between the hypothalamus and the pituitary were demonstrated by American neuroanatomist, Stephen Walter Ranson of Rush Medical College.

1920 *Allen Frederick Dwyer* born. An Australian orthopedic surgeon who devised an anterior spinal fusion with staples, screws and wire (Dwyer fusion).

1920 The Rideal–Walker test to determine the germicidal power of disinfectants was invented by English chemists, Samuel Rideal and J.T. Ainsley Walker.

1920 Puncture of the cisterna magna to obtain a sample of cerebrospinal fluid for diagnostic purposes (occipital puncture) was first carried out by American neurologist, James Bourne Ayer.

1920 Internuclear ophthalmoplegia in disseminated sclerosis (Lhermitte syndrome) was described by French neurologist, Jean Lhermitte.

1920 *Edward Donnall Thomas* born. An American hematologist and Nobel laureate (1990) who worked on bone marrow transplantation, developed tissue-typing, and the use of immunosuppressive drugs for the treatment of leukemia patients.

1920   A syndrome of dementia accompanied by pyramidal and extrapyramidal signs which usually occur after middle age (Creutzfeldt–Jacob disease) was first described by Hans Gerhard Creutzfeldt and a year later by Alfons Jakob.

1920   The hippuric acid synthesis test (where benzoic acid combines with glycol in the kidney to form hippuric acid) was used to test for renal functions by Émile Achard and Chapelle of Paris.

1920   Electrocardiographic changes in myocardial infarction were described by New York cardiologist, Harold Ensign Bennett Pardee.

1920   Wilfred Harris, a neurologist at St Mary's Hospital, performed alcohol injection of the Gasserian ganglion through the foramen ovale for treatment of trigeminal neuralgia.

1920   *Denton Arthur Cooley* born. An American cardiac surgeon working at the Texas Heart Institution in Houston who was a pioneer in open-heart and vascular surgery.

1920   An intermittent-flow machine (McKesson Machine) for anesthesia was introduced by American anesthetist, Ira McKesson of Toledo, Ohio.

1920   Use of mercurial diuretic (Novasurol) injections in treatment of cardiac failure were introduced by German physician, Paul Saxl.

Denton Arthur Cooley

1920   The increased malignant nature of embryonic or undifferentiated cells in a tumor was proposed by American pathologist, Albert C. Broders.

1921   Encephalitis lethargica as a cause of parkinsonism was demonstrated by French neurologist, Achille Alexander Souques.

1921   Carbon tetrachloride was introduced as treatment for hookworm by Maurice Crowther Hall of the United States Bureau of Animal Industry.

1921   Clinical use of 5% carbon dioxide with oxygen for anesthesia was introduced by Howard Wilcox Haggard and New Haven physiologist, Yandell Henderson.

1921   A detailed account of pelvic endometriosis was given by New York gynecologist, John Albertson Sampson.

1921 A radiological method of studying bronchiectasis by injecting bismuth through the bronchoscope (bronchogram) was devised by William Holmes Stewart and Henry Lowndes Lynah.

1921 Radiological visualization of the kidneys by injecting air into the retroperitoneal space (retroperitoneal pneumatography) was devised by Rossentein and Carelli.

1921 Optic atrophy, ophthalmoplegia and trigeminal neuralgia caused by a space-occupying lesion in the petrosphenoid space (Jacod triad) was described by French neurologist, Maurice Jacod.

1921 The failure or obstruction of the foramen of Luschka and Magendie giving rise to hydrocephalus (Dandy–Walker syndrome) was first described by American neurosurgeon, Walter Edward Dandy.

1921 *Angelo M. DiGeorge* born. An American pediatrician who described DiGeorge syndrome, characterized by congenital absence of the thymus and parathyroid glands, leading to recurrent infection.

1921 The contraceptive pill was developed from studies on the ovary by an Austrian biochemist, Ludwig Haberlandt.

1921 The amino acid methionine was discovered by American pathologist, John Howard Mueller, during his research on growth factors for microorganisms.

1921 The Westergren method for determining erythrocyte sedimentation rate (ESR) was devised by Swedish physician, Alf Wilhelm Westergren.

1921 The original nasogastric tubes were much improved by John Alfred Ryle, who covered the entire capsule tip with perforated rubber, thereby preventing damage to the gastric mucosa.

1921 *Grant Winder Liddle* born. An American endocrinologist who studied the adrenals, aldosterone, regulation of ACTH and MSH secretion, hormonal control, and corticosteroid therapy.

1921 The presence of antibodies in the blood of atopic or allergic individuals (Prausnitz–Küstner reaction) was shown by Otto Carl Willy Prausnitz, a British immunologist, and German gynecologist, Heinz Küstner.

1921 The first pericardiectomy was performed by Paul Hallopeau of Paris, France.

1921 *Sven Ivar Seldinger* born. An American radiologist who devised a modification of the percutaneous technique for arterial catheterization, which allowed the introduction of a catheter of larger diameter than the needle used for the initial puncture (Seldinger technique, 1953).

1921 The hydrogen carrier in cellular respiration, glutathione, was isolated by Frederick Gowland Hopkins of Cambridge University.

1921 Ergotamine was isolated from the fungus *Claviceps purpurea* by Karl Spiro and Arthur Stoll.

1921 *Amos Royston Robin Coombs* born. An English immunologist who devised the Coombs test for detecting red cell antibodies either on the red cell (direct), or in the serum (indirect) using rabbit anti-human globulin serum (Coombs serum).

1921 Necrosis of the epiphyses of the vertebrae leading to osteochondrosis in kyphosis (Scheuermann disease) was described by Danish radiologist from Copenhagen, Hoger Werfel Scheuermann.

1921 *Mahlon Bush Hoagland* born. A Boston biochemist who worked on cancer, liver regeneration and growth control, and confirmed Francis Crick's adaptor hypothesis.

1921 German-born pharmacologist, and physiologist, Otto Loewi of Strasburg discovered the first neurotransmitter, acetylcholine.

1921 *Arthur Beck Pardee* born. An American biochemist who (with Linus Pauling) worked on tumor metabolism and antibody reactions, and with Jacques Lucien Monod on the lac operon of *Escherichia coli*.

1921 Peutz–Jeghers syndrome, a familial disease due to an autosomal dominant trait manifesting as multiple polyps in the gastrointestinal tract associated with pigmentation of the mucosa and skin, was described by John Law Peutz of Holland.

1921 Costochondral junction syndrome, a painful swelling at the costochondral junction of the sternum, of unknown etiology, was described by Alexander Tietze, a surgeon from Breslau.

1921 A group of neurological cells within the central nervous system (oligodendroglia) was described and named by Spanish neurologist, Pio del Rio Hortega.

1921 Growth hormone was discovered by Herbert McLean Evans and Joseph Abraham Long.

1921 The first description of grasp reflex was given by Spanish neurologist, J.A.R. Barraquer of Barcelona.

1921 *Rosalyn Yalow née Sussman* born. An American biophysicist and Nobel laureate ((1977) who developed radioimmunoassay (RIA) for measuring minute amounts of biologically active substances, such as hormones and enzymes in blood.

1921 *Sir Michael Anthony Epstein* born. A professor of experimental pathology at the University of Bristol who discovered a new virus responsible for infectious mononucleosis (1964), the first found to be associated with cancer.

1921 Infantile acrodynia, consisting of agitation and muscular hypotonia of unknown etiology affecting infants (Pink disease) was described by Emil Feer of Erlangen.

1921 Iodized oil (lipiodol) was first used as a contrast medium in cerebral radiology by Jean A. Sicard.

1922 British biologist, Carl Hamilton Browning and R. Gulbransen discovered the phenomenon of therapeutic interference (drug interaction).

1922 The rickets preventing factor, vitamin D, was detected in cod liver oil by Elmer Verner McCollum at the Johns Hopkins Hospital in Baltimore.

1922 Sir Arthur Frederick Hertz of Guy's Hospital described a symptom complex occurring after gastroenterostomy (dumping syndrome).

1922

Robert Good (center right)

Robert Good born. A New York immunologist who showed the importance of the thymus in the immune system, advanced knowledge of the interaction between cellular and humoral immune responses, and wrote *Experiments of Nature*.

1922 *Roger Edward Collingwood Altounyan* born. A Syrian-born British physician who devised a method of delivery of drugs to the lungs via inhalation which became widely used as treatment for asthma (spinhaler).

Roger Altounyan

1922 *Stanley Cohen* born. An American neurologist and Nobel Prize winner (1986) who isolated nerve growth factor and epidermal growth factor.

1922 A rare condition with fever, chills, headache and vomiting (zincalism) was noted after a serious outbreak in Surrey, England

1922 Pioneer in the study of cancer, Sir John Bland Sutton published *Tumors, Innocent and Malignant*.

1922 Cavernous sinus syndrome, consisting of paralysis of the 3rd, 4th, 5th and 6th cranial nerves as a result of thrombosis of the cavernous sinus with involvement of its lateral wall, was described by Parisian neurologist, Charles Foix.

1922 *Hugh John Foster Cairns* born. A molecular biologist and virologist from Oxford University, England who pioneered study of the causes of cancer and demonstrated that it develops from a single cell by mutation of the DNA.

1922   Necrotic ulceration of the throat following the complete disappearance of polymorphonuclear cells in the blood (Schultz angina) was described by German physician, Werner Schultz of Berlin.

1922   Sphincteric fibers at the termination of the duodenum (Villemin sphincter) were described by French professor of anatomy at Bordeaux, Fernand Villemin.

1922   The Kahn test for diagnosis of syphilis was devised by Reuben Leon Khan, a bacteriologist at the University of Michigan School of Medicine.

1922   *Har Gobind Khorana* born. An Indian-born American biochemist and Nobel laureate (1968) who determined the sequence of nucleic acids in each of the 20 amino acids of the human body, and was one of the first to artificially synthesize a gene, from yeast and from *Escherichia coli*.

1922   The first documented outbreak of botulism occurred in Gairloch, Scotland.

1922   Erythrocytosis, caused by renal disease, was described by German physician, Felix Gaisbock.

1922   Insulin was isolated by Canadians, Frederick Banting and Charles Herbert Best, under the direction of John James Rickard Macleod.

1922   The delayed hypersensitivity reaction of the skin to horse dander was demonstrated on himself by R.A. Cooke.

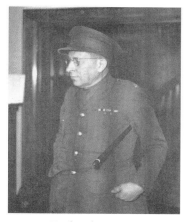

Frederick Banting

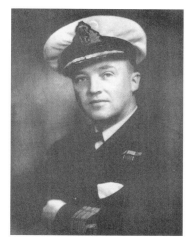

Charles Herbert Best

1922   One of the first journals in the United States devoted entirely to anesthesia, *Current Researches in Anesthesia and Analgesia* was founded by the physician, F. Hoeffer McMechan.

1922   Carcinogenicity of shale oil and lubricants was demonstrated by Archibald Leitch, director of the Cancer Hospital in London.

1923   Preparation of diphtheria toxin by treating with formalin was devised by Alexander Thomas Glenny and Barbara Hopkins.

1923   Thorvald Madsen began the first controlled trials on pertussis vaccine in the Faeroe Islands.

1923   The British Cancer Campaign was established by a surgeon at St Mark's Hospital, London, John Percy Lockhart-Mummery, with a donation from his patient Sir Richard Garton.

1923   The American Society of Regional Anesthesia was founded by Mauritius-born US professor of clinical surgery at New York University, Gaston Labat.

1923   The uncommon psychological disorder whereby the patient believes that familiar persons have been replaced by impostors (Capgras syndrome) was described by French psychologist, J.M.J. Capgras.

1923   A center in the upper part of the pons which rhythmically inhibits inspiration thereby allowing expiration, was described by English physician, Thomas William Lumsden.

1923   *D. Carleton Gajdusek* born. An American neurologist and Nobel Prize winner (1976) who worked on the causal agents in degenerative neurological disorders.

1923   The first valvotomy through a transventricular approach was performed by Elliot Carr Cutler of the Western Reserve University of Cleveland, Ohio.

Elliot Carr Cutler

1923   Frederick Grant Banting and John Mcleod won the Nobel Prize for Physiology or Medicine for the discovery of insulin.

1923   Acute tubular necrosis associated with myoglobinuria as a result of crush injury to soft tissues (Crush syndrome) was described by Seigo Minami of Tokyo.

1923   *Robert W. Goltz* born. An American dermatologist who described focal dermal hypoplasia syndrome, syndactyly and teeth abnormalities (Goltz syndrome).

1923   The fungus causing thrush, *Candida albicans*, was named by Christine Berkhout from the University of Delft.

1923   Amytal sodium was first synthesized.

1923   Surgical treatment for dislocation of the shoulder was performed by Arthur Sidney Blundell Bankart, a surgeon from Exeter, England.

1923 Andrew George Berkeley Moynihan of Leeds, England described chronic gastric ulcer as a precancerous state.

1923 Hemolytic streptococci were shown as the cause of scarlet fever by George Frederick Dick and his wife Gladys Rowena Dick of the Johns Hopkins School of Medicine.

1923 Genetic studies on sickle cell anemia were carried out by Clyde Graeme Guthrie and John Gardiner Huck of the Johns Hopkins Hospital, Baltimore.

1923 *Cardiotomy and Valvulotomy for Mitral Stenosis* was published in the Boston Medical and Surgical Journal by Elliott Carr Cutler of the Western Reserve University of Cleveland and Samuel Levine.

1923 Valuable work on hormones in ovulation was carried out by George Adelbert Doisy of St Louis who isolated the active principle of the ovarian hormone, estrogen.

1923 A form of bone atrophy, giving a spotted appearance to the distal bones on X-rays, accompanied by swelling and tenderness of the tissues overlying it (Sudeck atrophy) was described by Paul Sudeck, a surgical professor in Hamburg.

1923 Glucagon, a hormone in extract of pancreas which causes a rise in blood sugar, was discovered by John R. Murlin and C.P. Kimball at the University of Rochester.

1923 Sternal needle puncture for the study of bone marrow (bone marrow aspiration) was described by Carley Paul Seyfarth.

1923 *R. W. Senstaken* born. An American surgeon who designed an inflatable balloon for controlling hemorrhage from esophageal varices (Senstaken tube).

1923 The cardiac manifestations in systemic lupus erythematosus (SLE) were recognized by New York physician, Emanuel Libman, who published his findings with Benjamin Sacks (Libman–Sacks endocarditis).

1924 Heinrich Ewald Hering Jr described the branch of the glossopharyngeal nerve to the carotid sinus and its function.

1924 Classic papers on *The absorption, distribution and elimination of ether* were published by Howard Wilcox Haggard of Yale University.

1924 Systematic investigations of the pharmacological actions of the anti-asthmatic drug, ephedrine, were carried out by Chinese immunologist, Ko Kuei Shen.

1924 The whitish yellow spots sometimes seen in the iris of children with Down syndrome and occasionally in normal children (Brushfield spots) were described by London physician, Thomas Brushfield.

1924 Somatic antigens were first identified in cases of *Salmonella typhi* infection by Polish bacteriologist, Arthur Felix.

1924 H substance, similar to histamine and causing anaphylaxis symptom complex, was isolated by British cardiologist and physiologists, Sir Thomas Lewis and Ronald Thompson Grant.

1924 The fine particles of fat seen in the blood during the transport of fat (chylomicrons) were observed and named by Simon Henry Gage and Pierre August Fish of Washington, DC.

1924 The presence of amino acids in the urine and cystine crystals in the bone marrow of patients with cystinosis was demonstrated by Dutch pathologist, G.O.E. Lignac.

1924 The first description of the alpha rhythm in the electroencephalogram (Berger rhythm) was given by German neuropsychiatrist, Johannes Berger.

1924 Pulmonary embolectomy was successfully carried out by German surgeon from Heidelberg, Martin Kirschner.

1924 A contrast method in radiology with tetrabromophenolphthalein as an intravenous agent, to visualize the biliary tract (cholecystography), was invented by American surgeon, Evarts Ambrose Graham.

1924 Lymphadenopathy, leukemia and hypersplenism associated with rheumatoid arthritis (Felty syndrome), was described by American physician, Augustus Roi Felty of Johns Hopkins Hospital.

1924 *Sir James Whyte Black* born. An important figure in cardiovascular medicine who discovered prothenolol, the first betablocker which led to the development of propranolol.

1924 Three types of nerve fibers, A, B and C, were described by Nobel laureates, Joseph Erlanger and Herbert Spencer Gasser.

1924 Ephedrine was introduced into western medicine by C.F. Schmidt and K.K. Chen.

1924 Classical cesarean section, where the uterus is temporarily delivered from the abdomen and emptied, was revived by French gynecologist, Louis Portes.

1924 The bromosulphalein test for liver functions was introduced by American physician, Sanford Morris Rosenthal.

1924 A classic paper on ether, *The Absorption, Distribution and Elimination of Ether* was published by Howard Wilcox Haggard.

1925 The use of blood transfusion for treatment of shock due to burns was introduced by German physician, Gustav Riehl.

1925 *Entamoeba histolytica* was successfully grown in culture for long periods by William Charles Boeck and Jaraslav Drbohlav.

1925 Gordon Morgan Holmes provided the first record of surgical removal of an adrenocortical tumor, before that of English surgeon, Percy W.G. Sargent.

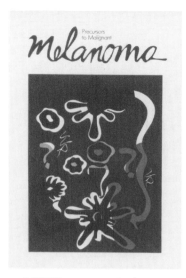

A WHO poster on Melanoma

1925 The causative organism of gonorrhea (*Neisseria gonorrhoeae*) was discovered by Albert Neisser, while he was a research assistant at Berlin Hospital.

1925 Visualization of the recesses of the anterior chamber of the eye, normally not seen with a slit lamp (gonioscopy), was devised by New York ophthalmologist, Manuel Uribe y Tronchoso.

1925 A specific test for venereal lymphogranuloma was devised by German dermatologist, Wilhelm S. Frei, which consists of an intradermal injection of antigen prepared from material containing the causative virus.

1925 An improved method of encephalography was developed by Leo Max Davidoff, a New York neurologist, with Cornelius D. Dyke.

1925 Surgical hernia following incision of the abdomen was studied by American surgeon Arthur Marriot Shipley, who described a method of closure.

1925 *Daniel Alagille* born. A French pediatrician who described multiple abnormalities associating neonatal cholestasis prolonged during childhood and adulthood, due to paucity of interlobular bile ducts (Alagille syndrome).

1925 The first successful treatment by surgical removal of parathyroid adenoma was performed by a Viennese surgeon, Felix Mandl.

1925 Cooley anemia (thalassemia major) a hereditary hemolytic anemia associated with bone changes in children, was described by American physician, Thomas Benton Cooley.

1925 An electric bone saw was constructed by New York surgeon, John Joseph Moorhead.

1925 A rare form of severe acute hemolytic anemia of unknown cause (Lederer anemia) associated with leucocytosis, enlarged spleen, reticulocytosis and pyrexia, was described by Max Lederer.

1925 Photomicrography was first applied to the study of bacteria and viruses in England by Joseph Edwin Barnard.

1925 The earliest cell line of white blood cells (myeloblasts) was observed and described by Charles Austin Doan and co-workers.

1925 *Robert Geoffrey Edwards* born. A British obstetrician and pioneer of in vitro fertilization who, in partnership with Patrick Steptoe, achieved the birth of the first 'test-tube baby'.

1925 Weber–Christian disease of non-suppurative nodular panniculitis associated with phagocytic ingestion of fat cells by macrophages was described by Frederick Parkes Weber from Temple University, Philadelphia.

1925 Bistovol (bismuth stovarsol) was prepared by C. Levadetti for treatment of syphilis.

1925 Diffuse thrombotic vascular lesions in arterioles and capillaries (thrombotic thrombocytopenic purpura) were described by American physician, Eli Moschcowitz.

1925 Relatively mild anemia due to a heterozygous thalassemia trait for a specific hemoglobinopathy (thalassemia minor) was described by F. Rietti.

1925 A new valvulotomy procedure was pioneered by London surgeon, Sir Henry Sessions Souttar, who introduced his fingers through the left atrium while splitting the mitral commissures.

1926 A report on the treatment of erysipelas with antistreptococci serum was given by American bacteriologist, Konrad E. Birkhaug.

1926 Oat cell carcinoma, a cancer of the mediastinum and hilum of the lung, so-called as the tumor consisted of small oval cells resembling oats, was described by London physician, William George Barnard.

1926 The grasp reflex in frontal lobe lesions was studied by P. Schuster and H. Pineas of Germany.

1926 The action of ergotamine on the uterus was studied by British pharmacologist, Sir John Henry Gaddum.

1926 *Aphasia and Kindred Disorders of Speech* was published by Sir Henry Head, a neurologist at the London Hospital and an expert in speech disorders.

1926 Selmar Ascheim and Bernhardt Zondek of Berlin found a substance in urine of pregnant women similar to gonadotropic hormone from the anterior pituitary, later named 'anterior pituitary-like hormone'.

1926 *David Hunter Hubel* born. A Canadian-born American neurophysiologist and Nobel laureate (1981) who studied cortical perception of visual stimulus.

1926 A variation of the fracture of the first metatarsal bone (Rolando fracture) was described by a surgeon from Milan, Silvio Rolando.

1926 Glaucosan for the relief of glaucoma was introduced by German ophthalmologist, Carl Hamburger.

1926 John Jacob Abel obtained the first crystalline form of insulin.

1926 Conservative treatment of sinusitis with irrigation was advised by Arthur Walter Proetz of St Louis.

1926 Aleksei Ivanovitch Abrikosov described Abrikosov tumor, a painless tumor occurring in the tongue, axilla and mandible (also known as granular cell myoblastoma).

1926 Yellow fever was shown to be a filterable virus by Max Theiler, a South African-born American.

1926 The concept of 'balanced anesthesia' was put forward by J.S. Lundy of the Mayo Clinic in Rochester.

1926 Adrenal insufficiency and hypothyroidism (Schmidt syndrome) was described by Martin Benno Schmidt of Germany.

1926 Cavernous sinus thrombophlebitis in relation to septicemia was described by American neurologist, Wells Phillips Eagleton.

1926 A pioneer of experimental carcinogenesis, Johannes Andreas Grib Fibiger from the University of Copenhagen, won the Nobel Prize for his discovery of the spiroptera carcinoma, and squamous cell carcinoma of the stomach (Fibiger tumor).

1926 An acute infection due to *Streptobacillus moniliformis* with fever, rash and polyarthritis (Haverhill fever) broke out in the Massachusetts township of the same name and was described by Edwin Hemphill Place, Otto Willner and L.E. Sutton.

1927 Gellhorn described infiltration of the perineum with anesthetic solutions to produce anesthesia during labor.

1927 Otto Butzengeiger of Germany discovered the anesthetic effects of Avertin.

1927 The onset of menstruation when estrogen stops acting on the epithelium was discovered by an American physician, Edgar V. Allen. A year later he isolated estrin.

1927 A description of similarities between skin vascular reactions to histamine (flare, local edema and vasodilatation) was given by British cardiologist, Thomas Lewis.

1927 An operation for extra-articular fusion of the sacroiliac joint was carried out by American orthopedic surgeon, Willis Cohoon Campbell.

1927 The Elman test, for quantitative analysis of serum amylase, was devised by American surgeon, Robert Elman.

1927 The first to observe the causative organism of lymphogranuloma venereum was Spanish dermatologist, José Antonio Gay-Prieto.

1927 Conclusive proof that the thyroid depended on the stimulating action of the anterior pituitary was given by Philip Edward Smith of California.

1927 The spectrophotometric method for determining hemoglobin in blood was developed by G.E. Davis and C. Sheard.

1927 South African physician A.C. Alport described hereditary hemorrhagic nephropathy associated with loss of vision and hearing (Alport syndrome).

1927 Viennese gynecologist, Walter Schiller, devised the Schiller test that visualizes suspected cancerous area of the uterine cervix after staining with iodine.

1927 Phosphocreatine, a substance in muscle contraction, was discovered independently by two groups of workers, Philip and Grace Eggleton of London, and Cyrus Hartwell Fiske and Yella-Pragada Subbarow of Boston.

1927 The first barbiturate routinely used for the induction of anesthesia, pernocton, was used in Germany by R. Bumm.

1927 The Speed operation, for recurrent anterior dislocation of the shoulder using a bone graft, was described by American surgeon, Kellog Speed.

1927 The Emmons method for determining cell diameter was devised by Canadian physician, Frank Williams Emmons.

1927 The first potent liver extract for oral administration in anemia was prepared by William Parry Murphy, George Richards and co-workers.

1927 German gynecologists, Selmar Aschheim and Bernhardt Zondek, found a marked development of the ovaries in animals while investigating the influence of the pituitary on sexual development, thus enabling them to diagnose early pregnancy.

1927 *Marshall Warren Nirenberg* born. A New York biochemist and Nobel laureate (1968) who worked out the sequence of amino acid codes needed to synthesize a protein.

1927 A modern clinical approach to congenital anatomical lesions of the heart was introduced by Maude Elizabeth Seymour Abbott of Canada in *Congenital Heart Diseases*.

1927 *Kenneth F. Fairley* born. An Australian physician from Melbourne who described a bladder washout test to determine the site of urinary infection (Fairley test).

1927 The use of needle puncture in hemopoietic diseases was popularized by Mikhail J. Arinkin of Germany.

1927 American scientist, Bret Ratner, carried out experiments on allergic sensitization in utero.

1927 Robert T. Frank and colleagues obtained the same potent hormone (follicle stimulating hormone) from the follicle, corpus luteum, placenta, and blood of pregnant women.

1927 Antonio Egaz Moniz from Portugal introduced radiological visualizization of cerebral circulation by injecting radio-opaque sodium iodide into the carotid artery (cerebral angiography).

1927 Leonard Stanley Dudgeon and C.V. Patrick carried out important cytological studies in detecting cancer of the cervix.

1927 A disorder of acute hemolytic anemia mostly in Mediterranean races following ingestion of the *Vicia faba* bean or the inhalation of its pollen was noted by L. Preti of Germany.

1927 Anterior wedge tarsectomy with triple fusion for drop foot (Lambrinudi operation) was described by an orthopedic surgeon at Guy's Hospital, Constantine Lambrinudi.

1928 Hypervitaminosis D, associated with metastatic calcification and renal calculi following high intake of irradiated ergosterol in experimental animals, was demonstrated independently by Pfannenstein, and Kreitmer.

1928 *James Dewey Watson* born. An American biologist from Chicago and Nobel laureate (1962) who discovered the structure of DNA in collaboration with Francis Harry Crick.

1928 Inhalation allergy to house dust was discovered by Dutch physician, Storm van Leeuwen.

1928 The specific hormone from the posterior lobe of the pituitary gland which causes contraction of the uterus (oxytocin) was isolated by American biochemist, Oliver Kamm and colleagues.

1928 A historical account of pulmonary cancer was given by R. Huguenin in *Cancer Primitif du Poumon*.

1928 W.H. Brown described the production of ectopic adrenocorticotropic hormone in a case of bronchial carcinoma.

1928 The ability of hemoglobin to combine reversibly with oxygen, thus enabling it to act as a transport agent of the gas from air to the tissues was shown by Joseph Barcroft of England, in his *The Respiratory Function of Blood*.

Barcroft gas manometer

1928 Irritable bowel syndrome, or spastic colon, was described by John Alfred Ryle, a physician at Guy's Hospital.

1928 The urea clearance test for renal functions was first devised by Paris physician, Leo Ambard, American

363

physician, Franklin Chambers McLean and San Francisco physician, Thomas Addis.

1928   Two cases of congenital absence of the vagina treated by plastic surgery (vaginal agenesis) were reported by American gynecologist, Carl Henry Davis of Milwaukee.

1928   Chicago physiologists, Andrew Conway Ivy and Erie Oldberg demonstrated that when acid is injected into the duodenum, a substance is released into the blood which causes the gallbladder to contract, later named 'cholecystokinin'.

1928   A local skin reaction to the filtrate of bacillus typhus culture (Schwartzmann phenomenon) was described by New York physician Gregory Schwartzmann.

1928   Clinical signs for diagnosis of congenital dislocation of the hip were described by George Perkins, professor of surgery from St Thomas' Hospital, in his *Signs by which to Diagnose Congenital Dislocation of Hip*.

1928   Male parthenogenesis was described by American zoologist and embryologist, Edmund Beecher Wilson.

1928   The role of the cervical smear in the diagnosis of cancer was described by American cytologists, George Nicholas Papanicolaou and Herbert Frederick Traut.

1928   The first series of infants suffering from hemorrhagic disease of the newborn was provided by R.S. Beveridge.

1928   *Daniel Nathans* born. An American microbiologist and Nobel laureate (1978) who pioneered the use of restriction enzymes to fragment DNA, and made the first genetic map of the SV40 viral DNA.

1928   *Norton David Zinder* born. An American geneticist who studied mutants of *Salmonella* and described bacterial transduction via a phage.

1928   John Parkinson and Evan Bradford described typical serial electrocardiographic changes of myocardial infarction.

1929   A single cannula technique for thoracoscopy was described by L.R. Davidson in New York.

1929   American microbiologist, Albert Bruce Sabin, devised a slide test for typing pneumococci.

1929   American physiologist, Arthur Grollmann, studied cardiac output in man using acetylene.

1929   Radium treatment for cancer was introduced into the UK.

1929   Jakob Erdheim, a physician in Vienna published a classic description of rupture of the aorta due to medionecrosis.

1929   Intravenous urography was introduced by German-born American urologist, Moses Swick.

1929   American physician, Cyrus Cressy Sturgis discovered the presence of an anti-pernicious anemia factor in the stomach, and advocated use of desiccated stomach as treatment.

1929   The National Radium Trust and the National Radium Commission were established in the UK through a Royal Charter.

1929   Mexican army surgeon, Miguel Garcia Marin, was the first to use intravenous ethyl alcohol for anesthesia.

1929   The suggestion that neurosis is a defect or failure in adjustment to the social environment and arises as a failure to defend the ego, was made by Viennese psychologist, Alfred Adler.

1929   A device to assist respiration by placing the patient in a chamber where alternate compression and decompression occur (iron lung) was invented by Philip Drinker of Harvard University.

1929   The association between achylia gastrica and pernicious anemia was described by American physician, William Bosworth Castle of Cambridge, Massachusetts who also used intravenous liver extract.

1929   A calorimetric method for estimating serum proteins was devised by Californian biochemist, David Morris Greenberg.

1929   Hematemesis due to post-emetic mucosal laceration of the lower end of the esophagus and gastric cardia was recognized by Boston pathologists, Kenneth G. Mallory and Konrad Weiss.

1929   Asthma, caused by the bites of bedbugs, was described by Sternberg in the *Journal of Allergy*.

1929   Evarts Ambrose Graham, professor of surgery at Washington University, St Louis, and Warren Henry Cole, made gallbladder visualization possible using chlorinated and brominated phenolphthalein.

1929   Nail–Patella syndrome, a hereditary disease due to a dominant trait, was described by K. Osterreicher of Germany.

1929   Percy William Leopold Camp used epinephrine in the form of an inhaler for asthma.

1929   Von Gierke disease, caused by an inborn error of glycogen storage and accompanied by hepatomegaly, was described in two children by Edgar Otto von Gierke of Germany.

1929   The association between polyuria of diabetes insipidus and the action of the posterior pituitary extract were noted by British pharmacologist, Ernest Basil Verney.

1929   The first photoelectric hemoglobinometer was made by C. Sheard and Arthur H. Sanford.

1929   *Gerald Maurice Edelman* born. A New York biochemist and Nobel laureate (1972) who studied and sequenced antibodies, postulated a three-dimensional structure and subunits, and described the immunoglobulin antibody.

1929 Detailed descriptions of the capillary basement membrane were given by Canadian physician, Leone McGregor.

1929 Reaction of a single motor neuron following its activation by a stimulus was demonstrated by Derek Denny-Brown, a New Zealand-born neurologist at Oxford.

1929 *Sir Roger G. Bannister* born. A British neurologist and athlete who studied the physiology of exercise, and edited *Brain's Clinical Neurology* until the late 1960s.

1929 Insulin shock treatment was used as treatment for schizophrenia by French physician, Manfred Joshua Sakel.

1929 Pyrexia was induced by means of a cabinet heated with electric light by W. Kahler and F. Knollmeyer.

1929 The ability of the vertebrate kidney to secrete foreign substances was demonstrated by Eli Kinnerly Marshall, an American pharmacologist from the Johns Hopkins Hospital.

1929 The process of loss of a segment of a chromosome (deletion) was described by American geneticist, Theophilus Shickle Painter and Joseph Hermann Muller.

1929 The antibacterial action of *Penicillium* mold was discovered by Sir Alexander Fleming while working at St Mary's Hospital, London.

1929 Danish biochemist, Carl Peter Henrik Dam, discovered anti-hemorrhagic factor (vitamin K) for which he shared the Nobel Prize for Medicine or Physiology with Edward Adelbert Doisy in 1943.

1929 Necrobiosis lipoidica diabeticorum, a degenerative disease of the skin in diabetes, was reported by Austrian dermatologist, Maurice Oppenheim.

1929 Morquio syndrome, an autosomal recessive disease leading to dwarfism, waddle gait and deafness, but not mental retardation, was described by Uruguayan pediatrician from Montevideo, Luis Morquio.

1929 Split skin grafts were introduced by plastic surgeon, Vitray Papin Blair.

1930 Electrocardiographic changes of Wolff–Parkinson–White syndrome were described by Paul Dudley White of Massachusetts General Hospital.

1930 The classification of nephritis, based on the hemorrhagic nature and nephrosclerosis, was proposed by American biochemist, Donald Dexter van Slyke and colleagues.

1930 The Lübeck disaster took the lives of a large number of children in Germany when BCG vaccination for tuberculosis was contaminated.

1930 The contractile effect of fresh semen on uterine muscle in vitro was demonstrated by two New York gynecologists, Raphael Kurzrok and Charles Lieb.

1930   Osteomalacia caused by vitamin D deficiency was described by English physician in China, John Preston Maxwell.

1930   Pseudo fractures seen on X-rays in osteomalacia (Milkman fractures) were described by American radiologist, Louis Arthur Milkman of Pennsylvania.

1930   The red cell index, mean corpuscular hemoglobin concentration (MCHC), and mean corpuscular volume (MCV), was proposed by American hematologist, Maxwell Myer Wintrobe.

1930   German dermatologist, Karl Theodore Fahr, described intracerebral calcification of the small vessels of the deep cortex and lenticular and dentate nuclei (Fahr disease).

1930   The first active cortical extract from the renal glands (corticosteroid) was prepared by Wilber Willis Swingle and Joseph John Pfiffner.

1930   The method of aspiration biopsy, for diagnosis of malignant infiltration of bone marrow, was used by H.E. Martin and E.B. Ellis.

1930   B. Shapiro of Germany started treating undescended testis (cryptorchidism) with an anterior pituitary-like substance isolated from the urine of pregnant women.

1930   The antithyroid properties of thiourea were identified by Julia and Cosmo Mackenzie of the Johns Hopkins Hospital, Baltimore while experimenting with products to induce intestinal suppression of bacterial flora.

1930   Vascular compression as a cause of trigeminal neuralgia was suggested by Baltimore neurosurgeon, Walter Edward Dandy, who performed partial resection of the sensory root of the trigeminal ganglion.

1930   Radiotherapy was added to surgery in the treatment of certain cancers.

1930   Bacille Calmette–Guérin vaccination (BCG) was introduced in France and Norway.

1930   An epidemic febrile infectious disease on the Danish island of Bornholm was described by Ejner Oluf Sylvest Sorenson as Bornholm disease.

1930   The forerunner of modern intrauterine device (IUD) was devised by a German gynecologist, Ernst Grafenberg.

1930   Estriol was obtained from urine by Guy Frederick Marrian of University College.

1930   Nobel laureate, Arne Wilhelm Tiselius of Stockholm, developed electrophoresis.

1930   The term arrhenoblastoma for an ovarian tumor was proposed by Robert Meyer of Berlin to denote the group of similar masculinizing tumors.

1930   A congenital variant of Oppenheim disease, consisting of kyphoscoliosis, contractures of the large joints and immobility of proximal joints with hypermobility of distant joints (Ullrich syndrome) was described by Otto Ullrich.

1930 The American Board of Obstetrics and Gynecology was established.

1930 The rickettsial cause of scrub typhus was demonstrated by M. Nagayo and colleagues, and they renamed it *Rickettsia orientalis*.

1930 H.B. Anderson reported the first case of hypoglycemia in a patient with an adrenal tumor.

1930 C.C. Wolferth described the 4th heart sound or atrial sound due to resistance to ventricular filling.

1930 Christian Heymans and coworkers located the peripheral chemoreceptors in the carotid and aortic bodies.

1930 Amniography was introduced by Thomas Orville Menees of Michigan.

1930 American biochemist, Harriet Isabel Edgeworth published a paper on the beneficial effects of ephedrine in myasthenia gravis.

1931 Rudolf Nissen in Basel did the first successful removal of a complete lung, followed by Cameron Haight at Ann Arbor in 1932.

1931 H. Schneider gave the first report of tick-borne encephalitis in Neunkirchen, Lower Austria.

1931 J.P. Peters and Donald Dexter van Slyke developed logarithmic dissociation curves for carbon dioxide in blood.

1931 J.H. Burn suggested a method for estimation of antidiuretic potency of posterior pituitary extract.

1931 Evarts Graham of Washington University School of Medicine, St Louis founded the *Journal of Thoracic Surgery*.

1931 J.A. Aeschlimann and M. Reinert synthesized an anticholinesterase and its antagonist, the depolarizing muscle relaxant, neostigmine.

1931 The chemical structure and function of vitamin A was established by Russian-born Swiss chemist and Nobel Prize winner, Paul Karrer.

1931 Maurice A. Cassidy suggested that abdominal carcinomatosis may be associated with the direct release of hormones.

1931 The term premenstrual tension was first used by New York gynecologist, R.T. Frank.

1931 Post-streptococcal arthritis following tonsillitis was noted as being due to an allergy to bacterial products rather than bacterial toxins, by Frederick John Poynton.

1931 *Hamilton Orthaniel Smith* born. An American molecular biologist and Nobel laureate (1978) who discovered endonucleases in bacteria that can split DNA of invading phage particles and inactivate them.

1931 American pathologist, M.M. Canavan, observed a form of familial degenerative disease of the white matter of the central nervous system in Jewish families (Canavan disease).

1931 Pale hypertension together with red hypertension, were noted by German physician, Franz von Volhard, a professor of Halle and Frankfurt.

1931 Shortwave diathermy was introduced by Erloin Schlieshake.

1931 Arthur Maurice Fishberg of Mount Sinai Hospital, New York classified nephritis into various forms, including focal glomerular nephritis and acute interstitial nephritis.

1931 Extradural anesthesia was introduced to obstetrics by Italian obstetrician from Milan, Achile Mario Dogliotti, who later founded the Italian Society of Anesthetics.

1931 *Jacques Francis Miller* born. A French–Australian immunologist who worked on leukemia in mice and found that the thymus gland is an important control in the immune system.

1931 A nail used for fixing fractures of the neck of the femur (Smith-Peterson nail) was designed by a Boston orthopedic surgeon, Marius Nygaard Smith-Petersen and colleagues.

1931 A catheter was injected into a living heart by Werner Forssman of Germany, who also performed the first angiography.

1931 Copper sulfate solution in the detection of sugar in blood and urine

(Benedict solution) was devised by Stanley Rossiter Benedict.

1931 A procedure for direct visualization of the spinal canal through lumbar puncture (myeloscopy) was pioneered by M.D. Burman of America.

1932 The first studies on the effect of unilateral lobectomy were performed independently by Canadian neurosurgeon, Wilder Graves Penfield, and J. Evans, W.C. German and J.C. Fox.

1932 H. Mauss and F. Mietzsch of Germany produced the acridine derivative, atebrine, or mepacrine.

1932 A rare disease due to excessive deposition of glycogen in all tissues (Pompe disease) was described by Dutch pathologist, Joannus C. Pompe.

1932 Crystals of the muscle protein, myoglobin, were isolated by Swedish biochemist, Axel Hugo Teodor Theorell, director of the Nobel Institute of Biochemistry in Stockholm.

1932 A crystalline form of the alimentary enzyme, trypsin, was obtained by American biochemist, John Howard Northrop of New York.

1932 Extra-articular bone-graft arthrodesis of the hip joint was developed by an Australian orthopedic surgeon, Hugh Compson Trumble.

1932 The term 'esophagitis' was first used in relation to pathology in the esophagus of patients with brain lesions by the American neurosurgeon, Harvey Williams Cushing.

1932 Cesare Gianturco, a radiologist from the Mayo Clinic in Rochester, Minnesota pioneered use of cinematography in the study of the gastrointestinal tract, with Walter Clements Alvarez.

1932 The Paul–Bunnel test for heterophilic antibodies was devised by American epidemiologist, John Rodman Paul and a physician from New Haven, Wallis Willard Bunnel.

1932 A classification for rectal carcinoma was proposed by London pathologist, Cuthbert Dukes (Dukes classification).

1932 A method of artificial respiration as first aid was described by Frank Cecil Eve of Hull, England.

1932 In his article Acute symptoms following work with hay in the *British Medical Journal*, J.M. Campbell described five cases of farmer's lung in Cumbria.

1932 Positive pressure arthrodesis as treatment for tuberculosis of the knee joint was introduced by John Albert Key, an orthopedic surgeon at Harvard University.

1932 The discovery that carcinoma of the breast can be produced in animals by estrone benzoate was made by French physician, Antoine Marcellin Lacassagne.

1932 A skin test to determine the presence of antibody in pneumococcal pneumonia (Francis test) was developed by an American pathologist, Thomas Francis.

1932 *Peter Vogt* born. A German-born American microbiologist from the University of Southern California who discovered oncogenes.

1932 Superior sulcus tumor of the apex of the lung, causing pressure on the chest wall, intercostal nerves and brachial plexus (Pancoast tumor) was described by American radiologist, Henry Khunrath Pancoast of Philadelphia.

1932 The study of nerve transmission was refined by Lord Edgar Douglas Adrian and New York neurophysiologist, Detlef Wulf Bronk.

1932 The term 'microangiopathic hemolytic anemia' was coined by William St Claire Symmers to denote the mechanical damage to red blood cells resulting in poikilocytosis or abnormally shaped red cells.

1932 Solomon Albert Hymen of the Beth David Hospital in New York gave a description of an artificial pacemaker in his experiments on the cardiac resuscitation of animals.

1932 Scottish neurosurgeon, Norman McOrmish Dott, performed the first planned operation for an intracranial aneurysm.

1932 Hexabarbitone was introduced as an intravenous anesthetic by Walther Scharpff and Helmut Weese.

1932 Pigmentation of the upper eyelid exophthalmic thyrotoxicosis (Jellinek sign) was described by Viennese physician, Stefan Jellinek.

1932 A comprehensive work on reflexes, *Reflex Activity of the Spinal Cord* was published by Sir Charles Scott Sherrington, an English professor of physiology.

1932 M. Holtzmann explained that the short PR interval and delta wave found in the ECG in Wolff–Parkinson–White syndrome, was due to preexcitation of the ventricle through an accessory or aberrant pathway.

1932 A measure of renal function (xylose excretion test) was devised by Ella S. Fishberg and Friedland.

1932 Regional ileitis (Crohn disease) was described by an American physician, Burril Bernard Crohn and colleagues.

1932 A method of arresting the longitudinal growth of bone by destroying the growth-plate at the growing end of the bone was reported, probably the first great advancement in the equalization of leg length.

1932 Sir Geoffrey Langdon Keynes introduced radium as a treatment for breast cancer.

1932 Nerve grafting for facial palsy was introduced by English neurosurgeon, Sir Charles Alfred Ballance.

1932 A demonstration of antigen-induced release of histamine from sensitized perfused guinea pig lung was published.

1932 A.R. Moritz, C.L. Hudson and E.S. Orgain demonstrated anastomotic channels between coronary circulation and adjacent tissues. They injected carbon particles into the coronary circulation and histologically demonstrated their appearance at the base of the heart.

1932 E. Bruusgaard provided the first proof that varicella was caused by contact with herpes zoster virus. He took vesicular fluid from herpes zoster patients to inoculate children who then developed varicella.

1932 Dutch physicians, Ernst Lacquer, E. Dingemanse and S.E. Jongh observed estrogenic activity in male urine.

1932 German physician, Carl Kaufmann used estrogenic hormones in treatment of amenorrhea.

1932 American physician, Carl Albert Dragstedt, demonstrated the release of histamine in anaphylactic reactions.

1933 D.R. Hooper of Johns Hopkins Hospital designed the first cardiac defibrillator with padded electrodes.

1933 Canadian biochemist, John Symonds Lyon Browne isolated estriol from placental tissue.

1933 L. Vajda of Germany suggested induction of artificial pneumoperitoneum as a form of collapse therapy in tuberculosis.

1933 Liverpool anesthetist, R.J. Minnitt developed the Minnitt apparatus for administering equal parts of nitrous oxide and air for obstetric anesthesia. It was approved for use by midwives in 1936.

1933 Boston surgeon, Robert Henry Aldrich used gentian violet for burns.

1933 Leo Eloesser of San Francisco performed the first bilateral lobectomy for bronchiectasis.

1933 The causative virus of St Louis encephalitis was isolated by a St Louis physicians, R.N. Mackenfuss, Charles Armstrong and Howard M. McCordock.

1933 John G.P. Cleland of Oregon provided a classic description of sensory innervation of the birth canal in relation to paravertebral and caudal block in obstetric anesthesia. His work formed the basis for regional obstetric anesthesia.

1933 Grantley Dick Read advocated correct mental attitude towards pregnancy and childbirth in his book *Natural Childbirth*. He published *Childbirth Without Fear* in 1944.

1933 M.W. Goldblatt described the presence of vasodepressor and smooth muscle stimulating factors, later named 'prostaglandins'.

Grantley Dick Read

1933 The International Union Against Cancer was inaugurated at the Cancer Congress at Madrid.

1933 The first work on experimental embryology and genetics in English was published by Nobel laureate and professor of physiology at Caltech, Thomas Hunt Morgan.

1933 Parrot-beaked nose, hypertelorism, cleft palate and congenital heart defects (Waardenburg syndrome) were described by Swiss ophthalmologist, Alfred Vogt and Dutch physician, Petrus Johannes Waardenburg.

1933 By anastomozing the heart to the vessels in the recipient animal's neck, Frank Charles Mann transplanted heterotrophic mammalian hearts.

1933 The first recorded case of a total removal of the entire lung for carcinoma of the bronchus was reported by American surgeon, Evarts Ambrose Graham.

1933   Richard Phillip Custer developed and promoted bone marrow aspiration as a diagnostic procedure.

1933   *Sir David John Weatherall* born. An English molecular geneticist who studied thalassemias and whose work greatly improved the clinical outcome and prediction.

1933   Pneumonectomy in a tuberculous patient for sarcoma of the lung was first performed by American surgeon, Howard Lilienthal.

1933   Dihydrotachysterol (AT10), obtained by ultraviolet irradiation of ergosterol, was introduced as treatment for rickets by Friedrich Holtz.

1933   Lumbar sympathectomy was first performed through an anterolateral extraperitoneal approach by René Leriche of Paris.

1933   William Dock of Brooklyn, New York, explained the first heart sound.

1933   K. David, E. Emanse, F. Freud and E. Laqueur isolated testosterone from the testicular tissue.

1933   A technique for recording internal body images at a predetermined plane using X-rays (tomography) was described by German physician, D.L. Bartelink.

1933   Norman Urquhart Meldrum and Francis John Worsley Roughton isolated carbonic anhydrase from tissues.

1933   A fibrinolytic substance from group A beta-hemolytic streptococcus was isolated by Baltimore physician, William Smith Tillet and R.L. Garner.

1933   Fetal hemoglobin was shown to be different from adult hemoglobin by Joseph Barcroft.

1933   The American Academy of Orthopedic Surgeons was founded.

1933   Greenfield disease, a fatal familial condition characterized by progressive loss of motor power with seizures, blindness, nystagmus and mental deterioration in children was described by London neuropathologist, Joseph Goodwin Greenfield.

1933   *Richard L. O'Connor* born. An American orthopedic surgeon who developed arthroscopy of the knee, and developed instruments for meniscectomy.

1933   Ascorbic acid (vitamin C) was synthesized by Polish chemist Tadeus Reichstein.

1933   Hyperinsulinism, a condition of abnormally low blood sugar with symptoms similar to insulin reaction in non-diabetic patients, was described by Seele Harris of America.

1933   A congenital hemorrhagic disease characterized by epistaxis and bleeding from the gastrointestinal tract with normal platelets (von Willebrand disease) was described by Finnish physician, Erik A. von Willebrand.

1933 A classification of pathogenic hemolytic streptococci based on serology and pathogenicity (Lancefield group) was proposed by a bacteriologist from the Rockefeller Institute in New York, Rebecca Craighill Lancefield.

1933 Derek Denny-Brown and Robertson designed a catheter, manometer and a moving strip of bromide paper to measure and record bladder and sphincter behavior.

1933 Additional features of oral, parotid and skin changes in Sjögren syndrome (keratoconjunctivitis sicca and xerostomia, enlarged parotid gland with polyarthritis) were noted by Henrik S.C. Sjögren, a Scandinavian neurologist.

1933 William Evans of the National Heart Hospital in London classified different types of stenosis and atresia of the aortic arch.

1934 *Bengt Ingemar Samuelsson* born. A Swedish biochemist who detailed the biochemical pathways of prostaglandins, discovered thromboxanes and showed how leukotrienes are slow reacting substances with a role in anaphylaxis in allergic diseases.

1934 The replacement of lateral ligaments with artificial ligaments in cases of knee injury was performed by Frederick Jay Cotton, a surgeon at Newport, Rhode Island.

1934 A closed-circuit method for cyclopropane anesthesia was devised by American anesthetists, Ralph Milton Waters and Erwin Rudolph Schmidt.

1934 A quantitative method of estimating urinary sediments was devised by San Francisco physician, Henry Gibbons.

1934 The virus of lymphogranuloma inguinale was cultivated by American microbiologist, Joseph T. Tamura, who experimented with its use in therapeutic inoculation.

1934 Iliac lymphadenectomy combined with irradiation in cases of cancer of the cervix (Taussig operation) was described by American gynecologist, Frederick Joseph Taussig.

1934 Phenylbutazone, an inherited biochemical disorder, was observed by Norwegian biochemist, Ivar Asbjorn Følling, who believed the cause of mental retardation was an inherited error of metabolism.

1934 *John A. Carney* born. An Irish pharmacist and physician who described gastric epithelioid leimyosarcoma, pulmonary chondroma and functioning extra-adrenal paragangliomas (Carney triad).

1934 The Griswold splint, formerly used for major fractures of tibia and fibula, was devised by American surgeon, Retig Arnold Griswold.

1934 American biochemist, Joseph Hyram Roe, devised a colorimetric test for fructose in urine and blood (fructosuria).

1934 American bacteriologists Albert Bruce Sabin and Arthur M. Wright isolated the herpes simiae virus (B virus) from the brain of a lab worker who died after being bitten by an infected monkey.

1934 Partial resection of the sensory root of the trigeminal ganglion as treatment of trigeminal neuralgia, was performed by Walter Edward Dandy, an American neurosurgeon from Johns Hopkins Hospital.

1934 A woman suffering from rheumatoid arthritis was shown to have a lessening of symptoms when pregnant by American biochemist, Edward Calvin Kendall, which led him to isolate hormones from the adrenal glands.

1934 Congenital metaphyseal dysostosis, consisting of mental retardation, dwarfism and metaphyseal widening of all the bones (Jansen syndrome) was described by Dutch orthopedic surgeon, Murk Jansen.

1934 The first clinical use of cyclopropane (trimethylene) in general anesthesia was by Alan Joan Styles.

1934 The reserve blood capacity of the inner organs was estimated by Joseph Barcroft as: liver 20%, spleen 16%, and skin 10%.

1934 The first X-ray diffraction photograph of pepsin was made by Irish crystallographer, John Desmond Bernal.

1934 Fracture of the radius accompanied by dislocation of the radioulnar joint (Galleazi fracture or dislocation) was described by orthopedic surgeon from Milan, Ricardo Galleazi.

1934 Inflammation of the temporal and other cranial arteries (temporal arteritis) was described by American physicians, Bayard Taylor Horton, T.B. Magath and George Elgie Broen.

1934 Ovarian tumor associated with ascites and pleural effusion (Meigs syndrome) was described by American professor of gynecology, Joseph Vincent Meigs.

1934 An external splint for the repair of fractured long bones (the Anderson splint) was created by American orthopedic surgeon Roger Anderson.

1934 The fragility of spherical red cells in hypotonic solution was studied in detail by Kansas physician, Russel Landram Haden.

1934 The production of renal hypertension by clamping the renal artery was shown by Harry Goldblatt, an American experimental pathologist, with J. Lynch and R. F. Hanzal.

1934 A microscopic study of coronary artery lesions was made by Timothy Leary of America, who concluded that the pathogenesis of the atherosclerotic lesions was related to disturbance of lipid metabolism.

1934 A generic classification of dermatophytes was proposed by American mycologist, Wilson Chester Emmons.

1934   Experimental transmission of the virus of Japanese encephalitis was shown by Hayashi.

1934   Gurvich and Yuniev at the Institute of Resuscitation in Moscow used direct current for external cardiac defibrillation.

1934   American physician Alvan Leroy Barach used helium for respiratory disease.

1934   Arthur E. Guedel of Cambridge City, Indiana introduced controlled respiration using ether for anesthesia.

1934   Rene Leriche and R. Fontaine used stellate ganglion block, or cervico-sympathetic thoracic block.

1934   A.F. Guedel, D.M. Treweek and M. Ralph Waters introduced controlled respiration in anesthesia and coined the term 'controlled respiration' in 1936.

1934   P. Frenckner introduced the spiropulsator, a prototype artificial positive pressure ventilator.

1935   Archibald introduced bronchial blockage with the use of a balloon for the control of secretions during pulmonary lobectomy.

1935   Tudor Edwards of the Brompton Hospital, London performed the first successful one-stage pneumonectomy for bronchiectasis, in Britain.

1935   M. Burger and W. Brandt discovered the humoral hyperglycemic action of glucagon.

1935   London physician, Hugh Leslie Marriot introduced continuous slow-drip flow blood transfusion.

1935   Mandelic acid was used in the treatment of urinary tract infections by Max Leonhard Rosenheim.

1935   Cecil, Nichols and Stainby discovered that blood from patients with rheumatoid arthritis caused bacteria to clump together, due to certain substances known as rheumatoid factors.

1935   Protonsil, the first antibacterial substance to give protection against streptococcal infection, was developed by German biochemist, Gerhard Domagk.

1935   An intradermal diagnostic skin test for sarcoidosis, using a saline suspension of sarcoid tissue (Kveim test), was devised by R.H Williams and D.A. Nickelson and was comprehensively described by Norwegian pathologist, Morten Ansgar Kveim in 1941.

1935   Claude Schaeffer Beck of America attempted to bypass diseased coronary arteries by implanting pectoral muscles onto the pericardium.

1935   The limitation of abduction in congenital dislocation of the hip was described by Charles Culloden Chapple (Chapple sign).

1935   Apicolysis, a method of collapsing the affected apical lobe of the lung by removal of the adjacent bony structure of the chest wall, was originally suggested by Carl Boye Semb of Scandinavia.

1935   *Surgical Diseases of the Chest* was written by American surgeon, Evarts Ambrose Graham.

1935   The Quick test to measure blood clotting time and monitor anti-coagulants, detect severe liver disease and vitamin K deficiency was devised by Armand James Quick and colleagues.

1935   The National Foundation for Infantile Paralysis, the first center in the world for research into polio, was established in America.

1935   The use of radioisotopes in the study of living tissues was initiated by a Hungarian-born professor of chemistry at Stockholm, Georg Charles von Hevesy.

1935   Threonine was isolated from hydrolysates of fibrin by William Cumming, an American biochemist.

1935   Hypophosphatasia, a hereditary disorder resembling rickets, was described by Chown of Winnipeg.

1935   C.H.J. Wrigley and Leonard Stanley Dudgeon pioneered work on sputum analysis of malignant cells for diagnosis.

1935   A laparoscope with a wide angle lens was used to perform liver biopsies by its inventor, H. Kalk.

1935   G.F. Cawhill discovered the radiological visualization of adrenal tumors by introducing air around the perinephric area.

1935   American cardiovascular surgeon, John Heysham Gibbon, and his wife, built a prototype heart–lung machine.

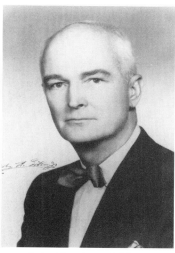

John Heysham Gibbon

1935   Synaptic transmission was suggested to be an electrical phenomenon rather than a chemical mechanism by Sir Carew Eccles, an Australian neurophysiologist.

1935   A maneuver for breech delivery that permitted spontaneous delivery of the baby, Bracht maneuver,

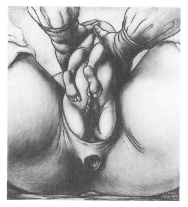

The Bracht maneuver

was designed by Berlin gynecologist and pathologist, Erich Franz Eugen Bracht.

1935 Stein–Leventhal syndrome, bilateral polycystic ovaries, was described by two American gynecologists, Irving Freiler Stein and Michael Leo Leventhal.

1936 *The Specificity of Serological Reactions*, the first large-scale study of chemical specificity in immunology, was published by Austrian-born American pathologist, Karl Landsteiner.

1936 A method for the localization of brain tumors with electroencephalography was developed by English physiologist, William Grey Walter.

1936 Atypical lymphocytes seen in infectious mononucleosis (Downy cells) were described by American hematologist, Hal Downy of Minneapolis.

1936 Micronodular lesions in the glomeruli of the kidney in diabetic nephropathy were described by Paul Kimmelsteil and Clifford Wilson.

1936 In studies on the treatment of pain relief British neurologist, W. Ritchie Russell, used intraspinal alcohol injections in cases of terminal cancer.

1936 A condition where younger red blood cells and nucleated forms are found in the peripheral blood, with a shift of erythopoiesis to the left (leuco-erythroblastic anemia) was described by Janet M. Vaughan of England.

1936 DNA in a pure state was obtained by Andrei Nikolaevitch Belozersky.

1936 A prototype for an artificial heart was developed by American biologist, Alexis Carrel and A. Lindbergh.

1936 Fat embolism due to fractured bones or as a result of orthopedic operations was observed by H.L. Davis and C.G. Goodchild.

1936 Cortisone was isolated independently by Nobel laureates, Tadeus Reichstein, Edward Calvin Kendall and Oskar Paul Wintersteiner.

1936 Peculiar spherical masses in the central portion of glomerular globules (Kimmelsteil–Wilson lesion) were described in eight patients with diabetes by German-American pathologist, Paul Kimmelsteil.

1936 The lymphatic spread of carcinoma of the prostate to the bones (Warren theory) was proposed by American physician, Shields Warren.

1936 G.H. Monrad-Krohn recognized the role of flicker mechanisms in precipitating epileptic fits, which led to a significant reduction in their numbers.

1936 William Bennett Kouwenhoven, an American professor of engineering, constructed a practical electrical defibrillator to treat the irregularity of the heart.

1936   The first blood banks were established in Moscow.

1936   J.A. Bargen and coworkers described autonomic diabetic neuropathy causing diarrhea.

1936   Alfred Blalock at Baltimore performed the first successful thymectomy for myasthenia gravis.

1936   W.R. Jordan first described neuropathic arthropathy, or Charcot joints, as a complication of diabetes.

1936   Swedish physician, Per Johannes Hedenius introduced use of heparin in blood transfusion.

1936   L. O'Shaughnessy of London introduced myocardial revascularization using omental grafts.

1936   F. Skorpil. E.R. Griffith made the first diagnosis and did the first surgical treatment for bronchiolo-alveolar carcinoma, and treated a second patient in 1943.

1936   Foundation of the American Society of Anesthesiologists.

1936   American physician, Clarence Elmer Sanders, devised a seesaw-bed for cardiovascular disease.

1937   French scientists, G. Unger and J.L. Parrot described the first antihistamine (933 F).

1937   P. Ayre described a new method (Ayre method) of endotracheal intubation and anesthesia in children, without valves and rubber

bags, for the circuit to be opened to the outside air.

1937   Rudolf Nissen did the first successful transpleural resection of esophageal carcinoma.

1937   H. Adler of Berlin showed the production of anti-acetyl choline substances by the thymus in myasthenic patients.

1937   Augustin Castelanos of Havana produced the first angiographic films of diagnostic quality in pulmonary stenosis and ventricular septal defect.

1937   Anatol Smorodinsev and colleagues in the Soviet Union produced the first human influenza virus vaccine.

1937   R.P. Martinova of the Soviet Union established the definite role of hereditary factors in predisposition to cancer of breast in women.

1937   British geneticist, Peter Alfred Gorer, discovered that the strongest histocompatibility locus, H-2, was responsible for the formation of blood cell antigens.

1937   John Streider of Boston made the first attempt at surgical correction of patent ductus arteriosus. His patient died of gastric dilatation a few days later.

1937   Magnetic resonance imaging (MRI) was developed to study atomic nuclei by Austrian–American physicist, Isidor Rabi and German–American physician, Polykarp Kusch.

1937 A contrast medium was first injected directly into the renal arteries by a Spanish physician, Reynaldo Dos Santos.

1937 An operation for resection of the duodenum and the head of the pancreas for carcinoma (duodeno-pancreatectomy) was introduced by American surgeon, Alexander Brunschwig.

1937 Q fever, named 'Q' to denote query as the causative agent was unknown, was observed by Edward Holbrook Derrick in Australia, after an outbreak of febrile illness amongst meat and cattle workers in Brisbane.

1937 Soviet scientist Vladimir P. Demikhov implanted the first artificial heart into an animal.

1937 The modern scientific explanation for fibrinolysis was given by Robert Gwyn Macfarlane.

1937 Electrically induced convulsions were given to mental patients by Lucio Bini and Ugo Cereletti in Italy.

1937 Research on drugs to combat urticaria, pruritis, hay fever and rhinitis began in France at the Pasteur Institute.

1937 Total pituitary failure as a result of post partum hemorrhage (Sheehan syndrome) was described by an English physician, Harold Leeming Sheehan.

1937 Claude Russel Brock described atelectasis and chronic pneumonitis of the middle lobe due to compression of the middle lobe bronchus (Brock syndrome).

1937 An extract of Bulgarian belladonna (deadly nightshade) was introduced as a treatment for post-encephalitic parkinsonism in England by F.J. Newahl and C.C. Fenwick.

1937 A disorder characterized by thrombocytopenic purpura and susceptibility to staphylococcal infection due to antibody deficiency (Wiskott–Aldrich syndrome), was described by German pediatrician, Alfred Wiskott.

1937 Target cells, in iron-deficiency anemia, were observed by Russell Landram Haden of Kansas and F.D. Evans.

1937 Factor VIII, antihemophilic globulin (AHG), effective in promoting coagulation in hemophiliacs, was isolated from the plasma of normal humans by Francis Henry Laskey Taylor and Jackson Arthur Patek.

1937 Four cases of internal carotid artery aneurysm were diagnosed using carotid angiography by Portuguese Nobel Prize winner, Egaz Moniz and Almeida Lima.

1937 The College of Obstetricians in London received its Royal charter to become the Royal College of Obstetricians and Gynaecologists.

1937 Orogenital ulceration (Behçet syndrome) was described by Turkish dermatologist, Halushi Behçet, who wrote *Syphilis and Related Skin Diseases*.

1937   The urographic appearance of the kidneys in renal papillary necrosis was described by G.W. Gunther of Stuttgart, Germany.

1937   X-ray diffraction was applied to the study of nucleic acids by English X-ray crystallographer, William Thomas Astbury.

1937   Myelofibrosis, a disease of adults, characterized by excessive production of fibrous tissue in the bone marrow, was discovered and described by R.A. Hickling.

1938   *Solomon Halbert Snyder* born. An American psychiatrist who investigated the biochemistry of nervous tissue, opiate receptors, and catecholamines from different areas of the brain.

1938   Sir Edward Charles Dodds produced the synthetic estrogen, stilboestrol.

1938   Rare renal hemangioma tumors were found by Elexius Thompson Bell, a professor of pathology at the University of Minnesota.

1938   The Laidlaw–Green hypothesis, that viruses arose from larger microorganisms due to their redundant parasitic mode of life, was proposed independently by Sir Patrick Playfair Laidlaw of Cambridge and R.P. Green.

1938   Sudden death in apparently healthy infants (cot death) was studied by A. Goldbloom and F.W. Wigglesworth of Canada.

1938   The first total replacement of the hip joint with an artificial hip joint made of steel was by English surgeon, Philip Wiles, at the Middlesex Hospital.

1938   *Physiology of the Nervous System*, published by John Farquhar Fulton from Yale University, contains the most comprehensive bibliography and author index on the subject.

1938   The plastic contact lens was introduced by Theodore E. Obrig, founder of the Obrig Laboratories.

1938   The metastatic lesions of prostate cancer were shown to cause elevation of serum levels of acid phosphatase by New York surgeons, Benjamin Stockwell Barringer and H.O Woodward.

1938   Histocompatibility genes were described by American geneticist, Georg Davis Snell of Massachusetts, during his research on the tissue transplant rejection reaction in mice.

1938   The protein nature of renin was suggested by Sir George White Pickering, an English professor of medicine, and Myron Prinzmetal, an American cardiologist.

1938   The Young operation, used for correction of hammer-toe and claw-toe, was devised by American surgeon, Charles Stephen Young.

1938   Charles A. Poindexter and M. Bruger demonstrated the statistical significance of a high cholesterol level in heart disease.

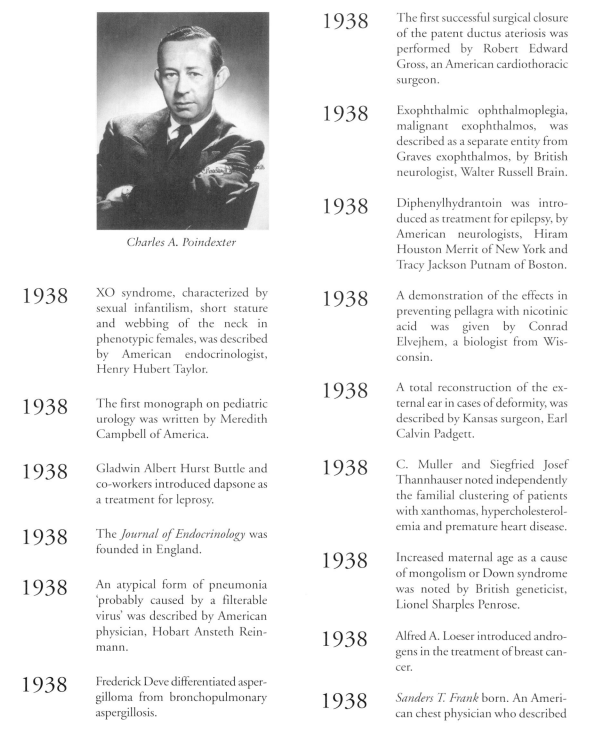

Charles A. Poindexter

1938   XO syndrome, characterized by sexual infantilism, short stature and webbing of the neck in phenotypic females, was described by American endocrinologist, Henry Hubert Taylor.

1938   The first monograph on pediatric urology was written by Meredith Campbell of America.

1938   Gladwin Albert Hurst Buttle and co-workers introduced dapsone as a treatment for leprosy.

1938   The *Journal of Endocrinology* was founded in England.

1938   An atypical form of pneumonia 'probably caused by a filterable virus' was described by American physician, Hobart Ansteth Reinmann.

1938   Frederick Deve differentiated aspergilloma from bronchopulmonary aspergillosis.

1938   The first successful surgical closure of the patent ductus ateriosis was performed by Robert Edward Gross, an American cardiothoracic surgeon.

1938   Exophthalmic ophthalmoplegia, malignant exophthalmos, was described as a separate entity from Graves exophthalmos, by British neurologist, Walter Russell Brain.

1938   Diphenylhydrantoin was introduced as treatment for epilepsy, by American neurologists, Hiram Houston Merrit of New York and Tracy Jackson Putnam of Boston.

1938   A demonstration of the effects in preventing pellagra with nicotinic acid was given by Conrad Elvejhem, a biologist from Wisconsin.

1938   A total reconstruction of the external ear in cases of deformity, was described by Kansas surgeon, Earl Calvin Padgett.

1938   C. Muller and Siegfried Josef Thannhauser noted independently the familial clustering of patients with xanthomas, hypercholesterolemia and premature heart disease.

1938   Increased maternal age as a cause of mongolism or Down syndrome was noted by British geneticist, Lionel Sharples Penrose.

1938   Alfred A. Loeser introduced androgens in the treatment of breast cancer.

1938   *Sanders T. Frank* born. An American chest physician who described oblique fissure of the ear lobe associated with coronary disease, hypertension and diabetes (Frank sign).

1938   The basis of modern pneumonectomy was established by Clarence Crafoord.

1938   W. Feldberg and C.H. Kellaway introduced the term 'slow reacting substance' for a material obtained from cobra venom and capable of contracting smooth muscle.

1938   A. Lezius of Heidelberg used cardiopneumopexy or suture of the lung to the heart, after removal of the pericardium, as treatment for coronary artery insufficiency.

1938   Indianapolis chemist, Rolla Neil Harger, invented the drunkometer for rapidly measuring alcohol content in expired air of a person suspected of intoxication.

1938   Herald Cox developed the first successful vaccine for *Rickettsiae*.

1938   Temple Fay used cryotherapy for carcinoma.

1938   P. Graffagnino and L.W. Seyler first used extradural lumbar block in obstetrics.

1939   C.F. Code showed the release of histamine during anaphylaxis in a guinea pig.

1939   English physician, Henry Stanley Banks, used sulfonamide for treating meningococcal meningitis.

1939   W.E. Ladd of Boston did the first successful staged operation for tracheoesophageal fistula.

1939   Boston thoracic surgeon, Oswald Sydney Tubbs, did the first successful closure of an infected ductus arteriosus.

1939   American physician, Isaac Starr, introduced the ballistocardiograph, a device used for recording the stroke volume of the heart.

1939   Ivor Lewis of University College Hospital, London did the first successful pulmonary embolectomy.

1939   C.J. Imperatori of New York did the first successful operation for congenital tracheoesophageal fistula (in the cervical esophagus) without esophageal atresia.

1939   A.A. Loeser and Paul Ulrich used testosterone in treatment of prostatic carcinoma.

1939   An effective vaccine against whooping cough was introduced by Pearl Kendrick and Grace Eldering.

1939   Visualization of opacified cardiac chambers by injecting contrast material through peripheral veins (ventriculography) was described by George Porter Robb and Israel Steinberg of America.

1939   A standardized form of curare, Incocostrin, was produced.

1939   A major review of coronary artery aneurysms was performed in 31 patients by N. Packard and H.F. Wechsler.

1939   René Jules Dubos, a French bacteriologist working in America, isolated one of the first antibacterial substances from *Bacillus brevis* and named it 'tyrothricin'.

1939   The Cancer Act was introduced in England to facilitate early diagnosis and rapid treatment.

1939   *Harold Elliot Varmus* born. An American molecular biologist and Nobel laureate (1989) who discovered oncogenes which can cause cancer.

1939   The vectorcardiogram was introduced into clinical medicine by Fritz Schellong of Germany.

1939   Radioactive isotopes were employed for the first time in treatment of leukemia by John Hundale Lawrence and co-workers.

1939   Alexander Fleming, I.H. Maclean and K.B. Rogers demonstrated how the advent of clinical chemotherapy with sulfonamides increased resistance in bacteria.

1939   The development of penicillin as an antibiotic followed the work of Howard Walter Florey and co-workers at the Sir William Dunn School of Pathology at Oxford, England.

1939   Transfusion of blood plasma was first described by American surgeon, Walter Low Tatum.

1939   Hailey–Hailey disease, a familial benign chronic pemphigus, was described by American dermatologists, William Howard Hailey and Hugh Edward Hailey.

1939   An operation to restore the function of the vocal cords was described by American surgeon in Seattle, Brian Thaxton King and New York otorhinologist, Joseph Dominic Kelly.

1939   *Susumu Tonegawa* born. A Japanese molecular biologist who used restriction enzymes and recombinant DNA techniques to study the origins of antibody diversity, and discovered that the number of antibody types far exceeds the number of cells responsible for their production.

1939   Refsum syndrome, a congenital condition consisting of retinitis pigmentosa, ataxia and peripheral neuropathy, was described by F. Thiebaut of Paris, France.

1939   James William Brown, a member of the editorial board of the *British Heart Journal* published *Congenital Heart Disease*, an important work which established cardiac surgery in England.

1939   O.M. Helmer and Irwin Henley Page discovered angiotensins.

1939   Antihistamine properties of aminoethanol derivatives were discovered by Nobel laureate, Daniel Bovet of the Pasteur Institute in Paris.

1939   The live yellow fever virus was attenuated by Max Theiler, an American virologist, whose work led to the development of the 17D vaccine for yellow fever.

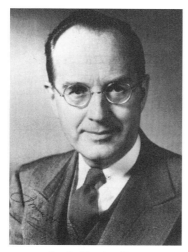

Irwin Henley Page

1940 The first description of 'a slow-reacting substance of anaphylaxis' giving rise to smooth muscle contraction, was given by American physician, Charles H. Kellaway.

1940 Dicoumarol, or warfarin, was isolated from sweet clover by Wisconsin biochemist, Karl Paul Link.

1940 The concept that specific genes control production of specific enzymes was developed by American geneticists, George Wells Beadle and Edward Lawrie Tatum.

1940 A method for the diagnosis of lymphogranuloma venereum by a complement-fixation test, was developed by American microbiologist, Clara M. McKee with G.W. Rake and M.F. Shaffer.

1940 A modern tourniquet was devised by English physician, L. Dougal Callander.

1940 *Joseph Leonhard Goldstein* born. An American molecular biologist and Nobel laureate (1985) who studied familial cholesterolemia and showed the missing receptor sites for low-density lipoprotein cholesterol in the liver of such patients.

1940 Impotence caused by thrombotic occlusion at the bifurcation of the aorta (Leriche syndrome) was described by René Henri Marie Leriche, a French professor of surgery at Lyons.

1940 The possibility of developing an artificial aortic valve was explored by American surgeon, Charles Anthony Hufnagel.

1939 The enzymatic nature of renin and its action on angiotensin were demonstrated by Eduardo Braun-Menendez from Buenos Aires and Argentinean Nobel Prize winner, Luis Frederico Leloir and colleagues.

1939 The Reid base line (anthropometric measurements) were defined by a Scottish anatomist, Robert William Reid, a demonstrator in anatomy at St Thomas' Hospital, London.

1940 A pure extract of penicillin from *Penicillium notatum* was produced by German-born British chemist, Sir Ernest Boris Chain.

1940 *Robin Weiss* born. An English molecular biologist and head of the Imperial Cancer Research Chester Beatty Laboratory, who worked on the role of retroviruses in causing cancer and on the HIV virus and its mechanism of entry into the cell.

1940   A congenital condition associated with dyschondroplasia, polydactyl, ectodermal dysplasia and cardiac malformations (Ellis–van Creveld disease) was described by British physician, Richard White Ellis and Dutch pediatrician, S. van Creveld.

1940   The influenza B virus was isolated independently by Thomas Francis and Thomas Pleines Magill.

1940   A description of blocking antibodies that arise during immunotherapy with pollen extracts was given by American physician, Mary Loveless.

1940   The causative bacteria of rheumatic fever (previously named, *Diplococcus rheumaticus* by Frederick John Poynton and Alexander Paine) was identified as Streptococcus group A by New York bacteriologist, Rebecca Craighill Lancefield.

1940   One of the first autoimmune diseases to be observed in humans, hemolytic anemia, was recognized by William Dameshek.

1940   Pethidine was used for obstetric analgesia.

1940   The first publication of *Anesthesiology,* the journal of American Society of Anesthesiologists.

1940   M. Danby and G.R. Biskind independently showed that androgens are inactivated in the liver.

1941   Canadian-born American urologist, Charles Brenton Huggins noted that metastatic carcinoma of the prostate responded positively to treatment with estrogenic substances.

1941   The first endowed chair of anesthesiology in the world was inaugurated at Harvard University, and Henry K. Beecher was appointed to it.

1941   Vernon Thompson of London did the first successful transpleural resection of carcinoma of the lower third esophagus.

1941   Australian immunologist, Sir Frank Macfarlane Burnet proposed a theory on immunological tolerance.

1941   The M.D. Anderson Tumor Institute at the University of Texas was established by the 47th Legislature of the State of Texas.

1941   Measurement of 17-ketosteroid levels in urine (ketosteroid excretion) was introduced as a diagnostic test for hypopituitarism by R. Fraser and P.H. Smith.

1941   An implant for fixing hip fractures (Jewitt nail-plate) was invented by Eugene Lyon Jewitt, an orthopedic surgeon from Orlando, Florida.

1941   The Ham test, hemolysis of red cells after incubation with acidified serum, for diagnosis of paroxysmal nocturnal hemoglobinuria and was devised by American physicians, G.C. Ham and H.M. Horack.

1941   The somatic symptoms of effort syndrome, or soldier's heart, were attributed to psychoneurosis arising from fear by the English cardiologist, Paul Hamilton Wood.

1941   The composition of biotin was established by American biochemist and Nobel laureate (1955) at Cornell University, Vincent du Vigneaud.

1941   The Hirst test to detect viruses or their corresponding antibodies was devised by New York physician, George Keble Hirst.

1941   A skin test for diagnosis of sarcoidosis was developed by Norwegian pathologist, Ansgar Morten Kveim, whose test bears his name.

1941   A method for the diagnosis of lymphogranuloma inguinale by means of a vesicular test was developed by American physician, Carlos Ottolina.

1941   Dihydrotachysterol was recommended as a treatment for hypoparathyroidism by Fuller Albright, the famous American endocrinologist.

1941   The increased risk of congenital heart disease and congenital cataracts during the first trimester of pregnancy was pointed out by Australian ophthalmologist, Sir Norman McAlister Gregg.

1941   Max Lederer described Baghdad spring anemia, an acute form of hemolytic anemia due to inhalation of pollen by atopic individuals.

1941   Bronchial asthma with recurrent pulmonary eosinophilic infiltration and polyserositis was described by Joseph Harkavy.

1941   The *Journal of Clinical Endocrinology* was founded in America.

1942   Hungarian scientist and Nobel laureate (1937), Albert Szent-Györgyi, demonstrated the action of the proteins actin and myosin (actomyosin) in bringing about muscle contraction.

1942   The cellular transfer of delayed cutaneous hypersensitivity and the role of mononuclear cells in the process of delayed hypersensitivity was described by American pathologist, Karl Landsteiner.

1942   An intrauterine electroencephalogram (EEG) of the fetus was recorded by D.B. Lindsley.

1942   Primary splenic anemia related to congenital hemolytic anemia (Wiseman syndrome) was described by American physician, Bruce Kenneth Wiseman of Ohio.

1942   *Robert Allan Weinberg* born. A pioneer in causes of cancer, acquisition of cancer-susceptible genes, and loss of tumor suppressor genes, who discovered the RbI suppressor gene responsible for a rare childhood cancer which affects the retina.

1942   The occurrence of shock in burns and trauma was investigated by American physician, Sanford M. Rosenthal.

1942   Curare was used as an anesthetic by Harold Randall Griffith and G. Enid Johnson of Canada.

1942   A pure form of cardiolipin was obtained from beef heart by Mary

Candace Pangborn, and was introduced as an agent for serological diagnosis of syphilis.

1942 *Richard De Forest Palmiter* born. An American molecular geneticist who produced the first transgenic mice by injecting human growth hormone into a mouse embryo.

1942 The first successful cardioesophageal resection for carcinoma of the cardia in England was performed by Claude Russell Brock.

1942 The introduction of Antergen by Swiss-born Italian pharmacologist, Daniel Bovet, and paved the way for the treatment of human allergic conditions.

1942 The concept of autoimmune disease was put forward by Ernest Witebsky from Germany, who proposed the postulate of autoimmune diseases.

1942 John McMichel and Peter Sharpey-Schafer at Hammersmith Hospital in London catheterized the right atrium in order to study heart failure and the effects of digoxin.

1942 English surgeon Alberto Francis Inclan introduced preservation of bone for bone graft by refrigeration.

1942 Geoffrey Langdon Keynes introduced thymectomy for myasthenia gravis.

1942 H.D. Adams and L.V. Hands of Boston did the first successful electrical defibrillation in a human.

1943 J. Garland suggested that herpes zoster may be due to reactivation of varicella virus acquired in earlier life.

1943 American pathologist, Elizabeth Machteld Sano used fibrin glue for skin grafting.

1943 The first rotating-drum artificial kidney was used to treat a patient by Dutch-born American physician, Willem Johan Kolff.

1943 English surgeon, John Chasser Moir, used ergometrine intravenously, before the delivery of the placenta in mothers.

1943 B. Stooky described brachial neuritis, due to lateral herniation of the cervical intervertebral disc.

1943 American biologists and Nobel laureates (1969), Salvador Edward Luria and Max Delbruck, showed that bacteria are capable of mutation.

1943 Herbert Frederick Traut and American anatomist, George Nicholas Papanicolaou, published *The Diagnosis of Uterine Cancer by Vaginal Smear.*

1943 The rejection reaction following autotransplantation of skin was described by English physicians, Thomas Gibson and Sir Peter Brian Medawar.

1943 A syndrome of cough and asthma accompanied by eosinophilia and X-ray changes in the lungs (tropical pulmonary eosinophilia) was described amongst the Indians by R.J. Weigarten.

1943 Penicillin was first used in the treatment of syphilis by John Friend Mahoney and colleagues, of the US Public Health Service.

1943 Section of supradiaphragmatic vagus nerves as treatment for duodenal ulcers was performed by Chicago surgeons, Lester Reynold Dragstedt and Frederick Mitchum Owens.

1944 Waldenström macroglobulinemia, dysproteinemia with raised IgM paraprotein in the serum and systemic effects of hyperviscosity of blood, was described by Swedish professor of medicine, Jan Gosta Waldenström.

1944 Type lll antigen of pneumococcus and its antigenic functions were shown by American bacteriologist, Theodore Oswald Avery.

1944 Hepatitis B (HBV), the virus responsible for serum hepatitis, was shown to be present in some batches of human pooled serum by Frederick Ogden MacCallum and Dennis John Bauer.

1944 Dextran was introduced as a substitute for plasma by Anders Johan Troed Gronwall and Bjorn Ingleman.

1944 One of the first units to treat and rehabilitate spinal injuries in England, Stoke Mandeville Hospital, which was founded by Sir Ludwig Guttman in Buckinghamshire.

1944 Intrathecal administration of penicillin in the treatment of pneumococcal meningitis was introduced by British neurologist, Sir Hugh Cairns and colleagues.

1944 Freda Pratt Bannister of Oxford helped to develop the direct laryngoscope and improved tracheal intubation.

1944 *The Psychology of Women, A Psychoanalytic Interpretation* was published by Helene Deutsch from the Vienna School of Medicine in Austria.

1944 *Surgery of the Hand* was published by Sterling Bunnell who established hand surgery as a specialty in the United States.

1944 H.T.J. Berk designed the first artificial kidney of therapeutic significance.

1944 A syndrome of diffuse interstitial pulmonary fibrosis leading to dyspnoea and clubbing (Hamman–Rich syndrome) was reported by American physician, Louis Virgil Hamman and American pathologist, Arnold R. Rich.

1944 American microbiologist and Nobel laureate, Selman Abraham Waksman, discovered streptomycin, and studied its value in the treatment of bacterial infections and especially in the treatment of tuberculosis.

1944 A fifth blood clotting factor was discovered by Paul Arnor Owren of Scandinavia, who named it 'Factor V'.

1944   American bacteriologist, Monroe Davis Eaton, identified the causative agent of atypical pneumonia as a filterable agent transmissible to rats (Eaton agent).

1944   Benjamin Minge Duggar from Wisconsin discovered the first tetracycline antibiotic, aureomycin.

1944   The Blalock–Taussig shunt, the first surgical operation for Fallot tetralogy, was performed by Alfred Blalock and Helen Taussig of Johns Hopkins Hospital.

1944   The TNM (tumor, node, metastasis) classification for cancer was proposed by P.F. Denoix of the Institut Gustav-Roussy in France.

1945   B. Johnson and co-workers developed the antibiotic bacitracin from *Bacillus subtilis*, and named it after Magaret Tracy, a patient from whom the bacillus was obtained.

1945   Jean Lenègre and Pierre Maurice of Paris produced the first intracardiac electrocardiogram. They used a catheter with a gold wire in its lumen.

1945   Karl Habel and John Franklin Enders cultivated the mumps virus in a chick embryo.

1945   R.D. Owen discovered and explained the occurrence of erythrocyte mosaicism in dizygotic twin cattle. His work led to the understanding of immunological tolerance.

1945   R.W. Rundles described autonomic neuropathy in diabetes causing abnormalities in blood pressure, sweating and skin temperature.

1945   The first clear evidence of the causal relationship between renal disease and erythrocytosis was provided by K.D. Fairley, who described cases caused by renal carcinoma and demonstrated its remission by removing the tumors.

1945   The histamine test for pheochromocytoma was devised by Grace Roth and Walter Kvale of America.

1945   The Coombs test to detect antigens in blood was devised by English immunologists, Robin Coombs, Arthur Ernest Mourant and Robert Russell Race.

1945   Albert Claude, an American cytologist, performed the first electron microscope study of the cell which showed the mitochondria and endoplasmic reticulum.

1945   An effective treatment for inversion of the uterus was proposed by James Vincent O'Sullivan, consisting of the application of hydraulic pressure through a vaginal douche to return the uterus to its normal position.

1945   F.S.H. Curd and co-workers synthesized paludrine, or proguanil, and tested it against avian malaria.

1945   The first vaccine for prophylaxis against dengue fever was prepared by Albert Bruce Sabin, the American microbiologist who developed the polio vaccine.

1945 A method of osteotomy for ankylosing spondylitis was described by Boston orthopedic surgeon, Marius Nygaard Smith-Petersen.

1946 Norepinephrine was shown to be the main transmitter of sympathetic nerve impulses by Swedish pharmacologist, Ulf Svante von Euler, who won the Nobel Prize 24 years later.

1946 Mephensin, an early tranquilizer and muscle relaxant, was discovered by F.M. Berger and Bradley of England during their search for a preservative for injections.

1946 Nitrofuranotoin, an oral urinary antibacterial compound developed from nitrofuran drugs was introduced by M. Dodd.

1946 Nitrogen mustard was introduced as treatment of Hodgkin disease by Alfred Gilman and Stanley Frederick Philips.

1946 The aspiration of gastric contents during general anesthesia in labor (Mendelson syndrome) was described by American obstetrician and gynecologist, Curtis Lester Mendelson.

1946 The National Health Service Act was passed in Britain by the Labour Party, which channeled money into the hospital system.

1946 Guido Fanconi, a Swiss professor of pediatrics at the University of Zurich, described renal tubular dysfunction (Fanconi syndrome) leading to aminoaciduria and cystic fibrosis of the pancreas.

1946 *Richard Axel* born. A New York geneticist and a pioneer in genetic engineering and cloning, who showed that DNA in chromatin can be cleaved at specific points by staphylococcal nucleases.

1946 J.B. Duguid proposed that the atheromatous plaques were essentially mural thrombi that had become incorporated into the vessel wall, in his modern theory of atherosclerosis.

1946 Frederick Stanley Phillips and Alfred Gilman discovered that nitrogen mustards could bring about regression of certain lymphomas and leukemias, in their landmark developments into cancer therapy.

1946 W.J.J. Gardener advocated controlled hypotension. This involved drawing blood from the radial artery until blood pressure is reduced to 80 mmHg, and the patient is afterwards retransfused.

1946 Willis Pott of the Children's Memorial Hospital, Chicago developed a new operation for tetralogy of Fallot (Potts operation) in very small infants whose subclavian artery is too small for anastomosis.

1946 H.M. Rogers noted the association between peptic ulceration and hyperparathyroidism.

1946 Karl Habel developed an experimental inactivated mumps vaccine and tested it on humans in 1951.

1946 Jacob Fine used peritoneal irrigation as treatment of acute renal failure.

1946 Claude Schafer Beck and colleagues of America used internal cardiac defibrillation countershock.

1946 Ivor Lewis of the North Middlesex Hospital, London developed a surgical technique for resection of carcinoma of middle-third of the esophagus.

1946 Adriani and Parmley used the saddle block technique of very low spinal anesthesia for forceps delivery.

1947 Establishment of the Faculty of Anaesthetists of the Royal College of Surgeons of England.

1947 O.T. Clagett of the Mayo Clinic did the first successful subclavian-aortic anastomosis for coarctation of aorta.

1947 E.J. Delorme of Edinburgh showed that hemorrhagic shock was better tolerated in cooled dogs than at normal temperatures.

1947 R.H. Franklin of London performed the first two successful operations in Britain for tracheo-esophageal fistula.

1947 The use of antihistamines to inhibit the reaction of the autonomic nervous system to physical stress in surgery was investigated by French surgeon H. Laborit at the Military Hospital in Paris.

1947 Stereotaxic surgery was first used as a treatment for Parkinson disease to produce discrete lesions in the basal ganglia by Ernest Adolf

Spiegel, H.T. Wycis, M. Marks and A. J. Lee of New York.

1947 The World Medical Organization, which coordinates work of various National Medical Associations, was founded at Ferney-Voltaire in France.

1947 The Nobel Prize was won by American biochemists, Carl Ferdinand Cori and Theresa Gerti Cori, for their work in isolating and crystallizing the enzyme, glycogen phosphorylase.

1947 A tiny electrical device which replaced the thermometer valve (transistor) was invented by John Bardeen, Walter Houser Brattain and William Bradford Shockley.

1947 Mildred Trotter gave the name 'caudal space' to the epidural space lying within the boundaries of the sacrum.

1947 George Eugene Moore introduced fluorescein, a radioisotopic agent, for diagnostic neuroradiology.

1947 Direct stimulation to the sinoatrial node of two patients who developed cardiac arrest during surgery, was applied by W.H. Sweet.

1947 A pioneer in neurosurgery, I. Caffey Adson, recommended the division of the scelenus anterior muscle for relief from symptoms of 'cervical rib syndrome'.

1947 In his book *Hearing*, American physiologist, Georg von Bekesy, wrote a modern study on the mechanism of the ear, and analyzed the manner in which it transmits sound to the brain.

1947 Understanding of color vision was developed by Edwin Herbert Land of Connecticut.

1948 Chlortetracycline (aureomycin) was obtained from *Streptomyces aureofaciens*, by Benjamin M. Dugger from Wisconsin.

1948 Czech obstetrician, Joseph Asherman, described intrauterine adhesions with amenorrhea and named it 'Asherman syndrome'.

1948 Direct injection of lumbar intervertebral discs with radio-opaque dye in orthopedics, was first carried out by Swedish orthopedic surgeon, Knut Lindblom.

1948 A fatal form of fibrosis of the endocardium leading to intractable heart failure (Davies disease) was described in children and young adults in Uganda by J.N.P. Davies.

1948 Malcolm H. Hargraves gave a description of neutrophil leukocyte phagocytozing nuclear material, characteristic of autoimmune/autoallergic diseases with antinuclear antibodies.

1948 The relationship between acromegaly and an increase in plasma growth hormone levels was demonstrated by Laurence Wilkie Kinsell.

1948 The physiological aspects of arthritis in knee joints were studied by British orthopedic surgeon, John Charnley, who developed a technique to fuse the bones of the knee.

1948 The routine use of rectal biopsy in proctology was established by the English surgeon, William Bahall Gabriel.

1948 A familial condition consisting of mental retardation, sexual precocity, hypertelorism, progeria and other features (Donohue syndrome) was described by Canadian pathologist, W.L. Donohue.

1948 New York surgeon, Charles Gardner Child, described one-stage pancreatoduodenectomy with preservation of external pancreatic secretion, for carcinoma of the duodenum (Child technique).

1948 Methotrexate was developed from aminopterin by Sidney Faber, a cancer scientist in the United States, as a folic acid antagonist in the treatment of leukemia.

1948 The diagnostic presence of L E cells in acute disseminated systemic lupus erythematosus was discovered by Malcolm MacCallum Hargreaves.

1948 The Coxsackie virus was isolated from the feces of two children during their acute phase of poliomyelitis in Coxsackie, New York, by American pathologist, G. Dalldorf and Grace Mary Sickles.

1948 The World Health Organization was established by the United Nations.

1948 A congenital form of hyperbilirubinemia (Rotor syndrome) was described by Arturo Rotor, a physician from the Philippines.

1948

Louis Klein Diamond

Exchange transfusion as treatment for erythroblastosis fetalis was introduced by Louis Klein Diamond.

1948 Cortisone was first tried for rheumatoid arthritis by Edward Calvin Kendall of Detroit, Michigan, with remarkable beneficial effects.

1948 Charles Dubost of Paris performed the first successful resection of an abdominal aneurysm and repair with a homologous graft.

1948 A scientific work on stress linking it to biological and pathological consequences in man was produced by Hans Selye, a Canadian physician of Austrian origin.

1948 The term 'effective blood volume' coined by J.P. Peters to refer to a component of blood volume to which volume regulatory systems in the body respond.

1948 J. Watson established the protective effect of fetal hemoglobin (Hb F) against sickling in sickle cell disease.

1948 Health was defined as the physical, psychological, and social well-being of the patient, and not just the absence of disease.

1948 B. Shapiro and E. Wertheimer demonstrated the active role of adipose tissue in metabolism.

1948 V.O. Björk developed a membrane oxygenator employing the principle of rotating discs to expose films of blood to oxygen. He perfected it 1952 and used it clinically in 1954.

1948 Robert Edward Gross and his colleagues did the first arterial homograft for restoring continuity during resection of aortic coarctation.

1948 The Marie Curie Memorial Foundation for cancer research was established.

1948 Fuller Albright and F C Reifenstein described renal tubular acidosis causing chronic hyperchloremic acidosis, nephrolithiasis, and recurrent urinary tract infection.

1948 Cameron Haight did the first successful operation for congenital tracheoesophageal fistula (within the thoracic esophagus) without esophageal atresia.

1949 San Francisco surgeon Emile F. Holman performed a radical operation to relieve pericardial constriction and free the right atrium.

1949 John Franklin Enders, Frederick Robbins and Thomas H. Weller successfully cultivated a strain of polio virus in human non-nervous tissues.

1949   The American College of Rheumatology proposed a functional classification for patients with arthritis.

1949   English pharmacologists William Paton and Eleanor Zaimus developed dexamethonium bromide as a ganglion blocking agent.

1949   C. E. Flowers, L. M. Hellman and R. A. Hingson used continuous extradural lumbar block in obstetrics.

1949   An illustrated book on the techniques of pulmonary resection was published by American surgeon, Richard Hollis Overholt.

1949   The molecular structure of penicillin was elucidated by Dorothy Crowfoot Hodgkin, an English biochemist who later received the Nobel Prize for Chemistry in recognition of her achievements.

1949   British neurologist, Sir Hugh Cairns, was the first to describe hydrocephalus following obstruction of the flow of cerebrospinal fluid secondary to tuberculosis meningitis.

1949   J.B. Duguid published his *Pathogenesis of Arteriosclerosis*.

1949   The British National Formulary (BNF) was first published.

1949   The causative fungus of histoplasmosis, was isolated from soil by American mycologist, Chester Emmons.

1949   German physician, Paul Furbringer, demonstrated the diagnostic value of the spinal tap, and described the Furbringer sign, in which a needle inserted into a subphrenic abscess moved with respiration.

1949   The *Treponema* immobilization test for the diagnosis of syphilis was devised by Robert Armstrong Nelson and Manfred Martin Mayer.

1949   Short-acting muscle relaxants were described by Daniel Bovet, an Italian pharmacologist (who was also the first to prepare antihistamines) and used clinically two years later in Italy and Sweden.

1949   Carl John Wiggers investigated asynchronous contractions of the left and right ventricles contributing to the components of the second heart sound.

1949   Familial cardiomegaly was described by William Evans of the National Heart Hospital in London.

1949   Kendall Brooks Corbin introduced artane, or benzhexol for the treatment of Parkinson disease.

1949   William B. Schwartz published his results on the effects of sulfanilamide on salt and water excretion in congestive heart failure.

1949   Australian psychiatrist, John Cade, published a paper on the value of lithium in treating manic depression.

1950   Sydney Farber and colleagues published their results on treatment of childhood leukemia with adrenocorticotropic hormone (ACTH) which stimulates the adrenal glands to increase natural steroid production.

1950 Claude S. Beck, a pioneer in open heart massage, used the electrical countershock method and direct cardiac massage to the exposed heart to stop intraoperative ventricular fibrillation.

1950 Wilfred G. Bigelow and coworkers at Toronto showed that, with progressive cooling, rectal temperature and oxygen consumption of the body had a linear relationship without the tissues incurring any oxygen debt.

1950 The first few cases of severe lymphopenia with extensive candida infection in infancy (combined immunodeficiency) were described in Switzerland.

1950 Methods of fractionation of proteins in human blood plasma were developed by Ewin J. Cohn and colleagues.

1950 Several articles appeared in the *Bulletin of the Johns Hopkins Hospital* on use of cortisone for diseases other than rheumatoid arthritis. These included treatment of asthma, drug hypersensitivity, systemic lupus erythematosis, polyarteritis nodosa, and eye diseases such as iritis and conjunctivitis.

1950 One of the most comprehensive historic accounts on obstetrics was given in the *Eternal Eve*, published by Harvey Graham.

1950 The newly invented polythene catheter, inserted through the brachial artery for catheterization, was used by J.A. Helmsworth and colleagues.

1950 Philip Showalter Hench, Edward Calvin Kendal and Tadeus Reichstein were awarded the Nobel Prize for Physiology or Medicine for their work on cortisone, and related compounds used in treatment of rheumatoid arthritis.

1950 The antibiotic, Nystatin, was isolated from *Streptomyces noursei*, obtained from soil in Virginia.

1950 Austin Bradford Hill and Richard William Shaboe Doll unambiguously demonstrated that cigarette smoking caused carcinoma of the lung in a paper in the *British Medical Journal*.

1950 *Alec John Jeffreys* born. An English molecular biologist and professor of genetics who developed the technique of DNA fingerprinting now used in forensic medicine.

1950 French pediatrician, Robert Debré, described 'cat scratch fever', characterized by fever and lymphadenopathy.

1950 Transformation of the mucosa of the esophagus into the columnar epithelium due to esophagitis, hiatus hernia or stricture was described by Australian surgeon, Norman R. Barrett, and known as 'Barrett epithelium'.

1950 A scientific study on the cause and mechanics of lumbar disc degeneration was carried out by Stein Freeberg and Carl Hirsh of Stockholm.

1950 Tuberculosis was successfully treated with streptomycin and para aminosalicylic acid (PAS) by British physician, Sir Austin Bradford Hill.

1950 A family physician from Cleveland, Lawrence Craven, noted that aspirin can prevent blood clotting in an article in *The Annals of Western Medicine and Surgery*.

1950 Ataxia, retinitis pigmentosa and abetalipoproteinemia (Bassen–Kornzweig syndrome) was described by Canadian-born American physician F.A. Bassen and New York ophthalmologist A.L. Kornzweig.

1950 An artificial femoral head for arthroplasty of the hip joint was devised by Jean and Robert Judet.

1950 The first suggestion of cardiac output as the primary regulator of renal sodium and water excretion was made by J.G. Borst and L.A. deVries.

1950 W.T. Beraldo proposed that plasma kinin may play a role in systemic anaphylaxis.

1950 Arthur Vineberg of Montreal performed the first operation on a human for myocardial vascularization using an internal mammary implant into a myocardial tunnel to stimulate anastomotic channels.

1950 V.E. Negus developed a hydrostatic bag (Negus bag) for treating pharyngeal diverticula.

1950 E.H. Wood developed an oximeter for cardiac catheter studies.

1950 J.C. Castello and E.J. de Beer showed the paralyzing effects of suxamethonium derivatives of choline esters of succinic acid.

1950 G.J. Rees and T.C. Gray divided anesthetic stages into triad, narcosis, analgesia and relaxation.

1950 The James Ewing Hospital for cancer opened at New York, and became the Ewing Pavilion in 1968.

1951 O. von Dardel and S. Thesleff of Sweden first used choline esters of succinic acid or suxamethonium for muscle relaxation.

1951 J. Bornstein and P. Trewhella demonstrated the phenomenon of insulin resistance.

1951 Welsh surgeon, Sir Clement Price Thomas, performed a successful pneumonectomy on King George IV.

1951 K. Campbell showed the occurrence of retrolental fibroplasia in babies exposed to high concentrations of oxygen.

1951 The first demonstration of the beneficial effects of a folate antagonist, aminopterin, in rheumatoid arthritis by R. Gubner and co-workers.

1951 Allergic granulomatosis involving the lung was described by J. Churg and L. Strauss in the *American Journal of Pathology*, and it was later named Churg-Strauss syndrome.

1951   *A History of Neurological Surgery*, edited by American neurosurgeon, A. E. Walker of Johns Hopkins Hospital in Baltimore was published.

1951   Mondor disease, superficial thrombophlebitis of the chest wall and the breast, was described by Henri Mondor, professor of clinical surgery in Paris, France.

1951   Alexander Lawson, C. Rimington and C.E. Searle synthesized the currently used antithyroid drug, carbimazole.

1951   Chlorambucil was first used for treatment of chronic lymphatic leukemia, by David Abraham, D. Galton and co-workers.

1951   Endocardial electrode pacing in heart block was first tried in animals by John C. Callaghan and Wilfred G. Bigelow.

1951   Harold Ridley, an ophthalmologist from St Thomas' Hospital in London, published a paper on intraocular acrylic lenses for use in cataract surgery.

1951   A method of allowing the blood from a cannulated artery to pass through tubing immersed in a cooling medium and to be returned to a vein (extracorporeal cooling), was described by J. Boerema and colleagues.

1951   Surgical anesthesia using 80% xenon and 20% oxygen was produced by Stephen C. Cullen and E.G. Gross.

1951   Max Theiler, a South African-born bacteriologist, was awarded the Nobel Prize for Physiology or Medicine for his work on yellow fever and immunity.

1951   The occlusion of the anterior spinal artery resulting in complex neurological signs was described as anterior spinal artery syndrome by Karl Beck of Germany.

1952   Congenital agammaglobulinemia, a sex-linked familial condition, was reported in a boy with recurrent infection by American pediatrician, Ogden C. Bruton.

1952   The water excretion test for adrenal function, was devised by L.J. Soffer and J.L. Gabrilov.

1952   Implantation of an artificial aortic valve in a patient was carried out at the Georgetown University Medical Center.

1952   A great London smog, associated with vastly increased death rates from chronic bronchitis, encouraged the passing of the Clean Air Act two years later.

1952   US virologist Jonas Edward Salk developed a killed vaccine against acute poliomyelitis.

1952   Coenzyme A, which takes part in the respiratory cycle, was discovered by American biochemist and Nobel laureate (1953), Fritz Albert Lipmann.

1952   The antibiotic, erythromycin, was obtained from *Streptomyces erythreus* from the soil in the Philippines by

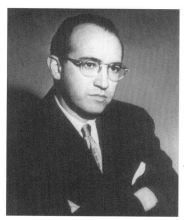

Jonas Edward Salk

James Myrlin McGuire and colleagues.

1952 Pituitary ablation or surgical removal as treatment for carcinoma of the breast was pioneered by Rolf Luft and Herbert Olivecrona.

1952 A revolutionary advance in the development of artificial joints was made by the Judet brothers of Paris who completely resected the femoral head of the hip joint, and replaced it with a new artificial head made of methyl methacrylate.

1952 American immunologist, Albert Coons, published his techniques on fluorescent labeled antibodies, following the work of Marrack on the attachment of visible dyes to antibodies.

1952 Selman Abraham Waksman, American microbiologist, received the Nobel Prize in Physiology for his work in the treatment of tuberculosis with streptomycin.

1952 A polio epidemic in Copenhagen led to the birth of intensive care when Bjorn Ibsen proved the benefits of artificial ventilation in treatment.

1952 Chlorpromazine was first used in the treatment of schizophrenia by David Clark and Joel Elkes.

1952 Christian disease, named after the patient in whom it was described, was recognized by Rosemary Peyton Biggs, who noted hemophilia B due to a lack of factor IX.

1952 The world's first sex change operation was performed on George Jorgenson, who later became known as Christine.

1952 Shortened PR interval and normal QRS on ECG, associated with paroxysmal tachycardia (Lown–Ganong–Levine syndrome), was described by three American cardiologists, Bernard Lown, William F. Ganong and Samuel Levine.

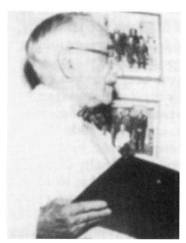

Selman Abraham Waksman

1952 The sodium-retaining factor in venous blood from the adrenal glands, aldosterone, was identified through chromatography by S.A. Simpson, J.F. Twit and P.G.G. Bush.

1952 J. Facquet of Paris performed left heart catheterisation by puncture of the left atrium. He used a bronchoscope to pass a needle into the left atrium through the wall of the left main bronchus.

1952 T.H. Weller and M.B. Stoddard isolated the varicella virus from samples taken from vesicles of patients with varicella.

1952 J. Gross and R. Pitt-Rivers isolated and purified triiodothyronine (T_3).

1952 H. King and H.B. Schumacker showed susceptibility to fulminant infections after splenectomy in infancy.

1952 Nalorphine was first used in obstetric analgesia.

1952 Charles Brenton Huggins and D.M. Bergenstal described bilateral adrenalectomy as treatment for disseminated carcinoma of the breast.

1952 Vincent du Vigneaud, E.A. Popenoe and H.C. Lawler discovered that lysine replaces arginine in the vasopressin of pigs, and determined the structure of oxytocin a year later.

1953 L.R. Reagan and colleagues in New Jersey did the first successful internal electrical defibrillation in acute coronary occlusion.

1953 G. Weber introduced fluorescence polarization to investigate the rotational properties of molecules.

1953 Maxwell Chamberlain of New York used segmental resection of the lungs for tuberculosis.

1953 Immune adherence, the attachment of human erythrocytes to microorganisms sensitized with antibody and complement, was coined by R.A. Nelson.

1953 Sir Peter Brian Medawar and coworkers proposed that immunological tolerance is not an all-or-none phenomenon, but varies from non-reactivity to normal reactivity.

1953 The concept of graft versus host reaction in transplantation medicine was put forward by M. Simonsen.

1953 The term 'neuroleptic' was applied to certain groups of drugs used in the treatment of psychoses by J. Delay, P. Denicker and Y. Tardieu.

1953 The first examination for Fellowship of the Faculty of Anaesthetists of the Royal College of Surgeons of England, was taken in London.

1953 The first pump oxygenator was successfully used on humans to close an atrial septal defect, by American cardiovascular surgeon, John Heysham Gibbon.

1953 A modification of the percutaneous technique for catheterization of the kidney, which allowed the introduction of a catheter of a diameter larger than that of the needle used for initial puncture, was devised by Swedish radiologist, Sven Seldinger.

1953 A report appeared in the *British Medical Journal* on use of isoniazid in treatment of tuberculosis.

1953 Ferdinand Perutz showed that the hemoglobin structure could be solved by comparing two or more X-ray diffraction patterns, one from pure protein and one from the protein with heavy atoms attached.

1953 O. Spuhler and H.U. Zollinger pointed out the association between prolonged analgesic use and chronic renal failure, analgesic nephropathy.

1953 Anthony Caplan described the combination of pneumoconiosis and rheumatoid arthritis, which caused well-defined X-ray opacities in the lungs of miners (Caplan syndrome).

1953 The first suggestion of volume-sensitive receptors in the arterial circulation was made by F.H. Epstein and coworkers, on patients with traumatic arteriovenous fistulae.

1953 The Schilling test for vitamin B_{12} absorption by oral administration of radioactive vitamin B_{12} and urinary excretion of radioactivity, was studied by American hematologist, Robert Frederick Schilling.

1953 Adenovirus was discovered by Wallace Prescott Rowe, and after further research further antigenic types and strains were found.

1953 Using the semiconductor transistor, American scientists, John Bardeen, Walter Houser Brattain and William Bradford Shockley, developed an implantable pacemaker.

1953 British biochemist, Sir Hans Adolf Krebs and German-born American biochemist, Fritz Albert Lipmann shared the Nobel Prize for Physiology or Medicine for their work on the citric acid cycle.

1953 Swiss microbiologist, Werner Arber, developed a technique for preparing bacteriophage.

1953 A paper elucidating the molecular structure of DNA was published by Nobel laureates, James Dewey Watson, a biologist from Chicago, and Francis Harry Compton Crick of Cambridge, England.

DNA strand

1953 Poulle Astroup devised the Astroup technique for measuring acid–base status in the blood.

1953 Mast cell granules as a significant source of released heparin were described by British physicians, James F. Riley and Geoffrey B. West.

1954 Visualization of the fetus in utero (fetoscopy) was achieved by introducing an instrument through the cervical canal by B. Westin.

1954 Menkes syndrome, an inborn error of leucine and isoleucine metabolism leading to mental deficiency, was described by American pediatrician, John H. Menkes.

1954 American bacteriologist, John Franklin Enders, American pediatrician, Frederick Chapman Robbins and American virologist, Thomas Huckle Weller were awarded the Nobel Prize for Physiology or Medicine for their work on the polio virus.

1954 Idiopathic hypercalcemia of childhood, was described by I. McQuarrie.

1954 Multiple adenomatous hyperplasia of the anterior pituitary gland, parathyroid glands and multiple tumors of the islands of Langerhans (Wermer syndrome), were described by New York physician, Paul Wermer.

1954 A Zeiss operating microscope was developed for use in eye and other surgery.

1954 The US Congress created and funded the Cancer Chemotherapy National Service Center to screen potential anti-cancer agents.

1954 Clarence Walton Lillehei performed the first open-heart repair for a child with Fallot tetralogy using his method of 'cross circulation' of the blood (passing blood from the patient through a human volunteer in order to oxygenate it). He later developed a mechanical pump oxygenator.

1954 Harold Hopkins, a British optical physicist, published details of the fiberoptic endoscope in *Nature*.

1954 Ultrasound was first used to record the continuous movement of the heart walls, by Inge Edler and Carl Helmuth Hertz.

1954 P. Huguenard defined drugs used in the treatment of psychoses as those which produce a cataleptic state, antagonize apomorphine, decrease sensitivity to catecholamines, and inhibit learned behavioral activity.

1954 Macleod syndrome, of abnormal radiotranslucency of one lung with no apparent clinical abnormality, was described by British physician, William Mathieson Macleod.

1954 A form of chronic intermittent jaundice with pigmented liver (Dubin–Johnson syndrome) was described by American pathologists, I.N. Dubin and S.B. Johnson.

1954 A successful renal transplant between identical twins was made by American surgeon and pioneer in this field, Joseph Edward Murray and co-workers, at the Peter Bent Brigham Hospital.

1954 The familial nature of Wiskott–Aldrich syndrome, due to an X-linked recessive trait, was shown by American pediatrician, Robert Aldrich.

1954 Treatment of ventricular septal defect by surgical closure was demonstrated by Herbert Edgar Warden and colleagues.

1954 C.G. Rob and H.H.G. Eastcott reported the first case of internal carotid artery reconstructive surgery (carotid endarterectomy).

1954 The first successful resection of ventricular aneurysm following myocardial infarction performed by C.P. Bailey in Philadelphia.

1954 The first statistical study of mortality rates in anesthesia was undertaken by Henry K. Beecher and D.P. Todd in the United States.

1954 Left heart catheterisation through a suprasternal puncture was performed in Lund by Stig Radner.

1954 Disturbances of pyridoxine metabolism due to isoniazid or isonicotinic acid hydrazide therapy was first demonstrated by J.P. Biehl and R.W. Vilter.

1954 L Pillemer and colleagues discovered properdin, a serum protein, mediating diverse phenomena such as lysis of red cells and bacteria, and protective against total body radiation.

1954 The side effects due to testosterone abuse, including prostatic hypertrophy found in weightlifters, were pointed out by US physician, John B. Ziegler.

1954 Mitral valvotomy with the use of a mechanical dilator inserted through the left atrium was performed in Paris by Charles Dubost.

1954 A technique for dilating stenosed pulmonary and tricuspid valves using a modified catheter was described by V. Rubio and R. Limson Lawson.

1955 Humphrey and Jacques demonstrated that serotonin is released from rabbit platelets in vitro through antigen–antibody reactions.

1955 Abdominal decompression as a method of pain relief in labor was introduced by a South African, O.S. Heyns. He applied negative pressure via a shell (Heyns bag) which could be controlled by the patient.

1955 Engström's ventilator for postoperative management was used by V.O. Björk, a Swedish cardiothoracic surgeon, founding the basis for future intensive care units.

1955 The humoral nature of the stimulation of erythropoiesis by anoxia was demonstrated by R. Schmid and A.S. Gilbertsen.

1955 Successful repair of four cases of dissecting aortic aneurysm by Michael Ellis DeBakey and Arthur Denton Cooley.

1955 Effectiveness of estrogens in the treatment of breast carcinoma was shown by O.H. Pearson and coworkers.

1955 Post-cardiotomy syndrome (Dressler syndrome) of pericarditis, pleurisy and fever following pericardiotomy, myocardial infarction, or trauma to the heart, was described by William Dressler of America.

1955 Excessive secretion of aldosterone leading to hypernatremia, hypertension and hypokalemic alkalosis (Conn syndrome) was described by American physician, Jerome William Conn.

1955 Hemolytic uremic syndrome, associated with renal failure, hemolysis and thrombocytopenia, was described by Swiss pediatrician, C. Gasser and co-workers at the University of Zurich.

1955 J.W. Cromwell and W.L. Read were the first to demonstrate that heparinization could prevent minute blood clots.

1955 The amino acid composition of bovine pancreatic ribonuclease was determined by American biochemists from Chicago, Stanford Moore and William Howard Stein.

1955 Autoimmune hemolytic anemia and thrombocytopenia (Evan syndrome), was described by American physician, Robert S. Evan of Seattle.

1955 The antibiotic, Novobiocin, was obtained from *Streptomyces spheroides*, from Vermont.

1955 Swedish biochemist, Hugo Teodor Theorell was awarded the Nobel Prize for Physiology or Medicine for discovery of some enzymes, heme protein and vitamins.

1955 J.W. Cromwell and W.L. Read were the first to demonstrate that heparization could prevent the formation of minute blood clots and low-dose heparin treatment for patients at high risk of embolism was introduced in the early 1970s.

1955 American biochemist, George Herbert Hitchings, synthesized the drug Azathioprine (Imuran).

1955 E.H. Kass demonstrated the value of 'clean-catch' mid-stream urine for detecting urinary tract infection.

1955 Large-scale polio vaccination was introduced.

1955 The first successful open-heart surgery.

1955 Zollinger–Ellison syndrome of recurrent peptic ulceration associated with non-insulin secreting islet cell tumors of the pancreas was described by two American surgeons at the Ohio State University, Robert Zollinger and Edwin Ellison.

1955 The congenital condition of agenesis of the spleen, situs inversus and cardiac abnormalities (Ivemark syndrome) was described by Björn Ivemark.

1955 Cronkhite–Canada syndrome, characterized by gastrointestinal polyposis and ectodermal changes including alopecia and nail and skin changes, was described by Leonard W. Cronkhite and W.J. Canada.

1955 Chlordiazepoxide was synthesized by Polish pharmacist, Sternbach in Cracow.

1956   B. Kisch observed the presence of secretory granules in the atrium of the heart.

1956   An autosomal recessive disease with skin rash, aminoaciduria, pellagra and cerebellar features (Hartnup disease) was described by D.N. Baron and colleagues.

1956   Paul Maurice Zoll applied external cardiac pacing for the first time in ventricular standstill in two patients.

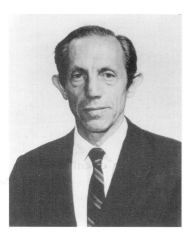

Paul Maurice Zoll

1956   Paul Charpentier and Simone Courvoisier published their results on trials of chlorpromazine for psychotic disorders.

1956   The role of the extracellular fluid volume in the control of aldosterone secretion in man was described by American physician Frederick C. Bartter, who also established the pathophysiology of the adrenogenital system.

1956   A marked fall in mortality from asthma was noted due to the introduction of the steroid (cortisone) group of drugs.

1956   A myasthenic reaction associated with small cell carcinoma of the bronchus (Eaton–Lambert syndrome) was described by American neurologists, E.H. Lambert and L.M. Eaton at the Mayo Clinic in Rochester.

1956   Hypo- and a-gammaglobulinemia syndromes, and the role of the thymus in immunodeficiencies, were described by American professor of pediatrics, Robert A. Good.

1956   The first factor common to both intrinsic and extrinsic pathways in blood clotting (Factor X) was discovered by T.P. Telfer, K.W. Densen and D.R. Wright.

1956   French-born American physician, André Frédéric Cournand, German physician, Werner Forssmann and American physician, Dickinson Woodruff Richards were awarded the Nobel Prize for Physiology or Medicine for their work on cardiac catheterization.

1956   DNA polymerase was discovered by American biochemist, Arthur Kornberg of New York, who also synthesized biologically active DNA for which he received the Nobel Prize.

1956   Use of D-penicillamine in the treatment of Wilson's disease was established by J.M. Walshe.

1956   An early description of placental bacteremia leading to shock (septic abortion) was given by William

Emery Studdiford, professor of gynecology at the New York University College of Medicine, and Gordon Watkins Douglas.

1956 External ophthalmoplegia, ataxia and areflexia due to a vascular cause (Miller Fisher syndrome) were described by Canadian neurologist, Miller Fisher.

1956 Cardiopulmonary resuscitation was first used.

1956 The radioimmunoassay technique was introduced by Samuel A. Berson and colleagues, and refined by American biophysicist, Rosalyn Yalow of New York, for which she was awarded the Nobel Prize for Physiology or Medicine.

1956 Ronald Kuhn used imipramine, the first tricyclic compound with antidepressant qualities, in successfully treating depression.

1956 The antibiotic, vancomycin, was obtained from *Streptomyces orientalis*, from soil in Borneo and Indiana.

1956 The twin-coiled artificial kidney was used by B. Watschinger and J. Kolff to treat two cases of uremia treated by hemiodialysis and ultra filtration.

1956 Cardiac involvement by coxsackie B virus was recognized in newborn infants in Johannesburg by S.N. Javett and colleagues.

1956 A sulfonylurea compound (tolbutamide) was introduced as treatment in diabetes by Helmut Maske of Germany.

1956 The first description of surgical aortic valvotomy was given by H. Swan and A. Korz.

1956 Use of biopsy capsules for peroral small intestinal biopsy was described by M. Shiner.

1956 Discovery of autoantibodies to thyroglobulin in patients with Hashimoto disease was made by Ivan. M. Roitt of Middlesex Hospital Medical School, London, and Deborah Doniach.

1957 Splitting of second heart sound due to a delayed pulmonary component in relation to the severity of pulmonary stenosis was explained by A. Leatham of London.

1957 Construction of the first electrometric apparatus for measurement of carbon dioxide in blood was made by R.W. Stow, R .F. Baer and B.F. Randall.

1957 Foundation of the Society for the Advancement of Anaesthesia in Dentistry (SAAD) in London.

1957 The role of the kidney in erythropoiesis was demonstrated by L.O. Jacobson and coworkers.

1957 Substitution of the amino acid valine for glutamic acid in the hemoglobin of patients with sickle cell anemia was described by Vernon Martin Ingram of England.

1957 Daniel Bovet of the Department of Chemical Therapeutics at the Pasteur Institute in Paris was awarded the Nobel Prize in Physiology or Medicine for his work on the treatment of allergies and development of sulfa drugs, and the way in which substances affect and interact with an invading organism.

1957 American virologist, Daniel Carleton Gajdusek, identified a form of spongiform encephalopathy (kuru) amongst the cannibal Fore tribe of Papua New Guinea.

1957 Ernest Witebsky of Germany described experimental autoallergic thyroiditis and the pathology and criteria of autoimmune diseases.

1957 The antibiotic Kanamycin was obtained from *Streptomyces kanamyceticus*, from soil in Japan.

1957 Glycoprotein with antiviral activity (interferon), was discovered by Scottish virologist, Alick Isaacs of Glasgow, and Jean Lindemann.

1957 A National Health Service survey in the USA indicated that almost 11 million people suffered from arthritis and rheumatism, of whom 10% were disabled and incapable of work.

1957 The flexible fiber optic endoscope was first used on a patient at Michigan University by South African gastroenterologist, Basil I. Hirschowitz.

1957 During their search for a carbonic acid inhibitor in the treatment of hypertension, F.C. Novello and J.M. Sprague synthesized chlorothiazide.

1957 A method of conservative treatment for congenital dislocation of the hip was introduced by a Czechoslovakian surgeon, Arnold Pavlik, using a harness with stirrups.

1957 Factor VIII was extracted from blood and used in treatment of hemophiliacs.

1957 Ancel Keys, director of the Laboratory of Physical Hygiene at the University of Minnesota, produced a paper on prediction of serum cholesterol responses in man to changes in fat in the diet.

1957 Myoclonic and akinetic seizures in children with a petit mal type of EEG (Lennox–Gastaut syndrome), was first described by French neurologist, Henri Gastaut.

1957 The problem of how DNA was synthesized simultaneously in opposite directions, but with corresponding opposite polarity was solved by Japanese biochemist, Reiji Okazaki, who discovered DNA–RNA fragments.

1957 A clinical description of corrected transposition of the great arteries, adequate to establish a diagnosis, was given by R.C. Anderson and colleagues.

1957 Masaki Watanabi of Japan published an atlas of arthroscopy.

1957 The term 'atralgesia', a process of induction of general analgesia as opposed to general anesthesia, was proposed by J.T. Hayward-Butt.

1957 An increase in fibrinogen degradation products in the blood was first observed by H. Stormorken.

1958 Pleural dialysis as a treatment for uremia was introduced by V. Gorlitzer, B. DeMorais and J. Hamburger.

1958 Cyclophosphamide was introduced into therapeutics by Herbert Arnold and co-workers.

1958 The first success of greisofulvin against fungal infection in humans was recorded by James Clark Gentles at Kings College Hospital, London.

1958 Edward D. Freis and colleagues published their findings on treatment of essential hypertension with chlorothiazide, which had less side-effects than previous drugs.

Edward D. Freis

1958 The Karolinska Hospital in Sweden applied the first generator implant for cardiac pacing.

1958 American biochemists and geneticists, George Wells Beadle, Joshua Lederberg and Edward Laurie Tatum, were awarded the Nobel Prize for Physiology or Medicine for their work on the role of genes in biochemical processes.

1958 Williams and Spencer used hypothermia to treat patients who sustained neurological damage following cardiac arrest.

1958 The repair of aneurysms using elastic dacron in modern arterial surgery was introduced by D. Emerick Szilagyi

1958 The acid perfusion test (Bernheim test) to differentiate esophageal pain from angina pectoris was devised by L.M. Bernheim and L.A. Baker.

1958 Transduction, basic to genetic engineering, was discovered by American geneticist, Joshua Lederberg, who shared the Nobel Prize in this year for his discovery.

1958 Zieve syndrome, jaundice, hyerlipidemia, fatty liver and hemolytic anemia related to alcohol intake, was described by American physician, Leslie Zieve.

1958 A simple endobronchial tube with a short bronchial cuff which could be placed in the left main bronchus so as to allow the collapse of the right lung and also allow free drainage was devised by R. Machray.

1958 Hairy cell leukemia was first described by B.A. Bouroncle, B.K. Wiseman and C.A. Doan.

1958   Mason Sones developed a method of opacifying coronary arteries for coronary angiograms, and recorded the images on a cine film.

1958   The first butyrophone, haloperidol, was introduced as a neuroleptic drug.

1958   Cardiopneumopexy or suture of the lung on to the heart, after removal of the pericardium, as treatment for coronary artery insufficiency was performed on 19 patients by F.R. Smith and colleagues at Seattle.

1958   Massive liver necrosis following halothane anesthesia was reported by R. Virtue and K.W. Payne.

1959   Left heart catheterisation through a puncture of the interatrial septum was performed by John Ross and coworkers at the National Heart Institute at Bethesda. They used a wide-bore catheter with a long needle through the inferior vena cava to reach the right atrium.

1959   An extensive and comprehensive study of the role of hereditary factors in predisposition to cancer of the breast in women was done by M.T. Macklin.

1959   A double-lumen endobronchial tube (Bryce-Smith tube) to conform to the anatomical shape of trachea and left bronchus was devised in England by R. Bryce Smith.

1959   The term 'neurolepsis' was coined by J. Delay, and J. De Castro and P. Mundeleer used the term 'neurolept analgesia' in the same year.

1959   Cardiac and renal involvement with pneumonia due to a virus (Lassa fever) was named after Lassa in Nigeria where the disease was first described.

1959   Hypoproteinemia due to loss of proteins through the gastrointestinal mucosa following a variety of diseases (protein losing enteropathy) was reported by Robert S. Gordon in *The Lancet*.

1959   American biochemist and geneticists, Arthur Kornberg and Severo Ochoa, were awarded the Nobel Prize for Physiology or Medicine for their work in elucidating the genetic code.

1959   Ferdinand Perutz elucidated hemoglobin's tetrahedral structure of four separate polypeptide chains, with four heme groups near the surface of the molecule.

1959   Polish chemist from Cracow, Sternbach, synthesized diazepam (Valium).

1959   Autohypnosis was pioneered by Maher-Loughman and Macdonald in London as a new form of asthma treatment, essentially preventive and consisting of self hypnosis.

1959   F. Mason Sones of Cleveland and Charles T. Dotter of Oregon devised a method of selectively visualizing coronary arteries by inserting a catheter into a major artery and passing it into the mouth of the coronary artery before injecting radio-opaque dye.

1959   Edward Donnell Thomas carried out entire body irradiation of leukemia patients, followed by marrow transfusion.

1959   The first recordings of electrical activity of the atrioventricular bundle in humans were made by Brian Hoffman.

1959   A preparation of cholecystokinin, which produced contraction of the gallbladder after intravenous administration, was made by J.E. Morpes and V. Mutt.

1960   Hungarian physicist and physiologist, Georg von Békésy, suggested the idea of implanting a miniature prosthesis in the inner ear or cochlea to overcome deafness.

1960   The first large series of cardiac resuscitation in 20 patients by American electrical engineer, William B. Kouwenhoven of Johns Hopkins University, and J. R. Jude and G. G. Knickerbocker. The following year they reported 24% long-term survival out of a total of 118 patients, and their results led to widespread use of external cardiac compression.

1960   The first subtotal parathyroidectomy for hyperparathyroidism secondary to uremia and renal failure was performed by S.W. Stanbury.

1960   The first flap valve was used in artificial heart studies by F.H. Ellis.

1960   The antibiotic, fusidic acid, was obtained from *Fusidium coccineum*, from monkey dung in Japan.

William B Kouwenhoven

1960   Erythrocytosis in polycystic kidneys was described by C. W. Gurney.

1960   The use of methotrexate and cyclophosphamide in the treatment of Burkitt lymphoma (a viral cancer) was introduced by Denis Parsons Burkitt of Enniskellen, Northern Ireland.

1960   George Mathe, at the Cancer and Immunogenetic Research Institute near Paris, pioneered the application of bone marrow transplantation for leukemia.

1960   The peak flow meter for clinical monitoring in asthma was introduced.

1960   The selective uptake of norepinephrine by sympathetic nerves was demonstrated, with the use of radioactive tracers, by Julius Axelrod of the American National Institute of Health.

1960   A progressive neurological disorder accompanied by postural hypotension, rigidity and tremor (Shy–Drager syndrome) was described by two American neurologists, George Milton Shy and Glen A. Drager.

1960   The existence of messenger RNA was confirmed by French biochemists, François Jacob and Jacques Lucien Monod of Paris in the *Journal of Molecular Biology*.

1960   The thalidomide tragedy led to governments insisting on formal drug safety and effectiveness testing before granting a product license.

1960   South Africans, C.A. Sleggs, P. Marchand and I.C. Wagner, recognized a definite association between exposure to asbestos and mesothelioma.

1960   American endocrinologist, Fuller Abright, noted the association between renal calculi and hyperparathyroidism.

1960   The clonal theory of antibody production and theories of immunological tolerance were developed by Sir Frank Macfarlane Burnet of Australian and British immunologist, Sir Peter Brian Medawar, which earned them the Nobel Prize. Burnet also identified the causative rickettsial organism in Q fever, *Coxiella burnetti*.

1960   The oral contraceptive pill became available to women.

1960   M.E. Hodes and colleagues published their preliminary results on using vincaleukoblastine (obtained from the Madagascar periwinkle) in treatment of leukemias. This later led to the development of vincristine, a powerful drug in such diseases.

1960   The clinical effectiveness in patients with post-encephalitic parkinsonism of L-Dopa was demonstrated by British neurologist, Oliver Sacks.

1960   Seymour Benzer, Alfred Day Hershey, Salvador Edward Luria and Max Delbruck established a group using bacteriophage as an experimental tool.

1961   Total hip replacement was performed by British orthopedic surgeon Sir John Charnley of the Manchester Royal Infirmary.

1961   A familial condition of medullary carcinoma of the thyroid, parathyroid adenoma and pheochromocytoma (Sipple syndrome) was described by American respiratory physiologist, John H. Sipple.

1961   The immunological nature of the thymus was demonstrated by French-born Australian immunologist, Jacques Albert Francis Pierre Miller.

1961   Application of ultrasonography for fetal examination in utero was first used by Ian Donald, professor of obstetrics at Glasgow University.

1961   A synthetic compound with anti-tuberculous activity in mice (ethambutol) was discovered by J.P Thomas and co-workers in America.

1961 Hungarian-born American physicist and physiologist, Georg von Békésy, was awarded the Nobel Prize for Physiology or Medicine for his work on hearing.

1961 The drug levadopa was successfully used in treatment of parkinsonism.

1961 The first attempt to prepare erythropoietin from renal tissue in vitro was made by Englishman, D.G. Pennington, who explained its role in the pathogenesis of anemia due to chronic renal failure.

1962 J. Berger and R. Duchinsky introduced flucytosine, the first synthesized antifungal agent.

1962 Thorpe and Waring developed one of the first cholesterol reducing drugs, atromid, or clofibrate.

1962 Bone scanning (radionuclide scintigraphy of the skeleton) was pioneered in orthopedic surgeon, C.H. Baur of Stockholm.

1962 The measles vaccine was developed by American bacteriologist and Nobel Prize winner, John Franklin Enders of Connecticut.

1962 Pulmonary disease due to exposure to cobalt or tungsten was described by A.O. Bech and M.D. Kipling.

1962 English molecular biologists, Francis Compton Crick, James Dewey Watson and the physicist, Maurice Hugh Frederick Wilkins were awarded the Nobel Prize for Physiology or Medicine for their work on the double helix structure of the DNA molecule.

1962 Increased mortality from asthma was found to be due to over-use of isoprenaline, which can seriously affect heart rhythms.

1962 Gastric parietal cell antibodies were demonstrated in nearly 80% of patients with pernicious anemia by K.B. Taylor and co-workers.

1962 Radical surgical management of scoliosis, using long metal rods placed deep in the muscle, was described by Harrington of Houston, Texas.

1962 The Royal College of Physicians of England issued a significant report on the dangers of tobacco, and rise in carcinoma of the bronchus as a result.

1962 G.G. Glenner and P. Berdal gave independent accounts of carotid body tumors secreting catecholamines.

1962 B. Lowen and R. Amarasingham developed a direct current capacitor capable of depolarizing the myocardium transthoracically.

1962 The use of lasers in medicine was made possible with the invention of a microlaser of 2.5 microns in diameter, by a Frenchman, Marcel Bessis.

1962 The antibiotic, Lincomycin, was obtained from *Streptomyces lincolnensis*, from soil in Lincoln, Nebraska.

1962   James Black and J.S. Stephenson published their pharmacological results on a 'new adrenergic beta-receptor blocking compound' (propranolol), designed specifically for angina and hypertensive patients.

1962   Rachel Carson published *Silent Spring* showing the effects of pesticides on wildlife. This led to a reduction in pesticide use and the banning of DDT.

1962   The first use of synthetic grafts during repair of congenital heart disease was by W. Klinner, M. Pasini and A. Schandig.

1962   A modification of Potts operation for tetralogy of Fallot, by anastomosing the ascending aorta and pulmonary artery was devised by David Waterston of Edinburgh.

1963   The New York Heart Association Functional Classification for patients with cardiac disease was proposed.

1963   The value of alternate-day glucocorticoid therapy in minimizing adrenal suppression was established by J.G. Harter and colleagues.

1963   The first report of the use of intravenous diazepam was given by H.H. Farb. He used it as a premedication for an interview in psychiatry.

1963   Arterial embolectomy through a balloon catheter was devised by Thomas Fogarty and colleagues.

1963   Lyman W. Smith of North Western Medical School, Chicago first used chymopapain to dissolve the nucleus pulposus of the intervertebral disc. He also pioneered use of ceramic plaster as a substitute for bone.

1963   Intrauterine transfusion of the fetus was pioneered by Albert William Liley of England.

1963   Frank J. Dixon discovered the role of antigen–antibody complexes in disease.

1963   The antibiotic, Gentamycin, was obtained from *Microspora purpurea*, from soil in Syracuse, New York.

1963   Joseph Murray and colleagues at the Brigham Hospital reported on the success of kidney transplants using the immunosuppressive drug, azathioprine.

1963   A report was published by the Shanghai Sixth People's Hospital on the first hand transplantation, on a 27-year-old man who subsequently became a table tennis champion!

1963   The American Heart Association ad hoc committee on dietary fat and atherosclerosis published a report on dietary fat and its relation to heart disease and stroke suggesting that a reduction in fat in the diet could reduce the incidence of heart disease but stating that there was 'no final proof' of the association.

1963   Anti-lymphocyte globulin was used experimentally to prolong the survival of transplanted skin allografts by M.F.A. Woodruff and A. Anderson.

1963 Hepatitis, encephalopathy and multi-organ failure in children following an acute mild illness (Reye syndrome) was described by an Australian physician of German origin, Ralph Douglas Reye.

Ralph Douglas Reye

1963 A method of applying electrodes through the vagina to record fetal electroencephalography was described by E. Huhner and P.A. Javinen.

1963 Molds and anti-*Thermosopora* IgG antibodies as a cause of farmer's lung were discovered by American microbiologist, Jack Pepys.

1963 Hypohyperparathyroidism, a condition of hypocalcemia, hyperphosphatemia and radiological bone changes in a girl patient, was described by J.M. Costello and C.E. Dent.

1963 A. Fleckenstein named calcium antagonists, a family of vasodilators which mimic the cardiac effects of calcium withdrawal.

1963 The first kidney transplantation was performed.

1963 Allan Macleod Cormack, a South African-born physicist, developed mathematical principles for the X-ray imaging of 'soft' biological tissue and confirmed its viability experimentally. He showed that by combining X-ray images it was possible to build up a picture of a slice through soft tissue.

1963 The operon, that coordinates expression from DNA to messenger RNA, was discovered and named by Frenchmen, François Jacob, Jacques Monod and Sydney Brenner.

1963 Australian neurophysiologist, Sir John Carew Eccles, English physiologists, Sir Alan Lloyd Hodgkin and Sir Andrew Fielding Huxley were awarded the Nobel Prize for Physiology or Medicine for their work on transmission of nerve impulses.

1964 C.T. Dotter and Melvin P. Judkins relieved atherosclerotic intraluminal obstruction of the iliofemoral arteries using a percutaneous catheter (angioplasty).

1964 A flexible fiber optic esophagoscope was described by P.A. LoPresti and A.M. Hilmi.

1964 The causative organism of infectious mononucleosis (Epstein–Barr virus) was discovered by London microbiologist, Sir Michael Anthony Epstein and Yvonne M. Barr.

414

1964   Heavy chain disease (HCD) was first described by Berlin-born American physician, E.C. Franklin and co-workers, in the *American Journal of Medicine*.

1964   Use of azathioprine for rheumatoid arthritis was reported by G.J. Galens and colleagues.

1964   Romano–Ward syndrome, an autosomal dominant disease with syncope, malignant ventricular arrhythmias and prolonged QT interval in the ECG, was described by O.C. Ward in the *Journal of Indian Medical Association*. C. Romano described it in the *Lancet* in 1965.

1964   A familial disorder consisting of hyperuricemia, choreoathetosis, mental retardation, cerebral palsy and compulsive self-mutilation (Lesch–Nyhan syndrome) was described by New York physician, Michael Lesch and William L. Nyhan.

1964   The previously unknown lipoprotein, Australia antigen, was detected by New York biochemist Baruch Samuel Blumberg.

1964   The importance of the house dust bug (*Dermatophagoides pteronyssinus*) in asthma was discovered by Voorhorst and colleagues in Holland.

1964   German-born American biochemist, Konrad Emil Bloch and German biochemist, Feodor Felix Konrad Lynen were awarded the Nobel Prize for Physiology or Medicine for their work on cholesterol.

1964   The US Surgeon General reported a rise in lung cancer as a result of growing cigarette consumption.

1964   John Hopewell and colleagues at the Royal Free Hospital published their results of kidney transplantations using the immunosuppressive drug, 6-mercaptopurine.

1964   Michael Hamilton and Eileen Thompson of the Chelmsford Hospital published their assessment of the role of blood pressure control in preventing the complications of hypertension.

1964   A failed attempt to carry out the first cardiac transplant with a xenograft (from a chimpanzee) was made by James Daniel Hardy.

1964   Pentazocaine, a narcotic analgesic and derivative of benzmorphinan, was first described by A.S. Keats and J.J. Telford.

1964   Antibodies to histones in patients with systemic lupus erythematosus were discovered by H.G. Kunkel and colleagues.

1965   The Barthel index for assessing daily activities was proposed by F.I. Mahony and D.W. Barthel.

1965   Prophylactic oophorectomy and ovarian radiation in breast carcinoma was first carried out by R. Nissen-Meyer.

1965   S. O. Freedman and P. Gold demonstrated the presence of tumor-specific antigens in human colonic cancer, through immunological and absorption techniques.

1965 Important studies by Burrows, Niden, Fletcher and Jones in London elucidated the respective roles of emphysema and chronic bronchitis in the development of airway obstruction in patients.

1965 Glutathione reductase deficiency, a cause of hemolytic anemia, was described by H.D. Waller, G.W. Lohr and Zysno Gerok.

1965 Lupoid hepatitis, active chronic hepatitis accompanied by markers of autoimmune disease, was described by I.R. Mackay, S. Weiden and J. Hasker.

1965 The effect of estrogen therapy in preventing atherosclerosis and osteoporosis in postmenopausal hormone replacement therapy (HRT), was first pointed out by Morris E. Davis.

1965 F. Avery Jones introduced carbinoxolone as a treatment for gastric ulcers.

1965 French biochemist, François Jacob and French microbiologist, André Lwoff were awarded the Nobel Prize for Physiology or Medicine for their work on the operon theory of DNA, the structure of genes, and virus synthesis.

1965 G.H. Green intensified the use of routine cytological examination for early detection of cervical carcinoma and preinvasive lesions.

1965 The role of acetylcholine in the transmission of nerve impulses was demonstrated by English physiologist, Wilhelm Siegmund Feldberg and British pharmacologist, Sir John Henry Gaddum.

1965 Barnett Rosenberg of Michigan State University discovered cisplatin, a dissolved form of platinum later shown to interfere with DNA prior to cell division, and effective in treatment of tumors of the ovary or testis.

1965 The loss of bone substance leading to spontaneous fractures secondary to long-term therapy with heparin, was first shown by G.C. Griffith and colleagues.

1966 Mitochondrial antibodies were demonstrated in 98% of patients with primary biliary cirrhosis, 31% with cryptogenic cirrhosis, and 28% with active chronic hepatitis, by Deborah Doniach.

1966 Sydney Farber and colleagues published their results on use of the antibiotic, actinomycin C, to treat Wilms tumor. This was later found to be effective in treating several other types of cancer.

1966 Increased risk of ischemic heart disease amongst the first degree relatives of those affected was established by J. Slack and K.A. Evans.

1966 The respiratory disease bagassosis was diagnosed using the precipitin reaction by Salvaggio and Seabury.

1966 Canadian-born American surgeon, Charles Brenton Huggins and American pathologist, Francis Peyton Rous were awarded the Nobel Prize for Physiology or

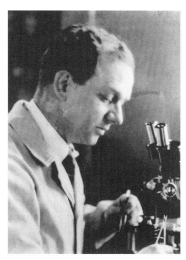

Francis Peyton Rous

Medicine for their work on cancer and its treatment.

1966   American, P.H. McDermott noted tachycardia, hepatomegaly, marked edema and enlarged heart in men who drink excessive amounts of beer (beer drinker disease).

1966   A characteristic soluble nuclear antigen (Sm antigen) in a patient called Smith was discovered by E.M. Tan and H.G. Kunkel, and found to be specific to patients with systemic lupus erythematosus.

1966   Use of ketamine in obstetric anesthesia was proposed by P. Chodoff and J. G. Stella.

1966   Spontaneous regression of certain cancers was observed and studied by Warren H. Cole.

1967   Prostaglandin receptors were found by V.R. Pickles.

1967   The first allotransplantation of the pancreas and duodenum, along with the kidney, in a case of diabetic nephropathy, was performed by W.D. Kelly and colleagues.

1967   The first pediatric heart transplant, from an anencephalic infant to a 3-week-old with cyanotic heart disease, was performed by A. Kantrowitz and colleagues at the Maimonides Downstate Medical Center, New York. The infant survived for over 6 hours after the procedure.

1967   The medical commission of the International Olympic Committee was established with a mandate to test for drugs in athletes.

1967   A description of a muscle relaxant in anesthesia, pancuronium or pavulon, was given by W.L.M. Baird and A.M. Reid.

1967   The founder of coronary artery bypass surgery, G. Rene Favaloro from La Plata, Argentina, performed the first coronary artery bypass on a woman.

1967   The work of Jean Baptiste Gabriel Dausset in the field of skin grafting, led to the procedure of tissue typing which greatly reduced the number of rejection reactions.

1967   Marburg disease, an acute febrile illness with high mortality similar to that caused by Ebola virus, was reported from Marburg in Germany.

1967   G.C. Rastelli and D.C. McGoon performed a successful operation for truncus arteriosis.

1967   Finnish-born Swedish physiologist, Ragnar Arthur Granit, American physiologist, Haldan Keffer Hartline and American biochemist, George Wald were awarded the Nobel Prize for Physiology or Medicine for their work on neurophysiology of vision.

1967   Patrick Steptoe published a monograph, *Laproscopy in Gynaecology*, which led to his partnership with Geoffrey Edwards in developing in vitro fertilization of human embryos.

1967   The term 'sick sinus syndrome' was coined by American cardiologist, Bernard Lown, who came across this condition when the sinus node failed to function after cardioversion for atrial fibrillation.

1967   DiGeorge syndrome, characterized by congenital absence of the thymus and parathyroid glands leading to recurrent infection, was described by American pediatrician, Angelo Mario DiGeorge.

1967   Intal (disodium cromoglycate) was discovered and first used in the United Kingdom by Roger Altounyan.

1967   German professor of gynecology at Jena, Ferdinand Frankenhauser, described the cervical sympathetic ganglion of the uterus.

1967   The first human heart transplant was performed in Cape Town by South African Christiaan Neethling Barnard.

1968   A modern technique of using an open skull flap in prefrontal leucotomy was used on patients at the combined neurosurgical unit of King's College, Guy's Hospital and Maudsley Hospital.

1968   A device for delivering precise radiation to brain tumors using cobalt-60 (Gamma helmet) was invented by Swedish physicists, Lars Leksell and Bjorn Larsson.

1968   Dizziness and the sensation of burning in the face and chest due to monosodium glutamate used in food (Chinese restaurant syndrome) was described by R.H.M. Kwok, in the *New England Journal of Medicine*.

1968   Halo traction for skeletal fixation of the injured spine was devised by Vernon L. Nickel, professor of orthopedics at the University of California, San Diego.

1968   Early experimental work on biofeedback mechanisms was carried out by N.E. Miller.

1968   The World Health Organization defined 'cardiomyopathy' as a condition involving the heart muscle, normally of unknown etiology, with cardiomegaly and heart failure.

1968   The first prenatal diagnosis of Down syndrome through amniocentesis was made.

1968   American biochemists, Robert William Holley and Marshall Warren Nirenberg, and Indian-born American molecular chemist, Har Gobind Khorana were awarded the Nobel Prize for

Physiology or Medicine for their work on the genetic code and amino acid synthesis.

1968   Naturally occurring opiate-like analgesic substances in the body (enkephalins) were discovered and named by German biochemist, Hans Walther Kosterlitz.

1969   An artificial heart made of silastic was inserted successfully into a calf.

1969   G.A. Kaiser introduced pig aortic valves fixed with glutaraldehyde in the evolution of artificial heart valve studies.

1969   A vaccine for hepatitis was introduced by American biochemist, Baruch Samuel Blumberg.

1969   Pre-natal diagnosis of Down syndrome was achieved.

1969   German biophysicist, Max Delbrück, American biologists, Alfred Day Hershey and Salvador Edward Luria were awarded the Nobel Prize for Physiology or Medicine for their work on viral genetics.

1969   The first successful in vitro fertilization of human gametes was carried out by Robert Geoffrey Edwards and Patrick Christopher Steptoe.

1969   Use was made of B and T lymphocytes by Ivan. M. Roitt of Middlesex Hospital Medical School, London and his colleagues.

1970   Multiple drug resistance in cancer therapy was first described by J.L. Biedler and H. Riehm.

1970   The term 'genetic engineering' coined by R.J.C. Harris.

1970   Suppressor lymphocytes of the immune system (T cells) were identified and described by Richard K. Gerson.

1970   Howard A. Temin published a paper on RNA-dependent DNA preliminaries in virions of Rous sarcoma virus.

1970   The use of a flow-directed balloon tip for cardiac catheterization (Swan–Ganz catheter) was devised by Harold James Charles Swan and William Ganz.

1970   IgE antibodies were identified in serum by Kimshige Ishizaka and co-workers in Denver, Colorado.

1970   The first neonatal intensive care unit was opened.

1970   David Baltimore of New York, announced his discovery of the enzyme reverse transcriptase which can transcribe RNA into DNA

Kimshige and Terry Ishizaka

419

without the involvement of DNA. The newly-formed viral DNA integrates into the infected host cell which may then be transformed into a cancer cell.

1970 Rifampicin was introduced for the treatment of tuberculosis.

1970 American pharmacologist, Julius Axelrod, British biophysicist, Sir Bernard Katz and Swedish pharmacologist, Ulf Svante von Euler were awarded the Nobel Prize for Physiology or Medicine for their work on the role and mechanism of action of neurotransmitters.

1971 A cure for the childhood cancer, acute lymphoblastic leukemia, was found by Donald Pinkel of St Jude's Hospital, Memphis. He used combined chemotherapy and radiotherapy.

1971 British biochemist and Nobel laureate, John Vane, showed that aspirin blocked the prostaglandin, thromboxane, which is responsible for blood platelet coagulation, and this was how aspirin was effective in preventing strokes.

1971 The report of the Yarborough Commission formed the basis of the 1971 National Cancer Act, signed by President Richard Nixon on 23 December. The aim of the Act was to make 'the conquest of cancer a national crusade'. Its initial allocation was 500 million dollars.

1971 American biochemist, Earl Wilbur Sutherland Jr was awarded the Nobel Prize for Physiology or Medicine for his work on cyclic AMP as a second messenger for many hormones.

1972 An association between smoking in pregnancy with smaller babies and higher perinatal mortality was shown by several group of workers including N.R. Butler, H. Goldstein and E.M. Ross.

1972

Map showing prevalence of Lyme disease
(courtesy of the National Institutes of Health)

The first few cases of recurrent polyarthritis (Lyme arthritis) were recorded in Old Lyme and Lyme communities of Connecticut.

1972 The British Association of Surgical Oncology was established, with Ronal W. Raven as its first president.

1972 An ultrasonic device to fragment kidney stones without causing bleeding (lithotripter) was invented by two Germans, Eisenberger and Chaussey in Munich.

1972 American biochemist, Gerald Maurice Edelman and British biochemist, Rodney Robert Porter were awarded the Nobel Prize for Physiology or Medicine for their work on antibody structure of human immunoglobulin.

1973 The late phase mechanisms of allergy were shown to be IgE mediated by J. Dolovich and colleagues.

1973 The protective property of omega-3 fatty acids against coronary heart disease, found fish, seal and whale meat consumed by Eskimos, was studied by J. Dyerberg and H.O. Bang.

1973 Isolation of cyclic endoperoxidase, an intermediate in prostaglandin synthesis, was made independently by M. Hamberg and D.H. Nugteren.

1973 'Cheese washer lung', an allergic condition due to *Penicillium caesi* spores in workers who removed mold from the surface of mature cheese, was described in Switzerland by Schlueter.

1973 Nobel laureate, Stanley N. Cohen and colleague, published a paper on construction of biologically functional bacterial plasmids.

1973 Elizabeth Stern of Canada reported a link between cervical cancer and the prolonged use of the contraceptive pill, which is associated with an increase in the incidence of cervical dysplasia.

1973 Computerized axial tomography (CAT) was invented by Sir Godfrey Newbold Hounsfield and Allan Macleod Cormack, in England and America independently.

1973 Austrian zoologists and ethologists, Karl von Frisch, Konrad Zacharias Lorenz and Dutch ethologist, Nikolaas Tinbergen were awarded the Nobel Prize for Physiology or Medicine for their work on animal behavior and adaptation to the environment.

1973 Further advances in work on enkephalins were made by American psychiatrist, Solomon Halbert Snyder, who demonstrated the presence of opiate receptors in nervous tissue.

1973 The first significant human leukocyte antigen (HLA) association with disease was found.

1974 A single assembly total prosthesis for hip replacement was introduced by Canadian surgeon, James Ennis Bateman of Toronto.

1974 Belgian-born American biologist, Albert Claude, English-born Belgian biochemist, Christian René du Duve and Romanian cell biologist, George Emil Palade were warded the Nobel Prize for Physiology or Medicine for their work on the substructure and biochemistry of cells.

1974 The first possible transmission of Creutzfeldt–Jacob disease from human to human was noted.

1975 Monoclonal antibodies were produced by an Argentinean-born immunologist, Cesar Milstein, while he was working at the Medical Research Council Laboratory of Molecular Biology in England.

1975   A spring loading device for skeletal fixation of the injured spinal cord was introduced by Marian Weiss from Poland.

1975   Southern blotting involving restriction digestion of the DNA and separation of its fragments by electrophoresis was invented by E.M. Southern. The same procedure applied to RNA is known as northern blotting. A similar procedure for identification of proteins is known as western blotting.

1975   American molecular biologist, David Baltimore, Italian virologist, Renato Dulbecco and American virologist, Howard Martin Temin were awarded the Nobel Prize for Physiology or Medicine for their work on viral genetics, reverse transcriptase, and the role of viruses in cancer.

1975   A WHO survey showed that death rates from breast cancer had not declined since 1900 and it was realized that surgery alone was not the answer.

1975   Robert Michael described the existence of calcium channels in cells.

1976   Increased risk of malignancy in coeliac disease was described by G.K.T. Holmes and colleagues.

1976   American biochemist, Baruch Samuel Blumberg and American virologist, Daniel Carleton Gajdusek were awarded the Nobel Prize for Physiology or Medicine for their work on the hepatitis B encephalopathy viruses, respectively.

1977   Lyme arthritis, characterized by short, recurrent attacks of asymmetric oligo-articular pain and swelling of the large joints, was reported by Steer, Malarista and Syndman in the *American Journal Arthritis and Rheumatism.*

1977   *Influenza: The Last Great Plague*, was written by William Ian Beadmore Beveridge, professor of anatomy and pathology at Cambridge University.

1977   The first scientific account of the Legionnaire disease epidemic in Philadelphia was given by David William Fraser who named the bacterium *Legionella*.

1977   J.F. Borel published his results on organ transplantation using the new immunosuppressant drug, cyclosporine, which markedly increased survival rates.

1977   Axel Ullrich published a paper on rat insulin genes: construction of plasmids containing the coding sequences.

1977   American pharmacologist, Ferid Murad, of Houston, analyzed how nitroglycerin and related vasodilating compounds act and discovered that they release nitric oxide which relaxes smooth muscle cells.

1977   H. Mohler and T. Okada showed that the tranquilizer, benzodiazeprine, acted on the neurotransmitter, GABA.

1977   French-born American physiologist, Roger Guillemin, Polish-born American biochemist, Andrew

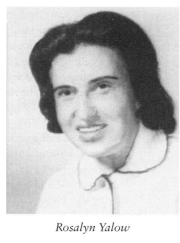

Rosalyn Yalow

Victor Schally and American biophysicist, Rosalyn Yalow were awarded the Nobel Prize for Physiology or Medicine for their work on the endocrine system.

1977 Aberration of the X chromosome was identified in Duchenne-type muscular dystrophy in a young girl by C. Verellen and coworkers.

1977 Living donors were used for the first time for pancreatic transplants at the University of Minnesota.

1977 Purified pneumococcal vaccine was used in immune compromised states such as splenectomy.

1977 Cyproterone acetate was used in the treatment of prostatic carcinoma by D.Y. Wang and R.D. Bulbrook.

1977 Erythropoietin was purified by T. Miyake and colleagues.

1978 The effectiveness and safety of captopil, an angiotensin convert-

ing enzyme inhibitor, in the treatment of hypertension in humans was demonstrated by H. Ondetti and colleagues.

1978 The efficacy of angiotensin converting enzyme inhibitor in the treatment of congestive heart failure, demonstrated by H. Gavras and colleagues.

1978 The term toxic shock to describe multisystem disease in seven children was first applied by J. Todd and colleagues.

1978 The cancer suppresser P53 gene was first observed by David Lane, a professor of oncology.

1978 English gynecologist and obstetrician, Patrick Christopher Steptoe and Robert Geoffrey Edwards achieved the first birth of a 'test-tube baby'.

1978 Harold Hopkins, an optical physicist, published a chapter on his invention of the modern urological endoscope, a modification of the Leitz cystoscope.

1978 American developmental geneticist, Edward B. Lewis, published his results on fruit fly genetics and mutations, in *Nature*. These results suggested mechanisms of development relevant to all organisms and pointed to causes for congenital deformities.

1978 American biologist, Daniel Nathans, shared the Nobel Prize for Physiology or Medicine with Hamilton Orthaniel Smith, a microbiologist from New York, and Werner Arber, a microbiologist from Switzerland, for their production of the first genetic map (of the SV40 virus).

1978 The argon laser, used in ophthalmology, was developed by a Frenchman, Gabriel J. Coscas.

1979 Percutaneous transluminal dilatation of stenozed renal arteries was performed as treatment for renal hypertension by Andreas R. Gruentzig and co-workers.

1979 Basil Hirschowitz published 'A personal history of the fiberscope', and published a monograph on its use since his early development of the instrument, a year later.

1979 South African-born American physicist, Allan Macleod Cormack and English electrical engineer, Sir Geoffrey Newbold Hounsfield were awarded the Nobel Prize for Physiology or Medicine for their development of computerized axial X-ray tomography scanning.

1979 WHO Global Commission document signed declaring the eradication of smallpox.

1979 Percutaneous transluminal coronary angioplasty was introduced by Andreas R. Gruentzig and W.E. Siegothaler.

1980 The Uniform Determination of Death Act was proposed by the Commission on Uniform State Laws. It stated that an individual who has sustained either irreversible cessation of circulatory and respiratory functions, or irreversible cessation of all the functions of the entire brain, including the brain stem, is dead.

1980 Epiphysitis of the calcaneus (Sever disease) described by a Boston Surgeon, James Warren Sever.

1980 The International Pancreas Transplant Registry was founded.

1980 German developmental geneticists, Christiane Nüsslein-Volhard and Eric F. Wieschaus published their results on fruit fly genetics in *Nature*. They examined and found that about 5,000 of the fly's 20,000 genes are important to embryonic development and about 140 are essential.

1980 The successful cloning of the human interferon gene and production of interferon in bacteria was achieved by Charles Weissmann from the University of Zurich.

1980 American pharmacologist, Robert F. Furchgott, of New York, suggested that blood vessels are dilated because the endothelial cells produce an unknown signal molecule that makes vascular smooth muscle cells relax. He called this the endothelium-derived relaxing factor (EDRF).

1980 The lack of receptors that bind LDL in cells of patients with familial hypercholesterolemia was noted by American molecular geneticists, Michael Stuart Brown of New York, and Joseph Leonard Goldstein of South Carolina.

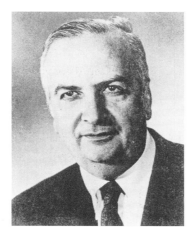

Baruj Benacerraf

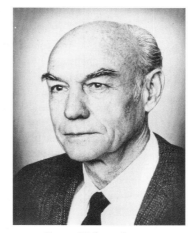

Roger Wolcott Sperry

1980   Heinrich Rohrer and Gerd Karl Binnig developed the first tunneling electron microscope.

1980   David Bottstein published a paper on construction of a genetic linkage map in man using restriction fragment-length polymorphisms.

1980   Samuel Epstein of the University of Illinois published a paper in *Nature* on environmental pollution and cancer, 'The fallacies of lifestyle cancer theories'.

1980   Data were published suggesting that heart disease was falling as a cause of death but that intake of fats had not changed. It was suggested that a reduction in infectious disease correlated with the decrease.

1980   Marcus de Wood of the University of Washington performed coronary angiograms on patients immediately after a heart attack and showed blockage of coronary arteries.

1980   Venezuelan–American immunologist, Baruj Benacerraf, shared the Nobel Prize for Physiology or Medicine with French immunologist, Jean Dausset and American geneticist, George Davis Snell for work on immune hypersensitivity, and tissue typing.

1980   David A. Robinson of Manchester identified *Campylobacter jejuni* as a cause of intestinal illness.

1981   Canadian-born American neurophysiologist, David Hunter Hubel, American neuroscientist, Roger Wolcott Sperry and Swedish neurophysiologist, Torsten Nils Wiesel shared the Nobel Prize for Physiology or Medicine for their work on understanding brain nerve function and vision.

1981   Alan Trounson and colleagues in Australia reported on the use of clomiphene in boosting harvestable eggs for in vitro fertilization.

1981   Sir Richard Doll published his authoritative book, *The Causes of Cancer* in which he suggested that 70% of cancers (other than those caused by tobacco) were related to diet.

1981   Frederick Sanger published a paper in *Science* on determination of nucleotide sequences in DNA.

1981   Walter Gilbert published a paper on DNA sequencing and gene structure.

1981   The genetic code for the B surface antigen of hepatitis B was discovered, and led to the production of the first genetically engineered vaccine approved by the US Food and Drugs Admini-stration in 1986.

1981   Uvulopalatopharyngoplasty, removal of the uvula, a portion of the soft palate and redundant tissues from the posterior wall, as treatment for obstructive sleep apnoea, was introduced by S. Fujita and coworkers.

1981   An exotoxin of *Staphylococcus aureus* causing toxic shock syndrome in menstruating women was identified by P.M. Schlievert and coworkers.

1981   Balloon dilatation of stenotic ductus arteriosus was first attempted by R.D. Corwin and coworkers.

1981   Acquired immune deficiency syndrome (AIDS) was recognized as a new disease entity and a full description including opportunistic infections and associated neo-plasms published. The first reports were published in the *Morbidity and Mortality Weekly Report* in June.

1982   Isolation of a new spirochete (*Borrelia burgdorferi*) from an *Ixodes* tick obtained from Staten Island, New York, by Burgdorfer. It was found to be the causative organism of Lyme disease later in the same year.

1982   An artificial heart was successfully transplanted into a human by American, Willem Kolff, keeping the patient alive for 112 hours.

1982   Stanley B. Prusiner, an American neurologist in San Francisco, isolated the scrapie-causing agent, the 'prion', unlike any other known pathogen as it consists only of protein and lacks the genetic material contained necessary for replication.

1982   Insulin was the first genetically engineered hormone to be approved by the FDA, and marketed by Eli Lilly.

1982   Swedish biochemists, Sune Karl Bergström, Bengt Ingemar Samuelsson and English pharmacologist, Sir John Robert Vane were awarded the Nobel Prize for Physiology or Medicine for their work on prostaglandins.

1982   Judy Chang and Yuet Wei Kan of the University of Southern California perfected a technique for diagnosing sickle cell anemia in the unborn fetus, the first prenatal screening test developed.

1983   The blood drawn from the umbilical cord was used for diagnosis of disease in the fetus (fetal diagnosis) by Fernand Daffos.

1983   Antiphospholipid syndrome (Hughes syndrome) Thrombosis, abortion and cerebral disease in the presence of lupus anticoagulant in the blood was described by G.R.V. Hughes in the *British Medical Journal.*

1983   The first genetic marker for Huntington chorea was discovered by James F. Gusella.

1983   J. Robin Warren of the Royal Perth Hospital in Australia observed unidentified curved bacilli (*Helicobacter pylori*) in biopsy specimens for patients with acute gastritis.

1983   The first removal of a gallbladder using laproscopy.

1983   The WHO published results from the Multiple Risk Factor Intervention Trial in which over 50,000 men had been selected and allocated to either intervention or control groups in relation to diet, lifestyle and heart disease in the 1970s. The results showed that death rates from heart disease did not differ between control and intervention groups.

1983   Familial hypertriglyceridemia of autosomal dominant origin was described by H.N. Neufield and U. Goldbourt.

1983   The gene marker for Duchenne muscular dystrophy was discovered by Kay Davies and Robert Williamson.

1983   American geneticist, Barbara McClintock, was awarded the Nobel Prize for Physiology or Medicine for providing the ultimate proof of the theory of heredity, through her work on maize.

1983   A new retrovirus, HIV, was isolated in Paris by a French molecular biologist, Luc Montagnier and colleagues at the Pasteur Institute.

1983   Successful treatment of alpha thalassemia with splenectomy was reported by P.L. de V. Hart and L. Eng.

1984   The first studies were published showing that the number of circulating T4 helper/inducer lymphocytes was markedly reduced in patients with AIDS.

1984   The first use of balloon valvuloplasty (for rheumatic mitral stenosis) was by K. Inoue, T. Owaki and coworkers.

1984   A transvenous catheter to deliver high energy direct electrical current for ablation of the aberrant pathway in Wolff–Parkinson–White syndrome was devised by F. Morady and M.M. Scheinmann.

1984   *Reshaping Life: Key Issues in Genetic Engineering,* was published by Australian immunologist, Sir Gustav Joseph Victor Nossal.

1984   The association between hepatitis B surface antigen and hepatocellular carcinoma was observed by Alfred M. Prince of New York Blood Center.

1984 The first surgery on a fetus before its birth was performed by William H. Clewall, a surgeon from the Colorado Health Sciences Center in Denver.

1984 Danish–English immunologist, Niels Kai Jerne, German immuno-chemist, Georges Jean Franz Köhler and Argentinean-born British molecular biologist, Cesar Milstein were awarded the Nobel Prize for Physiology or Medicine for their work on T-lymphocytes and specific antibody production (leading to modern monoclonal antibody production).

Niels Kai Jerne

1984 Prenatal screening for thalassemia in Cyprus led to a massive decrease in the number of children born with this disease.

1984 The fungus, *Pityrosporum ovale* was shown to be the main cause of dandruff.

1984 Robert Gallo of the National Cancer Institute showed that human immunodeficiency virus was responsible for AIDS, and destroyed the immune system of infected patients.

1984 J.S.H. Gaston suggested that infection may play a role in inflammatory arthritis.

1984 Australian physician, Barry J. Marshall, discovered, through self-experimentation, and identified *Helicobacter pylori* as the cause of gastritis and the probable cause of duodenal ulcers. He also noted remission in patients treated with antibiotics.

1985 The implantable defibrillator was approved by the American Food and Drug Administration.

1985 The gene marker for cystic fibrosis was discovered on chromosome 7.

1985 The presence of antiphospholipid antibodies that predispose patients to thrombotic events was pointed out by H. P. McNeil and co-workers.

1985 American molecular biologists, Michael Stuart Brown and Joseph Leonard Goldstein were awarded the Nobel Prize for Physiology or Medicine for work on cholesterol and low-density lipoproteins (LDL).

1985 Alpha inteferon was shown to have in vitro activity against hepatitis A virus by A. Vallbracht and co-workers.

1985   An automatic implantable cardio-verter–defibrillator was approved by the Food and Drug Administration.

1985   The role of oncogenes in the development of cancer was observed by M. Babacid.

1985   Cloning and expression of human erythropoietin gene was achieved by F.K. Lin and coworkers. Their work led to the therapeutic use of recombinant erythropoietin.

1986   An outbreak of thyrotoxicosis in the mid-western United States was caused by eating hamburger containing ground-beef thyroid.

1986   American biochemist, Stanley Cohen and Italian neuroscientist, Rita Levi-Montalcini were awarded the Nobel Prize for Physiology or Medicine for their work on growth factors.

Stanley Cohen

1986   A tiny television camera was added to the modern laparoscope, making a major advance in keyhole surgery.

1986   A new strain of *Chlamydia* that causes acute respiratory tract infection was discovered by J. Thomas Grayston of the University of Washington.

1986   John F. Kurtzke of Georgetown University School of Medicine in Washington provided evidence that multiple sclerosis was caused by a 'transmissible' agent.

1986   American pharmacologists, Louis J. Ignarro, of Los Angeles, concluded, together with and independently of Robert F. Furchgott, that EDRF was identical to NO. The gas and new drugs based upon it have been used to treat atherosclerosis, to reduce high blood pressure in infants (via inhalation), to treat penile dysfunction, to control artery dilatation and thus control blood pressure and prevent thrombi formation.

1986   Ernst August Friedrich Ruska, the inventor of the electron microscope, shared the Nobel Prize for Physics with two other workers on it, Gerd Karl Binnig and Heinrich Rohrer.

1986   The first series of successful heart transplants in newborns with hypoplastic left heart syndrome was presented by L. Bailey and colleagues.

1987   Single and dual-photon absorptiometry for bone measurement in osteoporosis were described by R.B. Mazess and colleagues.

1987   Evidence that red blood cells can be stored in a frozen state for periods as long as ten years was presented.

1987 Alpha gliadin antibody levels, as a serological test for coeliac disease, was introduced by C. O'Farrelly and colleagues.

1987 Japanese molecular biologist, Susumu Tonegawa was awarded the Nobel Prize for Physiology or Medicine for his work in proving that genes can change to produce a range or new antibodies.

1987 Implanting of cells from the adrenal gland into the brain as treatment was first proposed for treating Parkinson disease by Ignacio Navarro.

1987 The three dimensional structure of the major histocompatibility protein was elucidated by Jack Stromminger and Don Willy.

1987 Thrombolysis drugs were introduced for treatment of heart attack victims.

1987 Joseph Eschbach published a paper on correction of the anemia of end-stage renal disease with recombinant human erythropoietin.

1987 A protein that regulates the passage of calcium ions in and out of muscle cells during contraction and relaxation was identified by Kevin P. Campbell and Roberto Coronado.

1987 The first microscope image using positrons instead of electrons was published by James Van House and Arthur Rich.

1987 The first clinical use of recombinant human granulocyte–macrophage colony stimulating factor, was undertaken in 16 cases of acquired immunodeficiency syndrome with neutropenia, by J.E. Groopman and colleagues.

1987 The first long term follow up of percutaneous coronary angioplasty showing its benefits was done by A.R. Gruentzig and coworkers.

1987 The aphrodisiac yohimbine obtained from the bark of yohimbine tree was shown to be effective in erectile impotence of psychogenic nature by A. Morales and coworkers.

1987 Benefits of alpha inteferon in the treatment of chronic hepatitis C or non-A, non-B hepatitis were shown by J.H. Hoofnagle and coworkers.

1987 Specific synthesis of DNA in vitro via a polymerase catalyzed chain reaction was described by K.B. Mullis and F. Faloona. Their work revolutionized the approach to molecular genetics.

1988 An attempt to apply specific criteria to, and define the illness 'myalgic encephalitis' (ME), was made by G.P. Holmes and coworkers.

1988 The results of a study on intravenous streptokinase, oral aspirin, both or neither, among 17,187 cases of suspected acute myocardial infarction was published in *The Lancet*.

1988   P. Saikku of Finland published a paper in *The Lancet* providing serological evidence of an association of a new strain of *Chlamydia* with chronic heart disease and acute myocardial infarction.

1988   Alvin Feinstein, the editor of the *Journal of Clinical Epidemiology*, published an article on scientific standards in epidemiological studies that suggested there was a need for improvement in methodology.

1988   A. Ebringer published a paper suggesting the involvement of *Klebsiella* and *Proteus* bacteria in ankylosing spondylitis and rheumatoid arthritis, respectively.

1988   Scottish pharmacologist, Sir James Whyte Black, American biochemists, Gertrude Belle Elion and George Herbert Hitchings were awarded the Nobel Prize for Physiology or Medicine for their work on drugs for heart disease, leukemia, the anti-viral drug, acyclovir, and the anti-AIDS drug, zidovudine.

1988   German biophysicist, Robert Huber, shared the Nobel Prize for Chemistry in 1988 with Johann Deisenhofer and Hartmut Michel. He elucidated the antibody structure of the 'light chain' of the antigen binding site, the interaction between trypsin and trypsin inhibitor and studied glutathione peroxidase.

1988   The first primary myocardial disease, familial hypertrophic cardiomyopathy, to have a chromosomal locus for the defect mapped and identified was undertaken by J.A. Jarcho and coworkers.

1989   American molecular biologists and virologists, John Michael Bishop and Harold Elliot Varmus were awarded the Nobel Prize for Physiology or Medicine for their discovery of oncogenes.

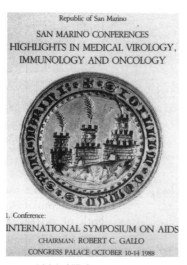

1998 AIDS symposium

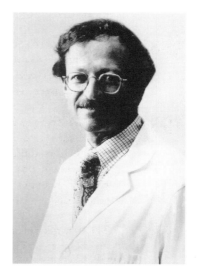

Harold Elliot Varmus

1989 Canadian biologist Sidney Altman, and Thomas Cech shared Nobel Prize for Chemistry for their work on transfer RNA, the amino acid carrier in protein synthesis.

1989 John R. Riodan published a paper on identification of the cystic fibrosis gene.

1990 American surgeon, Joseph Edward Murray and American physician and hematologist, Edward Donnall Thomas were awarded the Nobel Prize for Physiology or Medicine for their work on kidney transplantation.

1990 Thomas Starzl of the Veterans' Administration Hospital in Colorado published a survey of long-term survival of renal homograft patients, half-of whom had survived with immunosuppressive and steroid anti-rejection drugs.

1990 A study of 50 patients with 'intractable' peptic ulcer was published in *The Lancet* showing the effectiveness of antibiotic treatment in producing a cure.

1990 The American Society of Hypertension considered a report by R.S. Tuttle that suggested a role for the immune system and the beta receptor in the etiology and/or prevention of hypertension.

1990 R Michael Blaese undertook the first gene therapy treatment on two sisters with a rare disease, adenosine deaminase deficiency, by injecting them with a disabled virus containing the adenosine deaminase gene.

1990 Alpha inteferon was shown to have in vitro activity against hepatitis B virus, by R. Tur-Kaspa and co-workers.

1990 The first prospective controlled trial of alpha interferon against hepatitis C virus was described by L. Viladomiu and coworkers.

1991 German biophysicist, Erwin Neher and German electrophysiologist, Bert Sakmann were awarded the Nobel Prize for Physiology on Medicine for their work on electrical signals in single ion channels in membranes and development of the patch–clamp method to isolate small sections of membrane.

1992 American biochemists, Edmond Henri Fischer and Edwin Gerhard Krebs were awarded the Nobel Prize for Physiology or Medicine for their work on the role of phosphorylation–dephosphorylation in activation of glycogen phosphorylase by adenylic acid.

1992 The transmissibility of prions to mice, rats and hamsters was demonstrated by Stanley B. Prusiner of San Francisco.

1992 A. Shor and colleagues published a paper on detection of *Chlamydia* in coronary arterial fatty streaks and atheromatous plaques in recently deceased South African miners.

1992 Gary M. Williams and George T. Baker published a paper on the potential relationship between ageing and cancer showing that the risk of cancer increased substantially with age.

1993 British molecular biologist working in the USA, Richard Roberts and American molecular biologist, Phillip Allen Sharp were awarded the Nobel Prize for Physiology or Medicine for their work on introns in DNA (sections which do not contain any genetic information).

1993 The symptoms of chronic fatigue syndrome or 'myalgic encephalitis' (ME) were shown to be due to general fatigue rather than a myalgic disorder by R.H.T. Edwards and colleagues.

1993 British–Canadian biochemist Michael Smith, shared the Nobel Prize for Chemistry with Kary Banks Mullis for their work on site-specific mutagenesis, now used in altering the genetic code of organisms to produce useful proteins.

1993 The Eurogast Study Group provided results linking *Helicobacter pylori* with two thirds of stomach cancers.

1994 The first breast cancer gene, BRCA1 was identified.

1994 American pharmacologist, Alfred Goodman Gilman, shared the Nobel Prize for Physiology or Medicine with American biochemist, Martin Rodbell for their work on G proteins, intermediates in the pathway of cells in response to incoming signals.

1995 American developmental geneticist, Edward B. Lewis, shared the Nobel Prize for Physiology or Medicine with German developmental geneticist, Christiane Nüsslein-Volhard, and American developmental biologist, Eric F. Wieschaus, for their work on the functions that control early embryonic development.

1995 An internal review by the National Institutes of Health concluded that gene therapy had not yet proved clinically successful and that 'significant problems remain in all basic aspects of gene therapy'.

1995 Cholesterol-lowering drugs, such as Pravastatin, used in high blood pressure and heart disease patients were found not to act by lowering cholesterol but by thinning the blood and so preventing thrombus formation.

1995 J.D.H. Morris published a paper implicating the human wart virus in cancer of the cervix.

1995 Ron Breaker, Gerald Joyce and colleagues at the Scripps Research Institute in California succeeded in creating single strand DNA enzymes that can slice RNA.

1995 Stephen Safe published a paper on environmental and dietary estrogens in human health, asking if there was a problem.

1995 G.B. Clements and colleagues showed that the coxsackie virus attacks insulin producing cells in the pancreas and can lead to childhood diabetes.

1996 Australian immunologist and pathologist, Peter C. Doherty and Swiss immunologist, Rolf M.

Zinkernagel shared the Nobel Prize for Physiology or Medicine for their studies of the mechanism whereby the immune system distinguishes normal and viral-infected cells.

1996   Triple therapy drug treatment for AIDS patients was introduced.

1996   Shingo Murakami, a Japanese virologist, found traces of the herpes simplex virus in facial nerves of patients with Bell's palsy.

1996   Ishwarlal Jialal and Sridevi Devaraj of the University of Texas in Dallas showed that vitamin E supplements can reduce the level of interleukin-1b which promotes plaque formation and thus the vitamin may protect against heart disease.

1996   A second breast cancer gene, BRCA2, is discovered.

1996   Phyllida Brown published an article in *New Scientist* asking 'Can you Catch Heart Disease', on the involvement of *Chlamydia*.

1996   American neurologist, Stanley B. Prusiner's work on the prion received acceptance with the recognition of new variant Creutzfeldt-Jakob disease in Great Britain.

1997   American neurologist, Stanley Ben Prusiner, was awarded the Nobel Prize for Physiology or Medicine for his discovery of the disease-causing protein, the prion.

1997   Sandeep Gupta and colleagues showed elevated *Chlamydia* anti-

bodies in patients who had had a heart attack.

1997   Shah Ebrahim published an analysis of 125,000 participants from randomized trials of multiple risk factor interventions for preventing coronary heart disease which failed that changing diet had little or no effect on the incidence of heart disease.

1998   The Nobel Prize in Physiology or Medicine was jointly awarded to American scientists, Robert F. Furchgott of New York, Louis J. Ignarro and Ferid Murad of Los Angeles for their discoveries concerning nitric oxide as a signaling molecule in the cardiovascular system.

1998   The drug Viagra was introduced to treat impotence.

1998   Jaume Marrugat and colleagues at the Municipal Institute of Medical Research in Barcelona in Spain showed that women who suffer heart attacks are more likely to die than their male counterparts.

1998   Carl Hellerqvist and colleagues at the Vanderbilt University in Nashville showed that giving an experimental drug consisting of a polysaccharide form streptococci can block spinal cord injury in mice, allowing growth of new blood vessels.

1999   The malaria vaccine developed by Altaf Lal of the Centers for Disease Control in Atlanta successfully passed its first tests.

1999   The first drug was developed in Canada against the killer bacterium, *E. coli* 0157, that causes reduced hemolytic uremic syndrome and kidney damage.

1999   Children conceived by introcytoplasmic sperm injection have been shown to have higher rates of genetic abnormalities than children conceived naturally.

1999   Jennifer Elisseeff and colleagues at MIT have developed an injectable replacement for cartilage that hardens under bright light.

1999   Gerald Frenkel and Paula Caffrey of Rutgers University in Newark gave large doses of selenium to patients undergoing chemotherapy for ovarian tumors and showed that it prevented the tumors becoming resistant to treatment.

1999   Stephen Brown of the National Medical Laser Center in London described a new treatment for blocked arteries using laser light and 5-aminolaevulinic acid as a sensitizing chemical.

1999   David Humes and colleagues at the University of Michigan have developed an artificial kidney lined with living kidney cells which puts back essential molecules from the urine.

1999   Zemphira Alavidze and colleagues of the University of Maryland School of Medicine have found a way of using bacteriophages to infect and kill *Pseudomonas aeruginosa*, a bacterium responsible for most deaths of cystic fibrosis patients.

1999   Yong-Jun Liu and colleagues at the DNAX Research Institute in Palo Alto have purified cells from blood that produce large quantities of interferon.

1999   A cheaper drug combination for treatment of AIDS, hydroxyurea and ddI, is showing promising results in African trials.

1999   Patrick Brennan of the University College Dublin has provided evidence that ultrasound scans of the unborn fetus may stop cells dividing or cause some cells to commit suicide.

1999   A new inhalational drug, Zanamivir, was approved to fight flu, blocking the viral enzyme neuroaminidase so preventing flu virus from escaping the cell.

1999   The first HIV vaccine trial in Africa began using a weakened canarypox virus containing three HIV genes.

1999   Josef Penninger of the Ontario Cancer Institute showed that *Chlamydia* triggers an autoimmune disorder which can cause heart disease.

1999   Karin Nelson of the National Institutes of Health and Judith Grether of the California Birth Defects Monitoring Program suggested that inflammation during pregnancy, rather than lack of oxygen, can cause cerebral palsy in the newborn.

1999   Jan Walboomers of the Free University of Amsterdam and Michele

Manos of the Johns Hopkins University provided evidence that the human papilloma virus is present in 99.7% of all cases of cervical cancer.

1999   Günter Blobel of the Rockefeller University in New York was awarded the Nobel Prize for Physiology of Medicine for his discovery that proteins have intrinsic signals that govern their transport and localization in the cell. This research aids our understanding of the molecular mechanisms involved in many genetic diseases, such as cystic fibrosis or hyperoxaluria, and of the functioning of the immune system.